ABC of

Dermatology

Fifth Edition

EDITED BY

Paul K. Buxton
Consultant Dermatologist
Hampshire, UK

Rachael Morris-Jones
Consultant Dermatologist
Kings College Hospital
London, UK

WILEY-BLACKWELL

A John Wiley & Sons, Ltd., Publication

BMJ|Books

Library of Congress Cataloging-in-Publication Data

Buxton, Paul K.
ABC of dermatology / Paul K. Buxton, Rachael Morris-Jones. – 5th ed.
  p. ; cm.
  Includes bibliographical references and index.
  ISBN 978-1-4051-7065-9
  1. Dermatology–Handbooks, manuals, etc. 2. Skin–Diseases–Handbooks, manuals, etc. I. Morris-Jones, Rachael. II. Title.
  [DNLM: 1. Skin Diseases. WR 140 B991ab 2009]
  RL74.B88 2009
  616.5–dc22
                                                                                           2008034594

A catalogue record for this book is available from the British Library.

Set in 9.25/12 pt Minion by Newgen Imaging Systems Pvt. Ltd, Chennai, India
Printed and bound in Singapore by COS Printers Pte Ltd

1 2009

ABC of
Dermatology

Fifth Edition

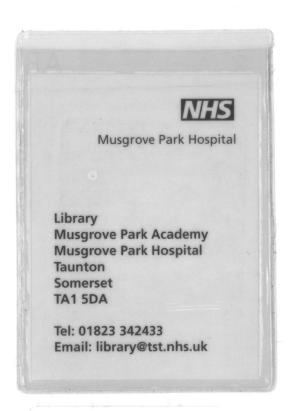

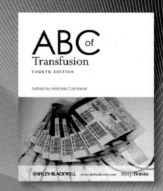
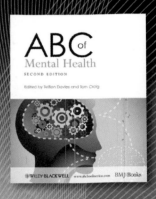
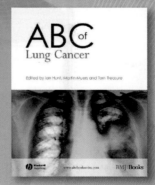
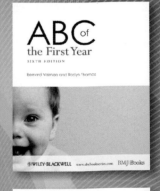
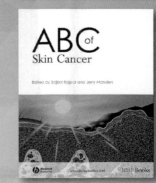
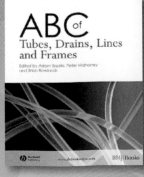

Contents

Contributors, vii

Preface, ix

Acknowledgements, x

1 Introduction, 1

2 Psoriasis, 11

3 Management of Psoriasis, 18

4 Eczema (Dermatitis) Including Management, 24

5 Urticaria and Angio-oedema, 36

6 Skin and Photosensitivity, 40

7 Inflammatory Dermatoses: Drug Rashes, 45

8 Inflammatory Dermatoses: Immunobullous and Other Blistering Disorders, 53

9 Inflammatory Dermatoses: Connective Tissue Disease, Vasculitis and Related Disorders, 60

10 The Skin and Systemic Disease, 67

11 Leg Ulcers, 78

12 Acne and Rosacea, 84

13 Bacterial Infections, 92

14 Viral Infections, 100

15 HIV and the Skin, 108

16 Fungal Infections, 115

17 Insect Bites and Infestations, 121

18 Tropical Dermatology, 128

19 Hair and Scalp, 137
Samantha Bunting, David Fenton

20 Diseases of the Nails, 144
David de Berker

21 Benign Skin Tumours, 153

22 Premalignant and Malignant Skin Tumours, 163

23 Practical Procedures, 172
Raj Mallipeddi

24 Lasers, Intense Pulsed Light and Photodynamic Therapy, 179
Alun V Evans

25 Dressings and Bandages, 184
Judy Davids

26 Formulary, 194
Karen Watson

Index, 201

Contributors

Samantha Bunting
Specialist Registrar in Dermatology
St John's Institute of Dermatology
St Thomas' Hospital
London, UK

Judy Davids
Dermatology Sister
Dermatology Department
Kings College Hospital
London, UK

David de Berker
Consultant Dermatologist
United Bristol Healthcare Trust
Bristol, UK

Alun V Evans
Consultant Dermatologist
Princess of Wales Hospital
Bridgend, UK

David Fenton
Consultant Dermatologist
St John's Institute of Dermatology
St Thomas' Hospital, London, UK

Raj Mallipeddi
Consultant Dermatologist
Cutaneous Laser and Surgery Unit, St John's Institute of Dermatology
St Thomas' Hospital, London, UK

Karen Watson
Consultant Dermatologist
Princess Royal University Hospital, Orpington, Kent, UK

Preface

The 5th edition of the *ABC of Dermatology* delivers a new look, a new approach and a new editor. The publishers and original editor are very grateful that Dr Rachael Morris-Jones has enthusiastically taken on this role – initially in conjunction with the original editor to ensure continuity.

The style and presentation of the ABC series has evolved over time and the *ABC of Dermatology* has embraced these changes in the new edition. Each chapter begins with a concise summary outlining the most important aspects to be covered. The chapters and content have been rewritten and the layout rationalized and where appropriate greater details of diagnostic techniques and specialized treatments are discussed. However, we have endeavoured to ensure that the successful formula of the previous editions has not been diminished but enhanced.

The challenge for the new edition has been to incorporate the latest scientific advances while maintaining a practical clinical approach.

Throughout the book we have striven to provide a basic understanding of pathological processes which explain the characteristic features of skin diseases. A straightforward approach to investigations and diagnoses in addition to the latest advances in the management of skin disease ensures the 5th edition of the *ABC of Dermatology* will be valuable resource for any medical or nursing practitioner.

There is no doubt that part of the appeal and interest of dermatology lies in the fact that it is par excellence a clinical specialty. There is an emphasis on making a clinical diagnosis through pattern recognition and medical detective work but at the same time utilizing modern diagnostic techniques offered by scientific advances.

There has been significant progress in our understanding of pathological mechanisms – particularly in the field of immunology – which are presented here in simple terms and can be used as starting point for the appreciation of complex interactions at the cellular level.

Equally challenging and important is the appreciation of how skin diseases present in the developing world. Those managing these conditions have been borne in mind throughout the book, particularly in relation to clinical diagnoses and simple treatments, mainly discussed in the chapter on tropical dermatology.

Within our global community there is increasing public awareness of general health issues in terms of disease prevention, potential triggers and the range of available treatments. Patients increasingly have access to more sophisticated healthcare systems closer to home and are able to access information through the internet. Public health campaigns aimed at the prevention of skin cancer are also raising awareness about the dangers of excessive sun exposure.

The skin is an excellent medium for research, providing a large accessible interface for the study of the immune system of the body, complex cellular interactions, drug/vaccine delivery and ultimately as a target for gene therapy which many believe will facilitate a cure for previously chronic and fatal skin diseases.

We trust this book will be a means of introducing the reader to a fascinating clinical discipline that is globally relevant to patients of all ages throughout the breadth and depth of clinical medicine.

Paul K. Buxton
Rachael Morris-Jones

Acknowledgements

We would very much like to thank our co-contributors whose expertise in specialist areas of dermatology has been invaluable in ensuring this new edition is right up to date and written by experts in their field. Dr Alun Evans, Consultant Dermatologist, Bridgend, UK (Lasers, Intense Pulsed Light and Photodynamic Therapy), Dr Raj Mallipeddi, Consultant Dermatologist, London, UK (Practical Procedures), Dr Samantha Bunting Specialist Registrar, London UK, and Dr David Fenton, Consultant Dermatologist, London, UK (Hair and Scalp), Dr David de Berker Consultant Dermatologist, Bristol, UK (Diseases of the Nails), Dr Karen Watson, Consultant Dermatologist, Kent, UK (Formulary) and Sister Judy Davids, Dermatology Sister, London, UK (Dressings and Bandages).

A large proportion of the illustrations come from Kings College Hospital, London, UK and we are indebted to the photography department for their excellent clinical images. Many of the images in the Hair and Scalp chapter have been provided by St John's Institute of Dermatology, St Thomas' Hospital, London, UK. Dr Stephen Morris-Jones, Consultant in Infectious Diseases, London, UK has kindly provided some of the new cutaneous infections illustrations for which we are very grateful. We have retained many of Dr Barbara Leppard's excellent illustrations in the Tropical Dermatology chapter. We are also indebted to Bernadette Byrne who is a Tissue Viability Sister working at Kings College Hospital, London, who provided many of the clinical illustrations for the chapter on Dressings and Bandages.

Many of the illustrations retained from previous editions come from the Victoria Hospital, Kirkcaldy and Queen Margaret Hospital, Dunfermline, Fife, the Royal Infirmary, Edinburgh and Paul Buxton's own collection. Some specific illustrations were donated by Dr Peter Ball (rubella) and Dr MA Waugh and Dr M Jones (AIDS). Miss Julie Close made the diagrams of the nail and types of immune response.

We would very much like to thank Dr Jon Salisbury (Consultant Histopathologist at Kings College Hospital) who has provided all the new histopathology skin section images for the book, which demonstrate so beautifully cutaneous disease at the cellular level. Equally, Dr Edward Davies (Consultant Immunologist, Kings College Hospital) who has provided the new direct immunofluoresence images which demonstrate so well the target antigens in the skin of immunobullous disease.

We owe a debt of gratitude to our colleagues in different dermatology departments and we would particularly like to thank the patients without whom there would be no dermatology. We are indebted especially to those who allowed us to use their pictures to demonstrate clinical skin diseases in this book.

CHAPTER 1

Introduction

Introduction

The aim of this book is to provide an insight for the non-dermatologist into the pathological processes, diagnosis and management of skin conditions. Dermatology is a broad specialty with over 2000 different skin diseases, the most common of which are introduced here. Pattern recognition is often the key to successful history-taking and examination of the skin, usually without the need for complex investigations. Although dermatology is a clinically orientated subject an understanding of the cellular changes underlying the skin disease can give helpful insights into the pathological processes. This understanding aids the interpretation of clinical signs and overall management of cutaneous disease. Skin biopsies can be a useful adjuvant to reaching a diagnosis; however, clinicopathological correlation is essential in order that interpretation of the clinical and pathological patterns is put into the context of the patient.

The interpretation of clinical signs on the skin in the context of underlying pathological processes is a theme running through the chapters. This helps the reader to develop a deeper understanding of the subject and should form some guiding principles that can be used as tools to help assess almost any skin eruption.

Clinically cutaneous disorders fall into three main groups.

1 Those that generally present with a characteristic distribution and morphology that leads to a specific diagnosis – such as chronic plaque psoriasis (Figure 1.1) and atopic eczema.

2 A characteristic pattern of skin lesions with variable underlying causes – such as erythema nodosum and erythema multiforme.

3 Skin rashes that can be variable in their presentation and/or underlying causes – such as lichen planus and urticaria.

A holistic approach in dermatology is essential as cutaneous eruptions may be the first indicator of an underlying internal disease. Patients may, for example, first present with a photosensitive rash

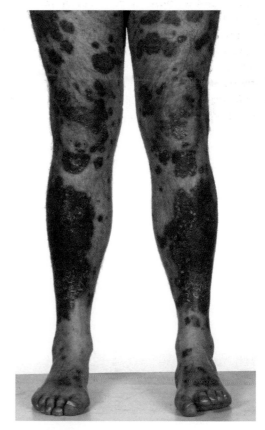

Figure 1.1 Extensive psoriasis.

ABC of Dermatology, 5th edition. Edited by P. K. Buxton and R. Morris-Jones.
© 2009 Blackwell Publishing, ISBN: 978-1-4051-7065-9.

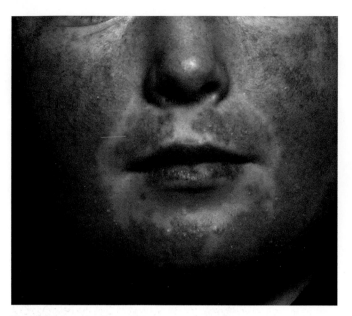

Figure 1.2 Lupus erythematosus.

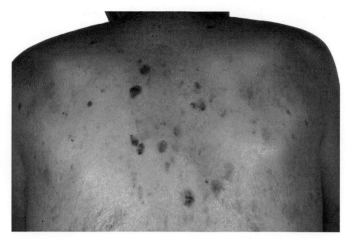

Figure 1.3 Seborrhoeic keratoses.

Box 1.1 **Dermatology history-taking**

- Where? Site of initial lesion(s) and subsequent distribution
- How long? Continuous or intermittent?
- Trend? Better or worse?
- Previous episodes? Timing? Similar/dissimilar? Other skin conditions?
- Who else? Family members/work colleagues/school friends affected?
- Symptoms? Itching, burning, scaling, or blisters? Any medication or other illnesses?
- Treatment? Prescription or over the counter? Frequency/time course/compliance?

on the face, but deeper probing may reveal symptoms of joint pains etc. leading to the diagnosis of systemic lupus erythematosus (Figure 1.2). Similarly a patient with underlying coeliac disease may first present with blistering on the elbows (dermatitis herpetiformis). It is therefore important not only to take a thorough history (Box 1.1) of the skin complaint but in addition to ask about any other symptoms the patient may have, and examine the entire patient carefully.

The significance of skin disease

Seventy per cent of the people living in developing countries suffer skin disease at some point in their lives, but of these 3 billion people in 127 countries do not have access to even basic skin services (Ersser & Penzer 2000). In developed countries the prevalence of skin disease is also high; up to 15% of general practice consultations in the United Kingdom are concerned with skin complaints. Many patients never seek medical advice and self-treat using over-the-counter preparations.

The skin is the largest organ of the body; it provides an essential living biological barrier and is the aspect of ourselves that we present to the outside world. It is therefore not surprising that there is great interest in 'skin care' and 'skin problems', with an associated ever-expanding cosmetics industry. Impairment of the normal functions of the skin can lead to acute and chronic illness with considerable disability and sometimes the need for hospital treatment.

Malignant change can occur in any cell in the skin, resulting in a wide variety of different tumours, the majority of which are benign. Recognition of typical benign tumours (Figure 1.3) saves the patient unnecessary investigations and the anxiety involved in waiting to see a specialist or wait for biopsy results. Malignant skin cancers are usually only locally invasive, but distant metastases can occur. It is important therefore to recognize the early features of lesions such as malignant melanoma and squamous cell carcinoma before they disseminate.

Underlying systemic disease can be heralded by changes on the skin surface, the significance of which can be easily missed by the unprepared mind. So, in addition to concentrating on the skin changes, the overall health and demeanour of the patient should be assessed. Close inspection of the whole skin, nails and mucous membranes should be the basis of routine skin examination. The general physical condition of the patient should also be determined as indicated.

The majority of skin diseases, however, do not signify any systemic disease and are often considered 'harmless' in medical terms. However, due to the very visual nature of skin disorders, they can cause a great deal of psychological distress, social isolation and occupational difficulties, which should not be underestimated. A validated measure of how much skin disease affects patients' lives can be made using the Dermatology Life Quality Index (DLQI). A holistic approach to the patient both physically and psychologically is therefore highly desirable.

Descriptive terms

All specialties have their own common terms, and familiarity with a few of those used in dermatology is a great help. The most important are defined below.

Macule (Figure 1.4). Derived from the Latin for a stain, the term macule is used to describe changes in colour (Figure 1.5) or

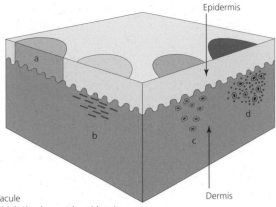

Macule
a) Melanin pigment *in* epidermis
b) Melanin pigment *below* epidermis
c) Erythema due to dilated dermal blood vessels
d) Inflammation in dermis

Figure 1.4 Section through skin.

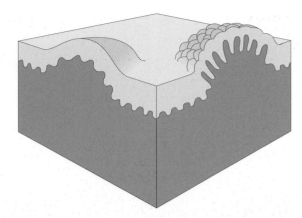

Figure 1.6 Section through skin with a papule.

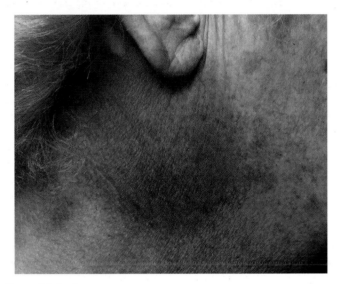

Figure 1.5 Erythema.

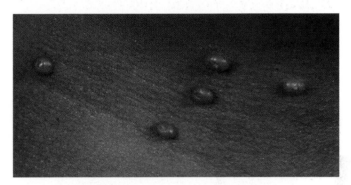

Figure 1.7 Papules.

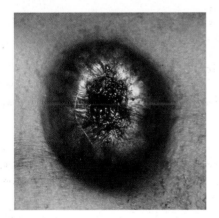

Figure 1.8 Nodule.

consistency without any elevation above the surface of the surrounding skin. There may be an increase in pigment such as melanin, giving a black or blue colour depending on the depth. Loss of melanin leads to a white macule. Vascular dilatation and inflammation produce erythema.

Papules and nodules (Figure 1.6). A papule is a circumscribed, raised lesion, of epidermal or dermal origin, 0.5–1.0 cm in diameter (Figure 1.7). A nodule (Figure 1.8) is similar to a papule but greater than 1.0 cm in diameter. A vascular papule or nodule is known as a haemangioma.

A plaque (Figure 1.9) is a circumscribed, superficial, elevated plateau area 1.0–2.0 cm in diameter (Figure 1.10).

Vesicles and bullae (Figure 1.11) are raised lesions that contain fluid (blisters) (Figure 1.12). A bulla is a vesicle larger than 0.5 cm. They may be superficial within the epidermis or situated in the dermis below it. The more superficial the vesicles/bullae the more likely they are to break open.

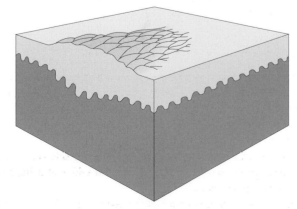

Figure 1.9 Section through skin with plaque.

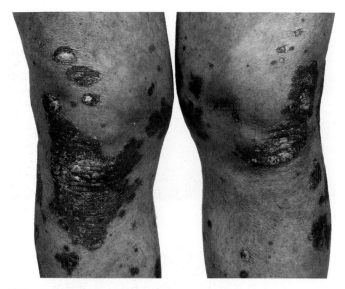

Figure 1.10 Psoriasis plaques.

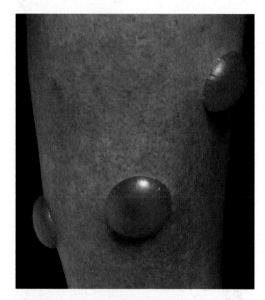

Figure 1.11 Acute reaction to insect bite: bullae.

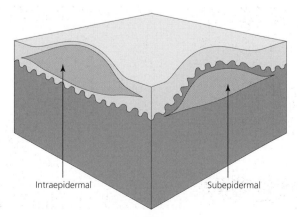

Figure 1.12 Section through skin showing sites of vesicle and bulla.

Intraepidermal   Subepidermal

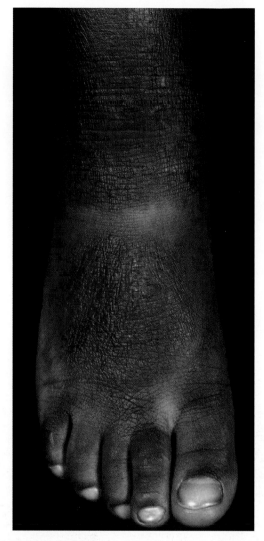

Figure 1.13 Lichen simplex.

Lichenification is a hard thickening of the skin with accentuated skin markings (Figure 1.13). It commonly results from chronic inflammation and rubbing of the skin.

Nummular lesions. Nummular literally means a 'coin-like' lesion (Figure 1.14). There is no hard and fast distinction from discoid lesions, which are flat disc-like lesions of variable size. The term is most often used to describe a type of eczematous lesion.

Pustules. The term pustule is applied to lesions containing purulent material – which may be due to infection – or sterile pustules (inflammatory polymorphs) (Figure 1.15) which are seen in pustular psoriasis.

Atrophy refers to loss of tissue, which may affect the epidermis, dermis or subcutaneous fat. Thinning of the epidermis is characterized by loss of the normal skin markings; there may be fine wrinkles, loss of pigment and a translucent appearance (Figure 1.16). In addition, sclerosis of the underlying connective tissue, telangiectasia or evidence of diminished blood supply may be present.

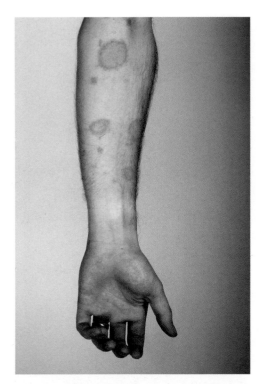

Figure 1.14 Nummular lesions.

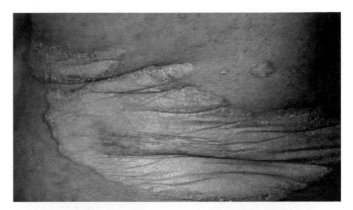

Figure 1.16 Epidermal atrophy.

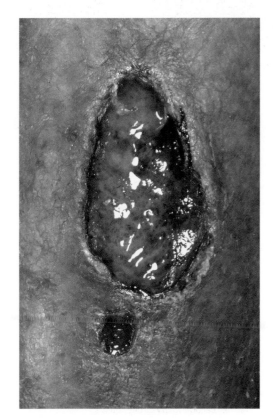

Figure 1.17 Ulceration.

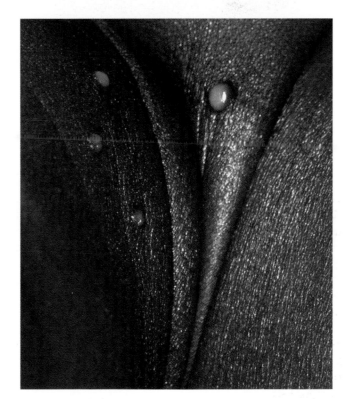

Figure 1.15 Sterile pustules.

Ulceration results from the loss of the whole thickness of the epidermis and upper dermis (Figure 1.17). Healing results in a scar.

Erosion. An erosion is a superficial loss of epidermis that generally heals without scarring (Figure 1.18).

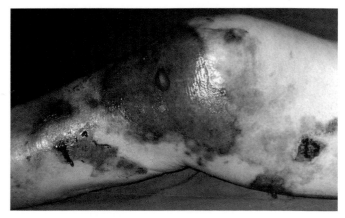

Figure 1.18 Bullous pemphigoid causing erosion.

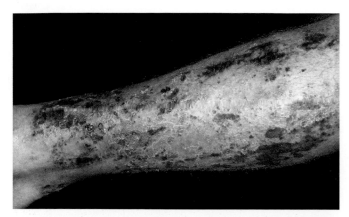

Figure 1.19 Excoriation of epidermis.

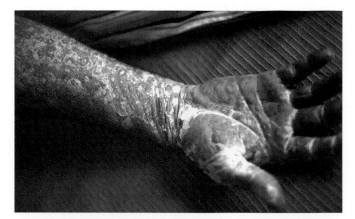

Figure 1.21 Desquamation.

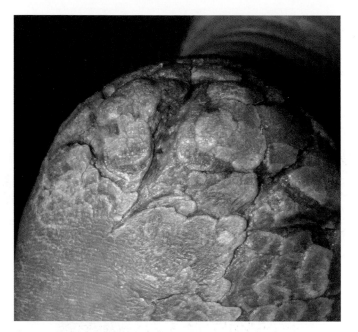

Figure 1.20 Hyperkeratosis with fissures.

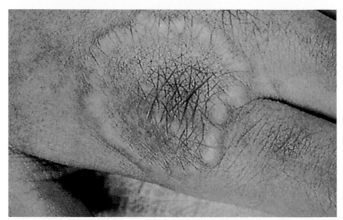

Figure 1.22 Ring-shaped annular lesion.

Excoriation is the partial or complete loss of epidermis as a result of scratching (Figure 1.19).

Fissuring. Fissures are slits through the whole thickness of the skin (Figure 1.20).

Desquamation is the peeling of superficial scales, often following acute inflammation (Figure 1.21).

Annular lesions are ring-shaped (Figure 1.22).

Reticulate. The term reticulate means 'net-like'. It is most commonly seen when the pattern of subcutaneous blood vessels becomes visible (Figure 1.23).

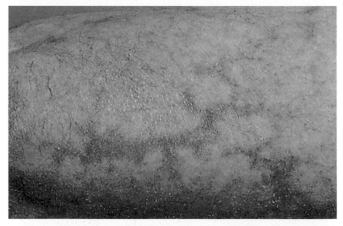

Figure 1.23 Reticulate changes.

Rashes

Approach to diagnosis

A skin rash generally poses more problems in diagnosis than a single, well-defined skin lesion such as a wart or tumour. As in all branches of medicine a reasonable diagnosis is more likely to be reached by thinking firstly in terms of broad diagnostic categories rather than specific conditions.

There may be a history of recurrent episodes such as occurs in atopic eczema due to the patient's constitutional tendency. In the case of contact dermatitis, regular exposure to a causative agent leads to recurrences that fit from the history with exposure times. Endogenous conditions such as psoriasis can appear in adults who have had no previous episodes. If several members of the same family are affected by a skin rash simultaneously then a contagious condition, such as scabies, should be considered. A common condition with a familial tendency, such as atopic eczema, may affect several family members at different times.

A simplistic approach to rashes is to classify them as being from the 'inside' or 'outside'. Examples of 'inside' or endogenous rashes are atopic eczema or drug rashes, whereas fungal infection or contact dermatitis are 'outside' or exogenous rashes.

Symmetry

As a general rule most endogenous rashes affect both sides of the body, as in the atopic child or a patient with psoriasis on the legs (Figure 1.24). Of course, not all exogenous rashes are asymmetrical. A chef who holds a knife in their dominant hand can have unilateral disease (Figure 1.25) from metal allergy whereas a hairdresser or nurse may develop contact dermatitis on both hands (Figure 1.26).

Diagnosis

- Previous episodes of the rash, particularly in childhood, suggest a constitutional condition such as atopic eczema.

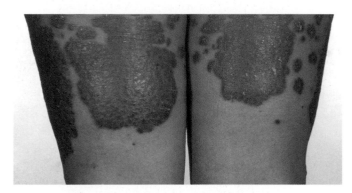

Figure 1.24 Psoriasis on both legs.

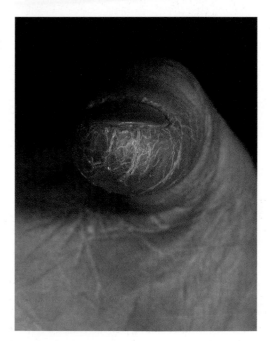

Figure 1.25 Irritant eczema on dominant hand of chef.

- Recurrences of the rash, particularly in specific situations, suggest a contact dermatitis. Similarly a rash that only occurs in the summer months may well have a photosensitive basis (Figure 1.27).
- If other members of the family are affected, particularly without any previous history, there may well be a transmissible condition such as scabies.

Distribution

It is useful to be aware of the usual sites of common skin conditions. These are shown in the appropriate chapters. Eruptions that appear only on areas exposed to sun may be entirely or partially due to sunlight. Some are due to a sensitivity to sunlight alone, such as polymorphic light eruption, or a photosensitive allergy to topically applied substances or drugs taken internally.

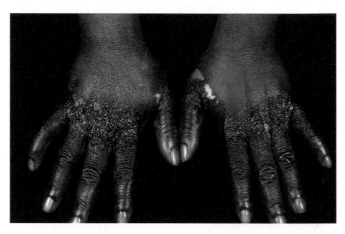

Figure 1.26 Bilateral contact dermatitis.

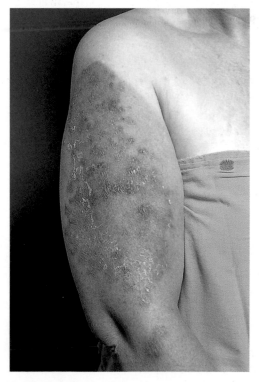

Figure 1.27 Allergic reaction producing photosensitivity.

Morphology

The appearance of the skin lesion may give clues to the underlying pathological process.

Changes at the *skin surface* (epidermis) are characterized by a change in texture when the skin is palpated. Visually you may see scaling, thickening, increased skin markings, small vesicles, crusting, erosions or desquamation. In contrast changes in the *deeper tissues* (dermis) can be associated with a normal overlying skin. Examples of changes in the deeper tissues include erythema (dilated blood vessels, or inflammation), induration (an infiltrated firm area under the skin surface), ulceration (that involves surface and deeper tissues), hot tender skin (such as in cellulitis or abscess formation), changes in adnexal structures and adipose tissue.

The *margin* or border of some lesions is very well defined, as in psoriasis or lichen planus, but in eczema it is ill-defined and merges into normal skin.

Blisters or vesicles occur as a result of:

- oedema (fluid) between the epidermal cells (Figure 1.28)
- destruction/death of epidermal cells
- the separation of the epidermis from the deeper tissues.

There may be more than one mechanism involved simultaneously.

Blisters or vesicles (Figures 1.29–1.33) occur in:

- *viral* diseases such as chicken pox, hand, foot and mouth disease, and herpes simplex
- *bacterial infections* such as impetigo
- *inflammatory disorders* such as eczema, contact dermatitis
- *immunological disorders* such as dermatitis herpetiformis, pemphigus and pemphigoid
- *metabolic disorders* such as porphyria.

Bullae (blisters more than 0.5 cm in diameter) may occur in congenital conditions (such as epidermolysis bullosa), in trauma and as a result of oedema without much inflammation. However, those forming as a result of vasculitis, sunburn or an allergic reaction may be associated with pronounced inflammation. Drug rashes can appear as a bullous eruption.

Induration is thickening of the skin due to infiltration of cells, granuloma formation, or deposits of mucin, fat, or amyloid.

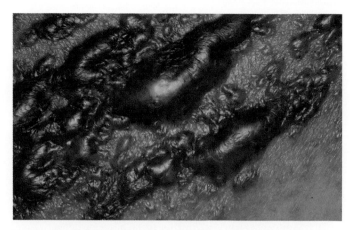

Figure 1.29 Vesicles and bullae.

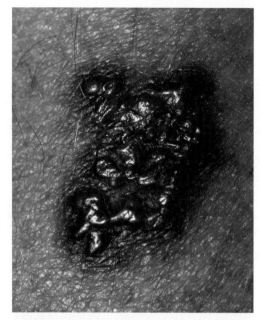

Figure 1.30 Herpes simplex.

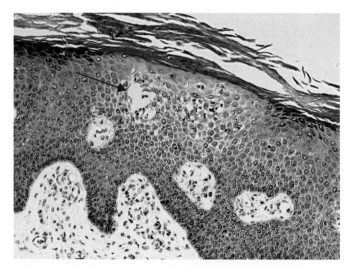

Figure 1.28 Eczema: intraepidermal vesicle (arrow).

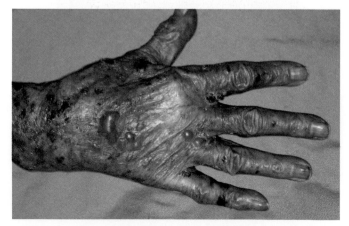

Figure 1.31 Bullous pemphigoid.

Inflammation is indicated by erythema, and can be acute or chronic. Acute inflammation can be associated with increased skin temperature such as occurs in cellulitis and erythema nodosum. Chronic inflammatory cell infiltrates occur in conditions such as lichen planus and lupus erythematosus.

Assessment of the patient

A full assessment should include not only the effect the skin condition has on the patient's life but also their attitude to it. For example, some patients with quite extensive psoriasis are unbothered whilst others with very mild localized disease just on the elbows may be

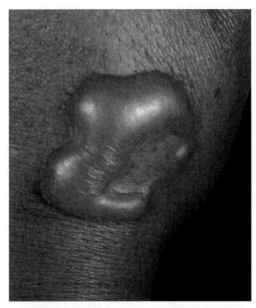

Figure 1.32 Bullous fixed drug eruption.

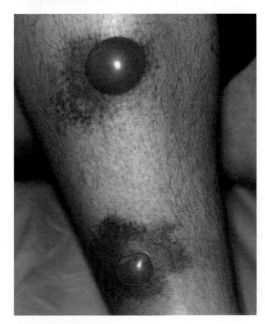

Figure 1.33 Insect bite reactions.

very distressed. Management of the patient should reflect their attitude as well as the clinical findings.

Fear that a skin condition may be due to cancer or infection is often present and reassurance should always be given to allay any hidden fears. If there is the possibility of a serious underlying disease that requires further investigation, then it is important to explain fully to the patient that the skin problems may be a sign of an internal disease.

The significance of occupational factors must be taken into account. In some cases, such as an allergy to hair dyes in a hairdresser, it may be impossible for the patient to continue their job. In other situations the allergy can be easily avoided.

Patients often want to know why they have developed a particular skin problem and whether it can be cured. In many skin diseases these questions are difficult to answer. Patients with psoriasis, for example, can be told that it is part of their inherent constitution but that additional factors can trigger clinical lesions (Figure 1.34). Known trigger factors for psoriasis include emotional stress, local trauma to the skin (Koebner's phenomenon), infection (guttate psoriasis) and drugs (β-blockers, lithium, antimalarials).

Skill in recognition of skin conditions will evolve and develop with increased clinical experience. Seeing and feeling skin rashes 'in the flesh' is the best way to improve clinical dermatological acumen (Box 1.2).

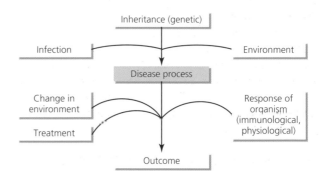

Figure 1.34 Possible precipitating factors in psoriasis.

Box 1.2 **Examination of skin lesions – key points**

Distribution
Examine all the skin for clues. For example, there are many possible causes for dry thickened skin on the palms, and finding typical psoriasis on the elbows, knees, and soles may give the diagnosis

Morphology
Are the lesions dermal or epidermal? Macular (flat) or forming papules? Indurated or forming plaques? Well defined or indistinct? Forming crusts, scabs or vesicles?

Pattern
The overall morphology and distribution of the rash. For example; an indeterminate rash may be revealed as pityriasis rosea when the 'herald patch' is found

Reference

Ersser SJ, Penzer R. Meeting patients' skin care needs: harnessing nursing expertise at an international level. *Int Nursing Rev* 2000; **47**: 167–73.

Further reading

Freedberg IM, Eisen AZ, Wolff K, Austen KF, Goldsmith LA, Katz SI. *Fitzpatrick's Dermatology in General Medicine*, 6th edn. McGraw-Hill, New York, 2003.

Hunter J, Savin J, Dahl M. *Clinical Dermatology*. Blackwell Publishing, Oxford, 2002.

Roxburgh AC, Marks R. *Roxburgh's Common Skin Diseases*. Oxford University Press, Oxford, 2003.

CHAPTER 2

Psoriasis

OVERVIEW

- The pathological features giving rise to lesions of psoriasis are explained, followed by description of the resulting changes in the skin.
- The clinical presentation of typical psoriasis including psoriatic arthropathy and nail changes are discussed.
- Factors causing psoriasis to appear including genetic predisposition, hormonal changes, stress and infection are discussed.
- Research into underlying immunological mechanisms has led to much more effective, specifically targeted treatments.
- The effect of psoriasis on the patient's life in terms of relationships, self-confidence and ability to come to terms with the disease and methods of management are discussed.

Introduction

Most practitioners are familiar with the clinical appearances of chronic plaque psoriasis, which is characterized by well-demarcated hyperkeratotic scaly plaques with an erythematous base. But why does psoriasis have these clinical features? The answer lies in changes at the cellular level.

Keratinocytes are the skin cells that predominate in the epidermis; they grow from the bottom (basal) layer and slowly migrate to the surface (Figures 2.1 & 2.2). This process of cell turnover takes about 23 days in normal skin. In patients with psoriasis cell turnover is rapidly accelerated, taking only 3–5 days for cells to reach the surface and accumulate in large numbers. This leads to one of the characteristic features of psoriasis, namely thickened skin due to scaling (hyperkeratosis). Keratinocytes normally lose their nuclei as they move to the skin surface; in psoriasis, however, they move so quickly that the cells retain their nuclei throughout the epidermis. Histologically this is parakeratosis.

The rapid production and turnover of cells means they do not differentiate normally to form keratinocytes. If the scale of psoriasis is gently scraped it comes off easily, revealing dilated blood vessels underneath – 'Auspitz sign'. The superficial and dilated blood vessels account for much of the erythema in psoriatic plaques. Indeed in some types of psoriasis there are widespread dilated cutaneous blood vessels leading to marked heat loss.

In addition, inflammatory polymorphs infiltrating the epidermis lead to swelling (oedema), inflammation and erythema. These inflammatory cells may occur in such large numbers that they form collections of sterile pustules at the skin surface. These are most commonly seen in palmoplantar pustulosis, a variant of psoriasis affecting the palms and soles.

The cellular abnormalities in the skin of patients with psoriasis can occur in the nails and many patients will therefore have additional nail changes.

Psoriatic nail dystrophy is characterized by:

- *onycholysis* (lifting of the nail plate off the nail bed) due to abnormal cell adhesion; this usually manifests as a white or salmon patch on the nail plate (Figure 2.3)
- *subungal hyperkeratosis* (accumulation of chalky-looking material under the nail) due to excessive proliferation of the nail bed that can ultimately lead to onycholysis
- *pitting* (very small depressions in the nail plate) which result from parakeratotic (nucleated) cells being lost from the nail surface
- *Beau's lines* (transverse lines on the nail plate) due to intermittent inflammation of the nail bed leading to transient arrest in nail growth
- *splinter haemorrhages* (which clinically look like minute longitudinal black lines) due to leakage of blood from dilated tortuous capillaries.

Clinical appearance

The main clinical features of psoriasis reflect the underlying pathological processes (as described above). Patients characteristically have the following features.

Plaques which are well-defined raised areas of psoriasis. These may be large or small, few or numerous, and scattered over the trunk and limbs (Figures 2.4 & 2.5).

Scaling may be very prominent causing plaques to appear thickened with masses of adherent and shedding white scales. Scratching the surface produces a waxy appearance – the 'tache de bougie' (literally 'a line of candle wax').

ABC of Dermatology, 5th edition. Edited by P. K. Buxton and R. Morris-Jones.
© 2009 Blackwell Publishing, ISBN: 978-1-4051-7065-9.

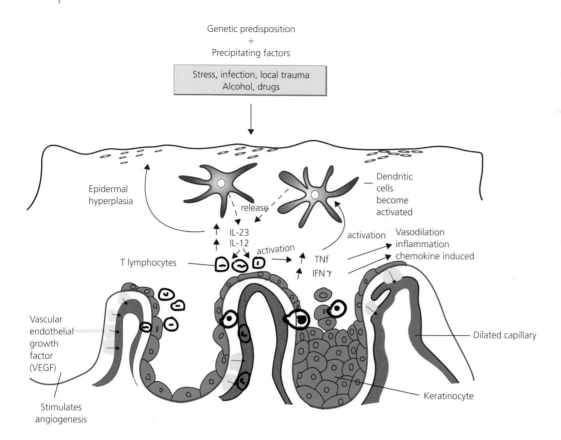

Figure 2.1 Pathophysiological mechanisms involved in the development of psoriasis.

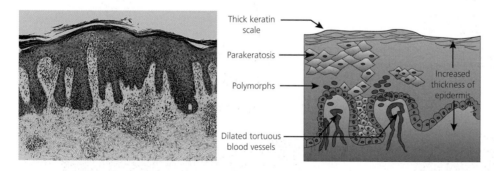

Figure 2.2 Increased epidermal proliferation.

Erythema or redness of the affected skin may be very marked, especially in the flexures. Erythema is a prominent feature in patients with erythrodermic psoriasis (who have more than 90% of their body surface involved).

Pustules are commonly seen in palmoplantar pustulosis where deep-seated sterile pustules are often the dominant feature. Pustules associated with plaques on the trunk and limbs are rare but can occasionally be seen if the psoriasis becomes unstable. Rarely pustules can appear at the edge of plaques on the trunk and limbs, which usually signifies unstable psoriasis.

The typical patient

Psoriasis is reported to affect approximately 2% of the US population. The median age of onset is 28 years, but it can present from infancy to old age, when the appearance may be atypical. The following factors in the history may help in making a diagnosis.

- Family history of psoriasis: 16% of the children will have psoriasis if a single parent is affected and 50% if both parents are affected.
- Trigger factors include stress, infections, trauma and childbirth.

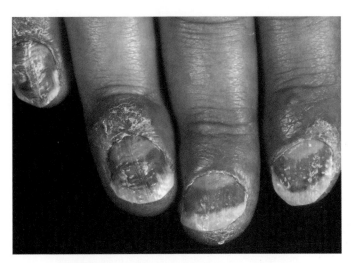

Figure 2.3 Pitting and onycholysis of the nails.

- Lesions may first appear at sites of minor skin trauma – Koebner's phenomenon.
- Lesions usually improve in the sun.
- Psoriasis is usually only mildly itchy.
- Arthropathy may be associated.

Clinical presentation

Classically psoriasis patients present with plaques on the elbows, knees, and scalp (Figure 2.6). Lesions on the trunk are frequently variable in size and are often annular (Figures 2.7–2.9). Psoriasis may develop in scars and areas of minor skin trauma: the so-called Koebner's phenomenon (Figure 2.10). This may manifest as hyperkeratosis on the palms associated with repetitive trauma from manual labour. Scalp scaling which affects 50% of patients can be very thick, especially around the hairline, but may be more confluent forming a virtual 'skull cap' (Figure 2.11). Erythema often extends beyond the hair margin. The nails show 'pits' and also

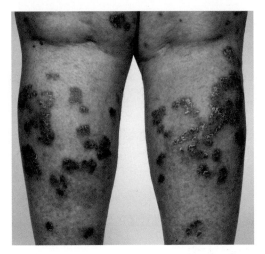

Figure 2.4 Small plaques.

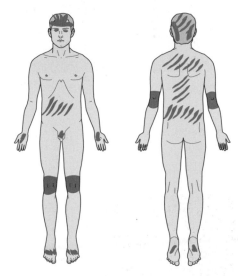

Figure 2.6 Common patterns of distribution in psoriasis.

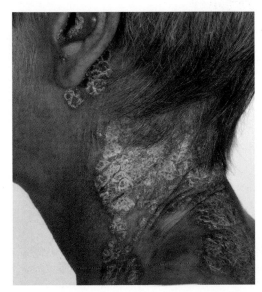

Figure 2.5 Large plaques.

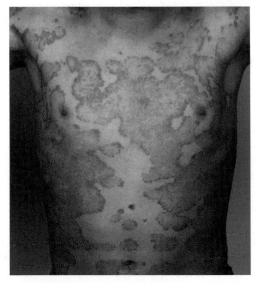

Figure 2.7 Generalized plaques.

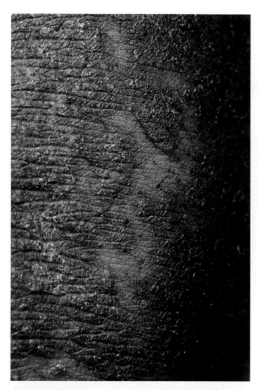

Figure 2.8 Psoriatic plaques.

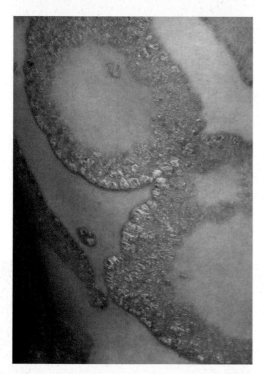

Figure 2.9 Annular plaques.

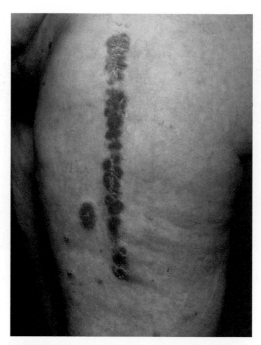

Figure 2.10 Koebner's phenomenon: psoriasis in surgical scar.

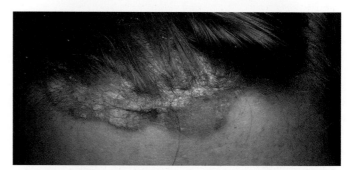

Figure 2.11 Scalp psoriasis.

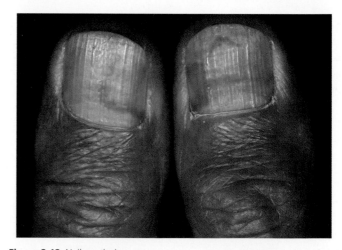

Figure 2.12 Nail psoriasis.

thickening with separation of the nail from the nail bed (onycholysis) (Figure 2.12).

Guttate psoriasis – from the Latin *gutta*, a drop – consists of widespread small plaques scattered on the trunk and limbs (Figure 2.13). Adolescents are most commonly affected and there

is often a preceding sore throat with associated group β haemolytic streptococcus. There is frequently a family history of psoriasis. The sudden onset and widespread nature of guttate psoriasis can be very alarming for patients; fortunately it usually completely resolves, but it can be recurrent or herald the onset of chronic plaque psoriasis.

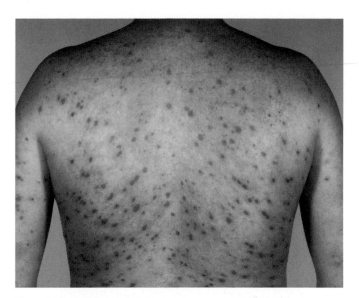

Figure 2.13 Guttate psoriasis.

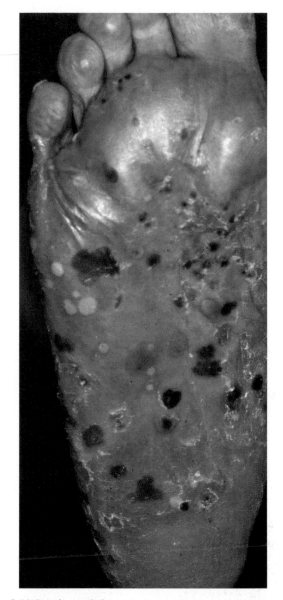

Figure 2.14 Pustular psoriasis.

Pustular lesions are sterile and usually occur as chronic deep-seated lesions on the palms and soles. There is surrounding erythema, and a brown discolouration and scaling usually develop (Figures 2.14 & 2.15). Most patients are smokers. Generalized pustular psoriasis is uncommon, and is usually an indicator of severe and unstable psoriasis. It may be precipitated by the use of oral steroids, or potent topical steroids. The pustules usually occur initially at the peripheral margin of plaques which are often sore and erythematous.

Acrodermatitis pustulosa is thought to be a variant of psoriasis that occurs in young children. Here pustules appear around the nails and the fingertips associated with brisk inflammation.

Flexural psoriasis produces well-defined erythematous areas in the axillae, groin and natal cleft, beneath the breasts and in skin folds. Scaling is minimal or absent (Figure 2.16). It needs to be distinguished from a fungal infection and if there is any doubt a specimen for mycology should be taken.

Napkin psoriasis in children may present with typical psoriatic lesions or a more diffuse erythematous eruption with exudative rather than scaling lesions (Figure 2.17).

Erythrodermic psoriasis is a serious, even life-threatening condition with confluent erythema affecting nearly all of the skin (Figure 2.18). Diagnosis may not be easy as the characteristic scaling of psoriasis is absent, although this usually precedes the erythroderma. Less commonly the erythema develops suddenly without preceding lesions. Increased cutaneous blood flow results in heat and water loss. Patients often feel systemically unwell and usually need admission to hospital.

It is important to distinguish between the *stable*, chronic, plaque type of psoriasis, which is unlikely to develop exacerbations and responds to tar, dithranol and ultraviolet treatment, and

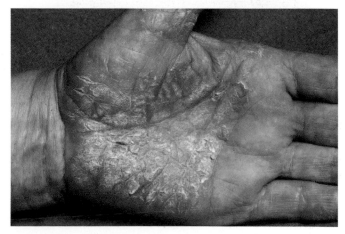

Figure 2.15 Psoriasis of the hand.

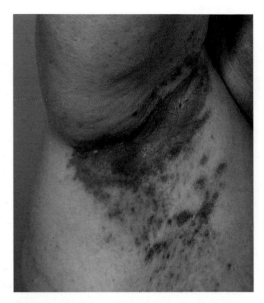

Figure 2.16 Flexural psoriasis.

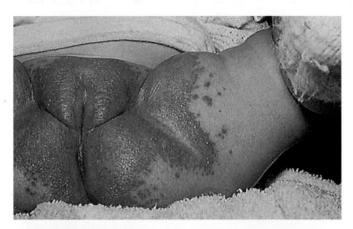

Figure 2.17 Napkin psoriasis.

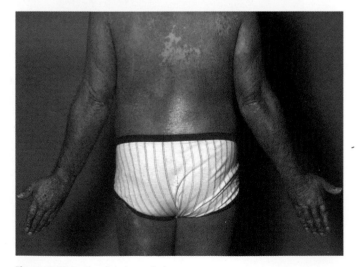

Figure 2.18 Erythrodermic psoriasis.

the more *acute* erythematous type, which is unstable and likely to spread rapidly. The use of tar, dithranol or ultraviolet light can irritate the skin and will make the psoriasis more widespread and inflamed.

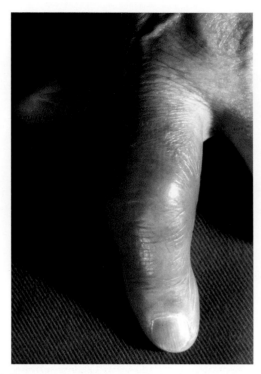

Figure 2.19 Acute arthropathy.

Joint disease in psoriasis

Psoriatic arthropathy is reported to affect 5–10% of patients with psoriasis (Figure 2.19), and of these 40% have a family history of psoriasis. Seronegative arthritis in the context of psoriasis is thought to be human leukocyte antigen (HLA) linked. Characteristically patients develop skin manifestations of psoriasis before joint involvement, but in 15% this is reversed. There are five recognized patterns of arthropathy associated with psoriasis (Box 2.1). The distal interphalangeal joints are most commonly affected (metacarpophalangeal joints are spared). The arthropathy is usually asymmetrical. The sex ratio is equal, however there is a male predominance in the spondylitic form, and a female predominance in the rheumatoid form (Figure 2.20). Arthritis mutilans is a rarer form where there is considerable bone resorption leading to 'telescoping' of the fingers. Radiological changes include a destructive arthropathy with deformity (Figure 2.21).

Psoriatic arthropathy usually waxes and wanes but can be severe enough to cause significant functional disabilities. Stiffness, pain and joint deformity are the most common manifestations.

Box 2.1 **Five types of psoriatic arthropathy**

1 *Distal interphalangeal joints* (80% have associated nail changes)
2 *Asymmetrical oligoarticular* (hands and feet, 'sausage-shaped' digits)
3 *Symmetrical polyarthritis* (hands, wrists, ankles, 'rheumatoid pattern')
4 *Arthritis mutilans* (digits, resorption of bone, resultant 'telescoping' of redundant skin)
5 *Spondylitis* (asymmetrical vertebral involvement, male preponderance)

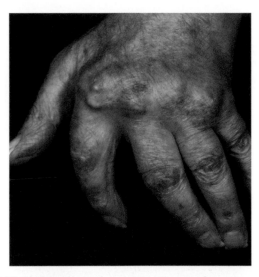

Figure 2.20 Psoriatic arthropathy.

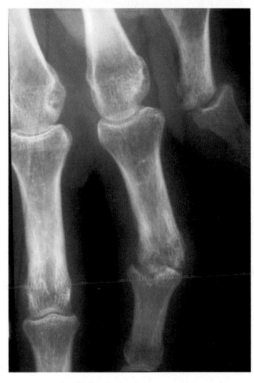

Figure 2.21 Acute arthropathy: X-ray signs.

Causes of psoriasis

Psoriasis is thought to be an autoimmune skin disease with an inherited genetic predisposition and immunological triggers. A psoriasis susceptibility locus (PSORS1) has been identified on chromosome 21 within the major histocompatibility complex. HLA-CW6 is the phenotype associated with psoriasis in 60% of patients, particularly those with early onset disease. HLA-B27, -B17, -CW6, -DR4, and -DR7 have been associated with psoriatic arthropathy. Immunological stimuli including β Haemolytic streptococcal infections and certain drugs (antimalarials, lithium and β-blockers) are known to trigger certain forms of psoriasis. Additional factors such as local trauma, general illness and stress are also thought to play a role. There is evidence that psoriasis occurs more readily and is more intractable in patients with a high intake of alcohol. Smoking is associated with palmoplantar pustulosis.

Both psoriatic arthropathy and Reiter's syndrome are associated with the presence of HLA B27. Reiter's syndrome is characterized by polyarthritis and the development of urethritis, inflammatory changes in the conjunctivae, and skin lesions including pustulosis hyperkeratosis of the soles.

At the cellular level there is increased T-cell activity in diseased skin, the cause of which is unknown. The activated T-cells lead to high levels of proinflammatory cytokines in the psoriatic lesions, especially gamma interferon (γ-INF) and tumour necrosis factor alpha (TNF-α). In turn, TNF-α increases keratinocyte proliferation and induces the SKALP/elafin gene, which is not expressed in normal keratinocytes. This gene is a marker of abnormal keratinocytes differentiation, a hyperproliferative epidermis and increased inflammation.

The cellular abnormalities found in psoriatic plaques are targeted by some of the novel biological therapies. TNF-α blockers include etanercept and infliximab. T-cell blockers include efalizumab and alefacept.

Further reading

Fry L. *An Atlas of Psoriasis*. Taylor and Francis, London, 2004.

Gordon KB, Ruderman E. *Psoriasis and Psoriatic Arthritis: an Integrated Approach*. Springer, Heidelberg, 2005.

Van de Kerkhof PC. *Textbook of Psoriasis*. Blackwell Publishing Ltd, Oxford, 2003.

www.bad.org.uk/healthcare/guidelines/psoriasis.asp

Management of Psoriasis

Introduction

An essential aspect of managing psoriasis is the early assessment of the impact the disease is having on the patient's life. Indeed managing psoriasis is as much a challenge for patients as it is for medical practitioners. Psoriasis is a chronic disease that may have a significant impact on the patient's quality of life. The appearance of the scaly plaques may cause social embarrassment, time needs to be set aside for the application of creams, and even if the skin is cleared recurrence is the rule. Assessing the impact of any skin disease on a patient's quality of life can be undertaken by using the validated Dermatology Life Quality Index (DLQI) score based on a questionnaire. A more specific survey for psoriasis patients is the Psoriasis Disability Index (PDI) which can also be used to assess the impact of the disease on the patient's life. The questionnaires embrace all aspects of life including work, personal relationships, domestic situation and recreational activities.

Patients often wish to know what has caused their psoriasis and are keen for a cure. However, the aetiology has not been fully characterized, and at present the disease can only be suppressed rather than eradicated. The current thinking on the underlying cause of psoriasis is that it is an inherited T-cell-mediated disease with an autoimmune profile that is affected by certain recognized trigger factors such as physical or emotional stress, local trauma to the skin (Koebner's phenomenon), infection (in guttate psoriasis) and drugs (β-blockers, lithium, antimalarials).

Management comprises topical preparations, phototherapy and systemic therapy (Table 3.1). Selection of the most appropriate

ABC of Dermatology, 5th edition. Edited by P. K. Buxton and R. Morris-Jones.
© 2009 Blackwell Publishing, ISBN: 978-1-4051-7065-9.

Table 3.1 Management of psoriasis.

Type of psoriasis	Standard therapy	Alternatives
Localized stable plaques	Tar preparations Vitamin D analogues Salicylic acid preparations Topical steroids	Dithranol/ichthammol TL-01 (UVB)
Extensive stable plaques	TL-01 (UVB) PUVA Acitretin PUVA + acitretin	Methotrexate Ciclosporin A Hydroxyurea Biological agents
Widespread small plaques	TL-01 (UVB)	Steroid with LPC
Guttate psoriasis	Moderate-potency topical steroids TL-01 (UVB)	Steroid with LPC
Facial psoriasis	Mild/moderate-potency topical steroid, vitamin D	Steroid with LPC
Flexural psoriasis	Mild/moderate-potency topical steroid + antifungal	
Pustular psoriasis of hands and feet	Moderate/potent topical steroids Potent topical steroid + propylene glycol ± occlusion	Acitretin Hand and foot PUVA
Acute erythrodermic, unstable/generalized pustular psoriasis	Inpatient management Short-term mild topical steroids	Methotrexate Acitretin Ciclosporin Mycophenolate mofetil

PUVA, psoralen with ultraviolet A; TL-01, narrow-band ultraviolet B; UVB, broad-band ultraviolet B; LPC, liquor picis carbis.

treatment for each patient should be tailored to the type of psoriasis, their age, general health, social and occupational factors, their level of motivation and the acceptability of the treatment to the patient. Some patients may start initially using simple topical therapy and then move to the stronger systemic agents if their disease is poorly controlled, whereas others may move from stronger treatments to simpler topical therapies once their disease is controlled.

Dermatology day treatment units

Dermatology day treatment units (DDTUs) facilitate the management of psoriasis patients, particularly in relation to topical therapy, phototherapy and administration of intravenous or subcutaneous injections. Benefits of the DDTU include compliance, monitoring, education, counselling/support, and an overall reduction in the patient's stress levels. Treatments not possible at home including short-contact dithranol and crude coal tar can be applied to psoriatic plaques by specialist nurses, phototherapy can be delivered in custom-built cabinets, and regular administration of biological therapy can be given by specialist dermatology nurses.

Rationalization of skincare services and a shift in the emphasis away from specialist units to primary care settings, however, means DDTUs are becoming less commonly or locally available.

Topical treatment

Topical treatments are those applied directly to the skin surface; they include include ointments, creams, tars, lotions, pastes and shampoo. The topical approach to therapy results in changes at and just below the skin surface (epidermis and dermis). Conventionally topical medicaments are applied directly to the diseased skin only, in contrast to moisturizers (emollients) which are usually applied more freely. In general, combination therapy is more effective than monotherapy, and change of therapy is superior to continuous usage. Hospital admission to manage stable chronic plaque disease with topical therapy is now extremely rare. Admissions to hospital are generally reserved for those with unstable disease.

The *advantages* of topical treatments:
- local effects only
- self-application
- safe for long-term use
- relatively cheap.

The *disadvantages* of topical treatments:
- time-consuming in extensive disease
- poor compliance (insufficient amounts and frequency)
- messy
- no benefit for associated joint disease
- tachyphylaxis (treatments become less effective with continuous use).

The majority of psoriasis patients with mild disease treat themselves using over-the-counter preparations. Those with moderate disease can be managed in the community, with guidance from the dermatologist. Patients with very extensive, recalcitrant or unstable psoriasis are usually managed in specialist dermatology centres.

Emollients act as a barrier to cutaneous fluid loss, relieve itching and help replace water and lipids, and therefore restore the barrier function of dry skin. Patients are able to purchase these over the counter, and personal preference and acceptability usually guide their choice. The regular application of emollients should be encouraged in all patients with dry/flaky skin.

Coal tar is obtained by distillation of bituminous coal. Many coal tar preparations are available for purchase over the counter and include ointments, pastes, paints, soaps, solutions and shampoo. Coal tar is keratoplastic (normalizes keratinocyte growth patterns), antipruritic (reduces itch) and antimicrobial. It can be used on stable chronic plaque psoriasis but will irritate acute, inflamed skin.

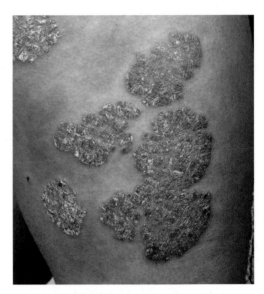

Figure 3.1 Plaques suitable for dithranol treatment.

Coal tar in combination with salicylic acid may be more effective for very thick plaques.

Ichthammol (ammonium bituminosulphonate) is a distillation of sulphur-rich oil shale. It has anti-inflammatory properties and is therefore suitable to use on 'unstable' or inflamed psoriasis. Various preparations can be purchased over the counter, including ichthammol ointment.

Dithranol (anthralin, Goa powder) originally derived from araroba trees, is now produced synthetically. Irritation and burning can occur if it comes into contact with normal skin, therefore careful application to psoriatic plaques is needed (Figure 3.1). Normal skin can be protected with petroleum jelly. Dithranol temporarily stains the skin/hair a purple-brown colour. Short/long contact dithranol can be applied by dermatology nurses to chronic stable plaques in specialist units. Dithranol creams can be applied by the patients themselves, left on for 30 minutes, then washed off. The strength is gradually increased from 0.1% to 3% as necessary. Strengths up to 1% can be purchased over the counter; higher concentrations are available by prescription only and are usually prescribed and managed via general practitioners.

Calcipotriol and *tacalcitol*, vitamin D analogues, are calmodulin inhibitors used topically for mild or moderate plaque psoriasis, and can be prescribed by general medical practitioners. Mild irritation can be experienced and after continuous use a plateau effect may be encountered with the treatment becoming less effective after an initial response. These preparations are therefore best used in combination with other topical agents. It is important not to exceed the maximum recommended dose as there is a risk of altering calcium metabolism.

Corticosteroids are an important adjuvant to the management of patients with psoriasis. These are prescription-only preparations and can be supervised by the general medical practitioner.

Corticosteroids help to reduce the superficial inflammation within the plaques. However, relapse usually occurs on cessation and tachyphylaxis is observed. Tachyphylaxis is thought to result from tolerance to the vasoconstrictive action of corticosteroids on cutaneous capillaries. Topical steroids should be applied to the affected areas of skin only once or twice daily. Manufacturers suggest that topical steroids should be applied sparingly but this is difficult for patients to quantify. Practitioners therefore advise the use of fingertip units (FTUs) as a guide. When steroid ointment/cream is squeezed out from a tube it comes out in a line: between the fingertip and the first skin crease is 1 FTU (approximately 500 mg) or enough to cover a hand-sized area of skin.

The strength of topical steroids is graded from mild to very potent. Prolonged use of very potent topical steroids should generally be avoided in the treatment of chronic skin diseases such as psoriasis. Mild/moderate topical steroids are safe to use on the face and flexural skin, and erythrodermic disease. Moderate or potent preparations can be used on chronic stable plaques on the body. Combination products seem to be amongst the most effective in the treatment of psoriasis, especially those containing salicylic acid, vitamin D, tar and antibiotics. Systemic corticosteroids should not be used to treat psoriasis.

Scalp psoriasis

Scalp psoriasis affects approximately 50% of patients; it can be one of the earliest skin sites affected. Scalp psoriasis is often difficult to treat due to the thick nature of the scales, and inaccessibility of the skin (due to hair getting in the way), and difficulty of self-application of treatment (Figure 3.2). Most patients need to treat the scalp regularly with products left on overnight (combinations of tar, salicylic acid, sulphur and emollient), tar-based shampoos and steroid-containing scalp applications. Treatment in the DDTU can be immensely helpful for difficult scalp psoriasis.

Ultraviolet (UV) treatment (phototherapy)

The mechanisms of action of phototherapy are complex. Evidence suggests that phototherapy reduces the antigen presenting capacity of dendritic cells, induces apoptosis of immune cells and inhibits synthesis and release of pro-inflammatory cytokines. The resultant cutaneous effects are those of topical immunosuppression and a reduction in dermal inflammation and epidermal cell turnover.

Phototherapy should be delivered in specialist dermatology units. It is suitable for psoriasis patients with extensive disease that has not cleared with topical therapy (Figure 3.3). Patients must be able to attend the phototherapy suite 2–3 times weekly on a regular basis for approximately 6–8 weeks. Contraindications to treatment include a history of previous skin malignancy and photosensitive diseases such as lupus, porphyria, albinism and xeroderma pigmentosum. A full drug history should be taken to ascertain whether the patient is taking any photosensitizing medication.

Phototherapy is usually delivered in vertical irradiation units (Figure 3.4). The dose and time of exposure to light is gradually increased as the treatment progresses. Patients apply a layer of emollient to their skin before standing inside the cabinet (this helps remove surface scale and aids UV penetration), they wear UV protective goggles (to protect against corneal keratitis and cataract formation) and 'sanctuary sites' (genitals) are covered.

There is an increased risk of developing cutaneous malignancies with increasing cumulative doses of phototherapy. How much phototherapy can be given safely will depend on the patient's skin type and the cumulative dose of UV received. In addition to the increased risk of cutaneous malignancy, premature ageing of the skin and multiple lentigines can result.

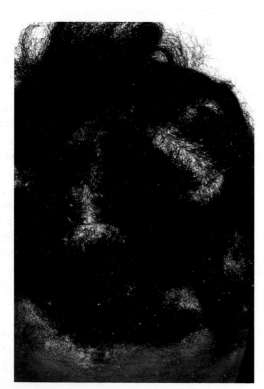

Figure 3.2 Scalp psoriasis.

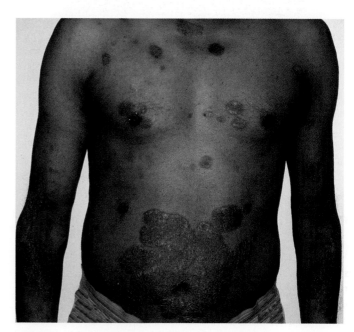

Figure 3.3 Psoriasis suitable for TL-01.

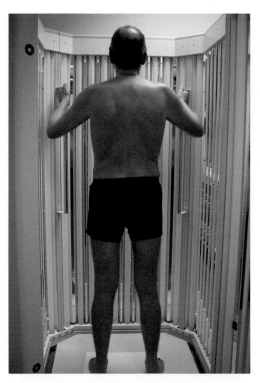

Figure 3.4 Psoralen with ultraviolet A (PUVA) cabinet.

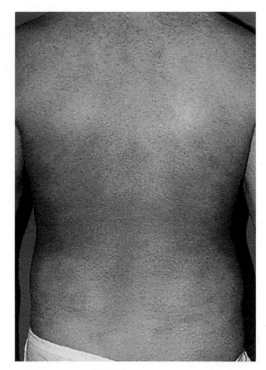

Figure 3.6 After phototherapy.

The total cumulative dosage is carefully monitored and kept as low as possible to reduce the risk of side-effects.

Two main types of phototherapy are currently available: ultraviolet B (UVB) and ultraviolet A with psoralen (PUVA). UVB phototherapy has advantages over PUVA as it can be used in children and during pregnancy, and does not require the wearing of UV-blocking glasses after treatment.

Ultraviolet B (UVB) is short-wavelength UV light and is administered three times weekly (20–30 treatments) for widespread psoriasis. Conventional broad-band UVB lamps emit wavelengths from 280 to 330 nm; these machines are largely being superseded by narrow-band UVB (TL-01) devices which emit ultraviolet light at 311 nm. TL-01 is more effective than broad-band UVB and there is a reduced risk of burning. The starting dose and subsequent increments (mJ/cm^2) for patients can be based on the MED (minimal erythema dose) which is the dose of UVB just sufficient to cause erythema (the patient's starting dose will then commence at 70% of the MED for psoriasis). Alternatively the patient's skin phototype (I–VI) can be used to guide the starting dose. The patient's phototype reflects the skin's tolerance to sunlight (type I very fair skin through to type VI black skin). UVB can be given in combination with tar (Goeckerman regimen) or dithranol (Ingram regimen) for chronic thick plaques of psoriasis. UVB in combination with oral acitretin can also increase the efficacy.

Ultraviolet A (UVA) is long-wavelength UV light (320–400 nm) and is given in combination with oral or topical psoralen (PUVA) twice weekly (20–30 treatments) for recalcitrant widespread thick-plaque psoriasis. There are two types of psoralen tablets: 8-methoxypsoralen (8-MOP) 0.6 mg/kg body weight, and 5-methoxypsoralen

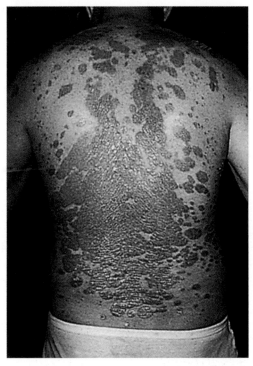

Figure 3.5 Before phototherapy.

Current estimates suggest that patients can be given approximately 200 individual treatments (<1000 J) of light safely within their lifetime. Consequently an individual patient's light 'quota' can soon be used up with a standard course comprising 20–30 treatments (Figures 3.5 & 3.6). Maintenance treatment with phototherapy is no longer recommended and rarely given for psoriasis.

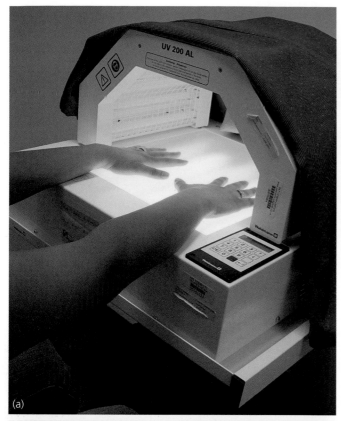

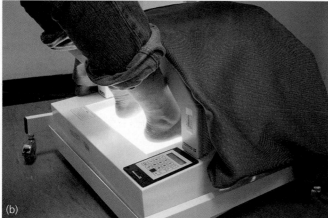

Figure 3.7 Hand (a) and foot (b) PUVA.

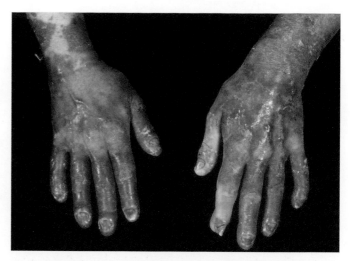

Figure 3.8 Severe psoriasis suitable for systemic therapy.

(5-MOP) 1.2 mg/kg taken 2 hours before treatment. 8-MOP is associated with a higher incidence of side-effects such as nausea, vomiting, pruritus and erythema. The MPD (minimum phototoxic dose) or skin phototype is used to determine the starting dose of UVA and the subsequent increments used (J/cm^2). Protective goggles are worn during the UVA exposure and sunglasses for 24 hours post treatment. Localized PUVA can be given to palmar/plantar psoriasis (Figure 3.7).

Systemic treatment

Systemic therapy for severe psoriasis should ideally be managed by experienced specialist dermatologists. The indications for systemic therapy include patients with unstable inflamed psoriasis (Figure 3.8), widespread disease that has failed to respond to topical/phototherapy regimens and concomitant psoriatic arthropathy. The first-line systemic agents in most dermatology centres are methotrexate and acitretin. Alternatives include ciclosporin, hydroxyurea, azathioprine and mycophenolate mofetil. Biological therapies (infliximab, etanercept, efalizumab, adalimumab) can be considered if patients have failed to respond or have experienced side-effects precluding the continued use of at least two systemic agents.

Methotrexate

Methotrexate is suitable for treating unstable erythrodermic/pustular psoriasis in the acute setting as well as maintenance for chronic plaque disease. Methotrexate reduces epidermal cell turnover by the inhibition of folic acid synthesis during the S phase of mitosis. Methotrexate is given once weekly as a tablet or injection. Conventionally, patients are given low doses initially that gradually increase until the psoriasis is 'sufficiently controlled' rather than clear. Maintenance doses of 7.5–15 mg weekly are usually adequate.

Side-effects

Methotrexate is hepatotoxic and therefore liver function tests must be measured before and during therapy. Routine liver biopsies for monitoring liver fibrosis have largely been superseded by measuring serum levels of procollagen III. Baseline procollagen III levels are measured and if these remain stable the patient is unlikely to have significant liver damage. However if the levels of procollagen III are persistently raised then a liver biopsy should be considered.

Myelosuppression can occur in patients taking methotrexate and its onset may be rapid or insidious. Patients should be monitored with regular full blood counts (FBCs). An initial test dose of 5 mg should be given on commencement of methotrexate followed by an FBC 1 week later to ensure there is no idiosyncratic marrow suppression. Folic acid supplements should be given (at least 5 mg weekly). Methotrexate is excreted in the urine and therefore the dose must be reduced in renal impairment. Aspirin and sulpho-namides diminish plasma binding. Interactions occur with several drugs including barbiturates, phenytoin, oral contraceptives and colchicine.

Acitretin

Acitretin is a vitamin A derivative that can be prescribed only in hospital in the UK. It is effective in treating chronic plaque psoriasis with approximately 70% clearance in 8 weeks. A synergistic effect has been observed with concomitant PUVA, when patients require less UV exposure to clear their psoriasis.

Side-effects

Most patients experience mucocutaneous symptoms including drying of the mucous membranes, crusting in the nose, itching, thinning of the hair, and erythema of the palms and nail folds. These are usually not severe and settle when treatment stops.

Hepatotoxicity and raised lipid concentrations occur in 20–30% of patients. Liver function tests and cholesterol/triglyceride concentrations should be carefully monitored. Acitretin can be metabolized to etretinate (half-life 70–100 days), which is terato-genic, and therefore women of reproductive age must use effective contraception during treatment and for 2 years afterwards.

Ciclosporin A

Ciclosporin A is an immunosuppressant widely used following organ transplantation. It is effective and suitable for the treatment of inflammatory types of psoriasis due to its rapid onset of action. Patients are given 3–5 mg/kg/day in two divided doses either for short courses or continuous use. The minimum dose required to control the psoriasis should be used.

Side-effects

These include renal impairment and hypertension. Baseline blood tests should include serum creatinine, urea, electrolytes and a glomerular filtration rate. Hypertension may be managed by reducing the dose of ciclosporin or giving the patient nifedipine. Transient nausea, gum hypertrophy and hypertrichosis may also be observed.

Hepatic metabolism of cyclosporin (via cytochrome P450) can be inhibited or induced by many different drugs. Drugs inhibiting ciclosporin metabolism include erythromycin, itraconazole, verapamil and diltiazem. Drugs increasing ciclosporin metabolism include rifampicin, phenytoin and carbamazepine.

Biological therapy

Biological therapy refers to substances derived from living organisms such as proteins or antibodies. Psoriasis is known to be T-cell mediated and cytokines such as tumour necrosis factor-alpha (TNF-α) and interferon-gamma (INF-γ) play a role. Biological therapies are currently directed against T-cells or specific inflammatory mediators such as TNF. The main biological agents currently used to treat severe psoriasis are infliximab, etanercept, adalimumab (TNF-α inhibitors) and efalizumab (T-cell inhibitor). Clinical guidelines exist to direct the usage of biological agents in patients with psoriasis, such as previous failure (lack of efficacy, adverse side-effects) with two systemic agents. Biologics are delivered by subcutaneous injection or intravenous infusion with frequencies varying from twice weekly to once per month, in either continuous or intermittent regimes. The main concern with these relatively novel agents is the resultant chronic immunosuppression leading to the potential increased risk of infections and tumours.

Further reading

Menter A, Griffiths CE. Current and future management of psoriasis. *Lancet* 2007; **370**: 272–84.

Weinberg JM. *Treatment of Psoriasis (Milestones in Drug Therapy)*. Birkhauser Verlag AG, Basel, 2007.

www.bad.org.uk/healthcare/guidelines/psorsites.asp

CHAPTER 4

Eczema (Dermatitis) Including Management

OVERVIEW

- What is eczema?
- Pathological changes in relation to clinical appearance.
- Classification of different types of eczema: endogenous and exogenous.
- Causes of contact dermatitis.
- Investigations in eczema.
- Management options.
- Occupational dermatitis.
- Causes and management of pruritus.

Introduction

Eczema or dermatitis are terms used to describe the characteristic clinical appearance of inflamed, dry, occasionally scaly and vesicular skin rashes associated with divergent underlying causes. The word eczema is derived from the Greek, meaning to 'boil over', which aptly describes the microscopic blisters occurring in the epidermis at the cellular level. Dermatitis, as the term suggests, implies inflammation of the skin which relates to the underlying pathophysiology. The terms eczema and dermatitis encompass a wide variety of skin conditions usually classified by their characteristic distribution, morphology and any trigger factors involved (Table 4.1).

Clinical features

Eczema is an inflammatory condition that may be acute or chronic. Acute eruptions are characterized by erythema, vesicular/bullous lesions and exudate. Secondary bacterial infection (staphylococcus and streptococcus) heralded by golden crusting may exacerbate acute eczema. Chronicity of inflammation leads to increased scaling, xerosis (dryness) and lichenification (thickening of the skin where surface markings become more prominent). Eczema is characteristically itchy and subsequent scratching may also modify the clinical appearance leading to excoriation marks, loss of skin surface, secondary infection, exudates and ultimately marked lichenification

ABC of Dermatology, 5th edition. Edited by P. K. Buxton and R. Morris-Jones.
© 2009 Blackwell Publishing, ISBN: 978-1-4051-7065-9.

Table 4.1 Classification of eczema.

Endogenous (constitutional) eczema	Exogenous (contact) eczema	Secondary changes
Atopic	Irritant	Lichen simplex
Discoid	Allergic	Asteatotic
Pompholyx	Photodermatitis	Pompholyx
Varicose		Infection
Seborrhoeic (see Chapter 16)		

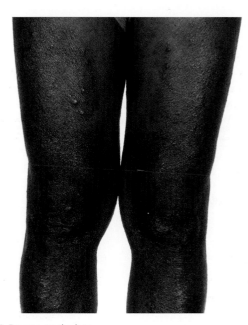

Figure 4.1 Eczema on the legs.

(Figure 4.1). Inflammation in the skin can result in disruption of skin pigmentation causing post-inflammatory hyper- or hypopigmentation. Patients often fear that loss of pigment is due to the application of topical steroids, but in the majority of cases it is due to chronic inflammation.

Pathophysiology

The underling causes of endogenous eczema are poorly defined, but genetic predisposition is common in patients with atopic eczema. In these patients there is an abnormality of T-helper (T_H)

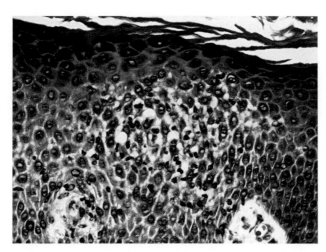

Figure 4.2 Histology of eczema.

lymphocytes, particularly the T_H-2 cells which are thought to play an important role in the disease. The abnormal T_H-2 cells interact with Langerhans cells causing raised levels of interleukins/IgE and a reduction in interferon (INF-γ) with resultant upregulation of pro-inflammatory cells. Defective skin barrier function and environmental allergen triggers have also been noted.

Pathology

The clinical changes associated with dermatitis are reflected accurately at the cellular level. There is oedema in the epidermis leading to spongiosis (separation of keratinocytes) and vesicle formation (Figure 4.2). The epidermis is hyperkeratotic (thickened) with dilated blood vessels and an inflammatory (eosinophil) cell infiltrate in the dermis.

Types of eczema

Eczema is classified broadly into endogenous (constitutional) and exogenous (induced by an external factor).

Endogenous eczema

Atopic eczema typically presents in infancy or early childhood, initially with facial and subsequently with flexural limb involvement (Figures 4.3–4.5). Eczema is intensely itchy, and even young babies become highly proficient at scratching, which can lead to disrupted sleep (for both patient and family), poor feeding and irritability. The usual pattern is for flare-ups to be followed by remissions, exacerbations being associated with intercurrent infections, teething and food allergies. In severely affected babies failure to thrive may result. In older children or adults, eczema may become chronic and widespread and is frequently exacerbated by stress. Atopic eczema is common, affecting 3% of infants; nonetheless 90% of cases spontaneously remit by puberty. Patients likely to suffer from chronic atopic eczema in adult life are those who have a strong family history of eczema, who present at a very young age with extensive disease and who have associated asthma (Figure 4.6).

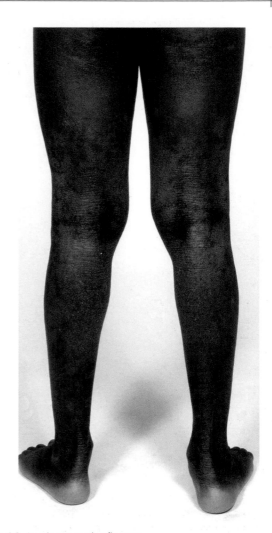

Figure 4.3 Atopic eczema leg flexures.

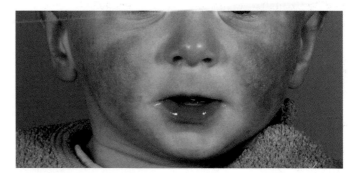

Figure 4.4 Facial eczema.

Pityriasis alba is a variant of atopic eczema in which pale patches of hypopigmentation develop on the face of children. Juvenile plantar dermatosis is another variant of atopic eczema in which there is dry cracked skin on the forefoot in children (Figure 4.7).

Eczema herpeticum is herpes simplex viral infection superimposed onto skin affected by eczema (usually in atopics). There is frequently a history of close contact with an adult with herpes labialis (cold sore). Eczema herpeticum is a serious complication of eczema that may be life-threatening, and therefore early intervention with

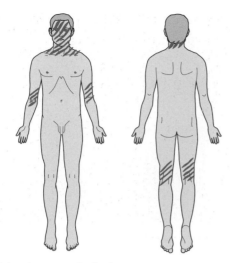

Figure 4.5 Atopic eczema: distribution

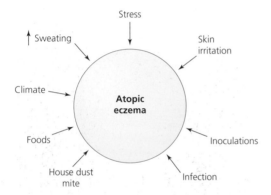

Figure 4.6 Factors leading to development of atopic eczema.

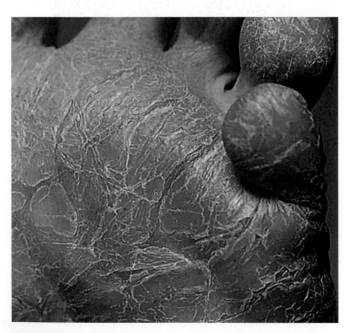

Figure 4.7 Plantar dermatoses.

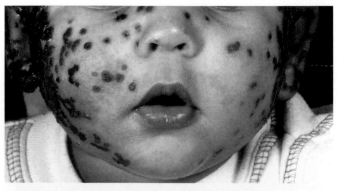

Figure 4.8 Eczema herpeticum.

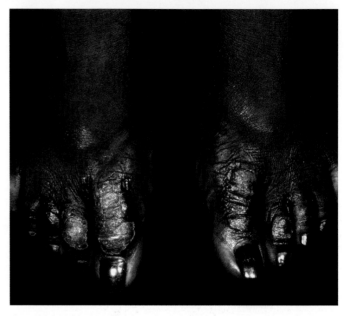

Figure 4.9 Lichen simplex.

systemic aciclovir is essential under the guidance of a dermatology specialist (Figure 4.8).

Lichen simplex is a localized area of lichenification produced by rubbing (Figure 4.9).

Asteatotic eczema occurs in older people with a dry skin, particularly on the lower legs. The pattern on the skin resembles a dry river-bed or 'crazy-paving' (Figure 4.10).

Discoid eczema appears as intensely pruritic coin-shaped lesions most commonly on the limbs (Figure 4.11). Lesions may be vesicular and are frequently colonized by *Staphylococcus aureus*. Males are more frequently affected than females.

Pompholyx eczema is itching vesicles on the fingers, palms and soles. The blisters are small, firm, intensely itchy and occasionally painful (Figure 4.12). The condition is more common in patients with nickel allergy.

Venous (stasis) eczema is a common insidious dermatitis that occurs on the lower legs of patients with venous insufficiency. These

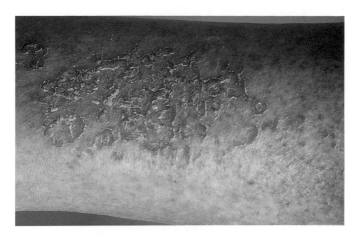

Figure 4.10 Asteatotic eczema.

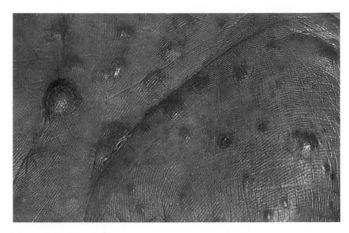

Figure 4.12 Pompholyx eczema.

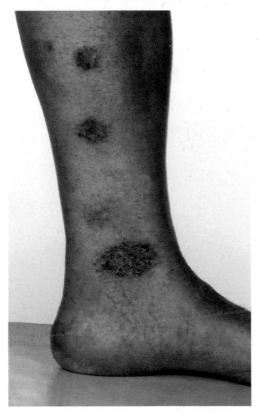

Figure 4.11 Discoid eczema.

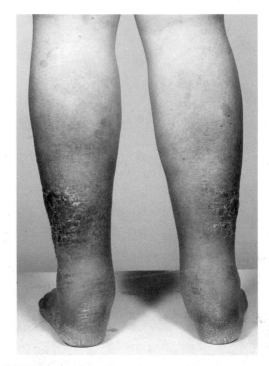

Figure 4.13 Venous eczema.

patients have back-flow of blood from the deep to the superficial veins leading to venous hypertension. In the early stages there is brown haemosiderin pigmentation of the skin especially on the medial ankle, but as the disease progresses skin changes can extend up to the knee (Figure 4.13). Patients typically have peripheral oedema and ulceration may result. The mainstay of management is compression (see Chapter 11).

Investigation of endogenous eczema

Skin swabs should be taken from the skin if secondary bacterial or viral infection is suspected (Figure 4.14). The swab should be moistened in the transport medium before being rolled thoroughly on

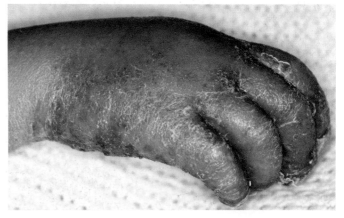

Figure 4.14 Infected eczema.

the affected skin, coating all sides of the swab to ensure an adequate sample is sent to the laboratory. A significant growth of bacteria reported with its sensitivity and resistance pattern can be useful in guiding antibiotic usage. Nasal swabs should be performed in older children and adults with persistent facial eczema, to check for nasal *Staphylococcus* carriage. If a secondary fungal infection is suspected then scrapings or brushings can be taken for mycological analysis.

Routine blood tests are not necessary, but an eosinophilia and raised immunoglobulin E (IgE) level may be seen. RAST (radioallergosorbent testing) looks for specific IgE levels against suspected allergens such as aeroallergens (pollens, house dust mite, animal dander) and foods (egg, cow's milk, wheat, fish, nuts, soya proteins).

Skin biopsy (usually a punch biopsy) for histological analysis may be performed if the diagnosis is uncertain. Beware unilateral eczema of the areola which could be Paget's disease of the nipple (Figure 4.15).

Varicose eczema (leg ulcer) patients should have their ABPI (ankle brachial pressure index) measured before compressing their legs with bandages. The ABPI is the ratio of their arm to ankle systolic blood pressure.

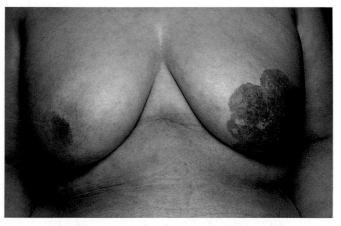

Figure 4.15 Paget's disease of the nipple: beware unilateral 'eczema'.

Exogenous eczema

Contact dermatitis

Contact dermatitis can result from allergic or irritant reactions in the skin (Box 4.1). Cutaneous contact allergy is not inherent but acquired due to exposure to environmental or occupational allergens (Figure 4.16). In general the more a person is exposed to a potential allergen (quantity and frequency) the more likely they are to develop an allergy. Patients with abnormal skin barrier function (e.g. those with eczema) are more likely to develop contact dermatitis and suffer from irritant reactions than those with normal skin. Patients develop an allergic skin reaction at the site of sensitization to an allergen and then on subsequent exposure at a distant skin site develop eczema simultaneously at previous sites of allergy.

Clinical features
The clinical appearance of both allergic and irritant contact dermatitis may be similar, but there are specific changes that help in differentiating them. An acute allergic reaction tends to be intensely itchy and results in erythema, oedema and vesicles. The more chronic lesions are often lichenified. Irritant dermatitis may be itchy or sore, and presents as slight scaling, erythema and fissuring.

The distribution of the skin changes is often helpful in identifying the underlying cause (Figure 4.17). For example, an itchy rash

---

Box 4.1 **Common contact allergens**

- Nickel/cobalt (jewellery, clothing, wristwatch, scissors, cooking utensils) (Figure 4.18)
- Perfumes, Balsam of Peru (fragrances)
- Formaldehyde, parabens, quaternium (preservatives)
- Paraphenylenediamine (PPD) (permanent hair dyes, temporary tattoos, textiles) (Figures 4.19 & 4.20)
- Ethylenediamine (adhesives, medications) (Figure 4.21)
- Chromates (cement, leather) (Figure 4.22)
- Mercaptobenzothiazole, thiurams (rubber gloves, shoes)
- Neomycin, benzocaine (medicated ointments) (Figure 4.23)
- Lanolin (wool alcohol, emollients, medicated ointments)

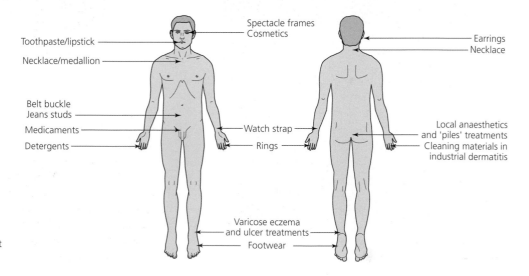

Figure 4.16 Common sources of contact dermatitis.

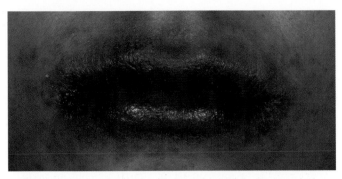

Figure 4.17 Contact dermatitis on the lips secondary to topical aciclovir allergy.

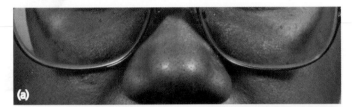

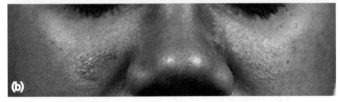

Figure 4.18 (a,b) Contact dermatitis to nickel spectacle frames.

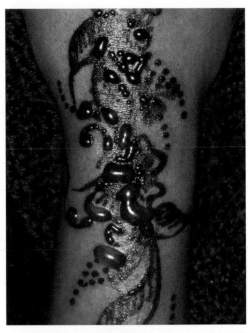

Figure 4.20 Acute PPD allergy in 'henna' tattoo.

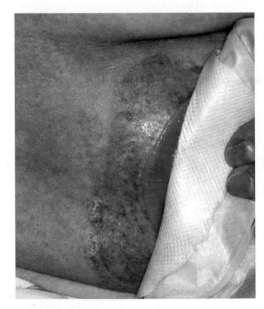

Figure 4.21 Contact allergy to stoma dressing.

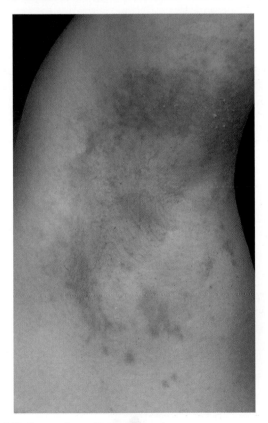

Figure 4.19 Contact dermatitis to clothing dye.

on the waist may indicate an allergy to rubber in the waistband of underclothing, a metal fastener or clothing dyes. An allergy to medications used for treating leg ulcers is a common cause of persistent dermatitis on the lower leg. Hand dermatitis can result from glove allergies (rubber, latex) or irritation from sweat under gloves. Periorbital dermatitis may result from nickel allergy (spectacle frames), fragrance allergy (cosmetics) or eye drops (containing neomycin). An irritant substance often produces a more diffuse eruption such as physical irritation to the skin caused by air conditioning.

Allergic contact dermatitis

The characteristics of allergic dermatitis are:
- previous exposure to the substance concerned
- 48–96 hours between contact and the development of changes in the skin
- activation of previously sensitized sites by contact with allergen at a distant skin site
- persistence of the allergy for many years.

Immune mechanisms

Allergic dermatitis results from a type IV delayed hypersensitivity reaction in the skin. Specific antigens (usually proteins) penetrate the epidermis, combine with a protein mediator and are then picked up by Langerhans cells. This causes T lymphocytes

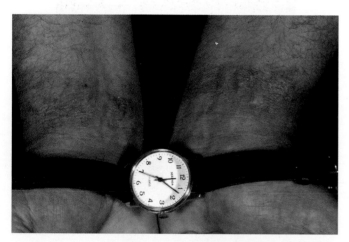

Figure 4.22 Contact dermatitis to leather in watch strap.

in regional lymph nodes to become sensitized to the antigen. On subsequent exposure to the antigen an allergic reaction occurs, due to accumulation of sensitized T lymphocytes at the site of the antigen with a resultant inflammatory response. This takes 48 hours and is amplified by interleukins that provide a positive feedback stimulus to the production of further sensitized T lymphocytes (Figure 4.24).

Irritant contact dermatitis

This may be chemical or physical, has a less defined clinical course and is caused by a wide variety of substances with no predictable time interval between contact and the appearance of the rash. Physical irritants include air conditioning, prosthetic limbs, personnel-protective clothing and repetitive mechanical trauma. Chemical irritants include detergents, solvents and acids. Dermatitis occurs soon after exposure and the severity varies with the quantity, concentration and length of exposure to the substance concerned. Previous contact is not required, unlike allergic dermatitis where previous sensitization is necessary.

Photodermatitis

Photodermatitis is caused by the interaction of light and chemicals absorbed by the skin. It can result from (a) drugs taken internally, such as sulphonamides, phenothiazines, tetracycline and voriconazole or (b) substances in contact with the skin, such as topical antihistamines, local anaesthetics, cosmetics and antibacterials. Phytophotodermatitis results from contact with plant material, often containing forms of psoralens (poison oak, common rue, lime juice, celery), and sunlight causing an allergic contact dermatitis. Patients with chronic actinic dermatitis (chronic eczema on sun-exposed skin) are allergic to sunlight but in addition they

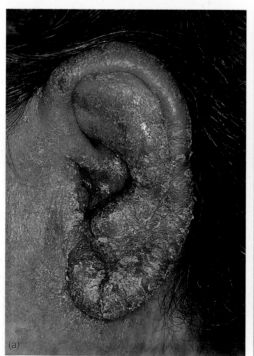
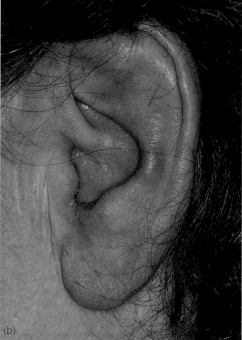

(a)   (b)

Figure 4.23 Allergic response to topical neomycin (left). After stopping ointment (right).

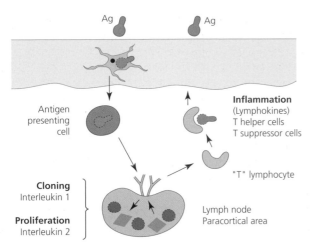

Figure 4.24 Immunological response leading to contact dermatitis.

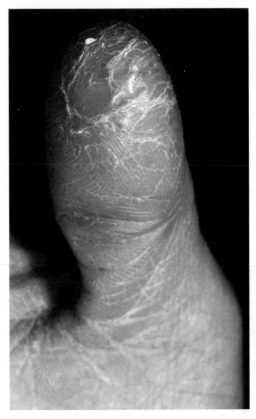

Figure 4.26 Irritant hand eczema in a chef.

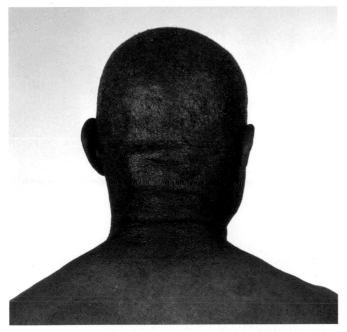

Figure 4.25 Chronic actinic dermatitis.

may be allergic to compositae plants (daisy, sunflower family) (Figure 4.25).

Occupational dermatitis

In the workplace employees may have contact with allergens or irritants that can result in dermatitis. If an individual has an atopic tendency to develop eczema they are at increased risk of developing an occupational dermatitis. Secondary bacterial infection can play a role once dermatitis has occurred. Therefore contact dermatitis, atopic eczema and infection may all be superimposed. For example, a student nurse or trainee hairdresser is exposed to water, detergents and other factors that will exacerbate any pre-existing eczema. The skin then becomes broken due to scratching and secondary infection occurs.

An occupational dermatitis is likely if:
• the dermatitis first occurred during a specific employment and had not been present before
• the condition generally improves or clears when away from the workplace
• there is exposure to known irritant/allergic substances and personnel-protective measures are inadequate.

Persistence of dermatitis away from the workplace may occur in occupational dermatitis if the allergen is also present at home (e.g. rubber in gloves), if there is secondary infection, and if there are chronic skin changes. The morphology of the skin eruption itself will be indistinguishable whatever the cause of the eczema.

Occupational irritant contact dermatitis can be acute or chronic. Acute reactions are usually associated with a clear history of exposure to a chemical or physical irritant. Chronic irritant dermatitis can be harder to assess as it develops insidiously in many cases. Individuals involved in frequent 'wet work' such as nurses, cleaners, chefs and those looking after small children can develop irritant hand dermatitis from repeated exposure to water (Figure 4.26). Initially transient inflammation may clear, however with each successive episode the damage becomes worse with an escalation of inflammatory changes that eventually become chronic and fixed. Once chronic damage has occurred the skin is vulnerable to any further irritation, so the condition may flare up in the future even after removal of the causative factors. Individuals with atopic eczema are particularly liable to develop chronic irritant dermatitis and secondary infection is an additional factor.

Occupational allergic contact dermatitis occurs as an allergic reaction to specific substances. There is no immediate reaction on first exposure, but after repeated exposure a cell-mediated inflammatory response develops. Some substances are highly sensitizing such as epoxy resin whilst others need prolonged exposure over many years to trigger allergy such as cement. In addition to the capacity of the substance to produce an allergic reaction, individuals also vary considerably in the capacity to develop allergies.

Contact urticaria is an immediate-type sensitivity reaction that can occur to certain food proteins and latex glove allergy. Chefs may develop allergies to foods proteins (usually on their non-dominant hand as knives are usually held in the dominant hand) that can result in contact urticaria, or a more chronic irritant contact dermatitis.

Investigation of contact dermatitis

A full detailed history is essential if the potential irritant or allergen is to be identified. Dermatology specialists should particularly assess those with a suspected occupational dermatitis as the investigations and subsequent results could affect the patient's future employment and possible compensation claims.

In relation to suspected occupational dermatitis the exact details of the patient's job should be taken in careful detail. Occasionally an 'on-site' visit to the workplace may be required. For example, a worker in a plastics factory had severe hand dermatitis but the only positive result on patch testing was to nickel. On visiting the factory it became clear that the cause was a nickel-plated handle that he used several thousand times a day. It is also important to assess the working environment because exposure to damp (on an oil rig) and irritants (dry air in aircraft cabins) can result in skin irritation.

Patch testing

Patch testing is used to determine which substances are causing a contact dermatitis. The concentration used is critical to ensure a low false negative/positive rate. The optimum concentration and best vehicle have been ascertained for most common allergens. The standard series contains a 'battery' of tests that encompasses the most common allergens encountered. Additional specialist 'batteries' (dental, medicaments, metals, perfumes etc.) may also be available in some specialist dermatology centres. It is important that patch testing is managed by experienced dermatologists to ensure the most appropriate tests are performed, in the correct manner (timings and dilutions), interpreted correctly (irritant or allergic reactions) and then any relevance sought.

The test patches are usually placed on the upper back (sites marked) and left in place for 48 hours then removed and any positive reactions noted (Figures 4.27 & 4.28). A further examination is carried out at 96 hours to detect any late reactions (Figure 4.29). Patients need to visit the unit 3 times in one week, be off systemic immunosuppressants and have an area of clear skin (usually the upper back) on which to perform the tests. Although rare, sensitization may occur as a consequence of exposure to an allergen through patch testing.

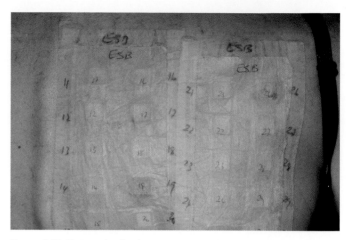

Figure 4.27 Test patches in place.

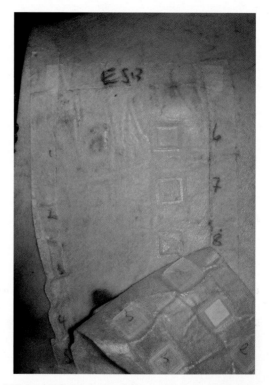

Figure 4.28 Patches being removed after 48 hours.

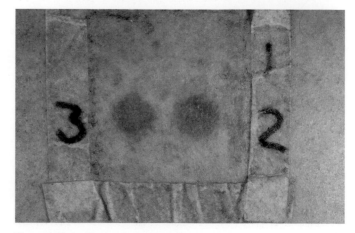

Figure 4.29 Positive patch test reactions.

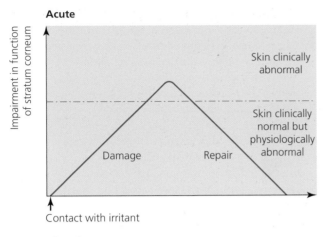

Acute

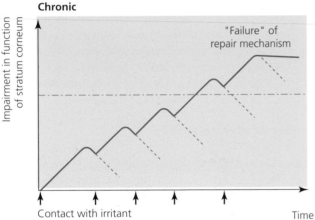

Chronic

Figure 4.30 Progression of acute and chronic dermatitis.

General management of eczema

We must always remember to treat the patient and not just the rash. Many patients suffer considerably with their eczema whilst others seem less concerned. Many parents of children with atopic dermatitis are hoping for a quick 'cure' by the removal of triggers such as foods, but in the majority this is not the case. Management of atopic eczema patients should therefore include adequate time to discuss the aims of therapy and its limitations, namely suppression rather than cure of the disease. Exogenous eczema may be transient and 'cured' after identification and avoidance of trigger factors (Figure 4.30).

Practitioners need to have realistic expectations about what patients can tolerate in terms of acceptability of topical formulations as some are greasy and smelly. Patients need to be physically capable and able to find the time to apply their own creams.

Many simple treatments can be purchased and applied by the individuals themselves without the need to consult a medical practitioner. Treatments usually start with simple emollients and mild topical steroids, but with increasingly recalcitrant disease stronger therapies such as systemic immunosuppressants may be needed.

Patients with dry skin conditions have ready access to a wide range of *emollients* (moisturizing creams) over the counter. In general the oilier the cream the better its emollient properties, but patients tend

to prefer lighter creams. Moisturizers should be applied repeatedly throughout the day in generous amounts. Emollients help to restore barrier function and reduce itching.

Normal soap contains surfactants which disrupt the lipid barrier and cause drying of the skin. *Aqueous cream* and *emulsifying ointments* are useful soap substitutes. Antibacterial moisturizing washes are available for those prone to secondary bacterial infections. Bath oils may be added to the water, or used as a shower wash. Soothing and descaling shampoo can be useful for dry, flaky and itchy scalps.

Topical steroids – frequency and quantity. Topical steroids continue to be the mainstay of treatment for active eczema. Many patients are wary of using topical steroids as they are worried about skin thinning. We need to reassure patients that under careful medical supervision steroids should be safe and are highly effective. Ointments rather than creams should be used whenever possible (creams are more likely to cause irritation and have a higher risk of inducing contact allergies). Steroids should be applied once or twice daily to the affected skin only. One fingertip unit (a line of ointment from the tip of the finger to the first skin crease) is a sufficient amount to treat a hand-sized (palmar and dorsal surface) area of affected skin. Strength and frequency should be tailored to the severity and skin sites affected. Generally they should be used twice daily on affected skin.

Topical steroids –potency. Very low potency steroids such as hydrocortisone may be purchased over the counter and used to treat mild eczema. For moderate to severe disease the current approach is to prescribe potent topical steroids (mometasone, betamethasone, fluocinolone acetonide) for short periods followed by steroid 'holidays' rather than using daily low-potency steroids, which rarely clear the eczema. For acute dermatitis start with a potent topical steroid for a few days or weeks and then reduce to a lower potency once the disease is controlled. Lower-potency topical steroids should be used on the face and groin areas (hydrocortisone, clobetasone butyrate).

Immunomodulators in topical formulations are relatively new and their use should be prescribed and supervised by an experienced dermatological practitioner. Tacrolimus (0.03% for children aged 2–15 years, 0.1% for adults) and pimecrolimus (1%) are applied twice daily to the affected skin. As yet the long-term safety data are unavailable for these topical calcineurin inhibitors and there is a theoretical risk of increased malignancies. Consequently their use should be limited to those whose condition has failed to respond adequately to first-line treatment (topical steroids). Usage should be for short periods only and not continuous.

Occlusion of topical therapy with bandages, body suits, 'wet-wraps' and dressings can be very helpful in the management of chronic eczema (see Chapter 25). Before occlusion the practitioner should ensure the eczema is not infected. Patients and their carers should be taught how to apply these occlusive aids which are generally worn overnight. Occlusive therapy helps to relieve symptoms of itch, keep emollient creams on the skin and 'drive' topical therapy through the epidermis. The potency of topical steroids is enhanced 100-fold by occlusion, so only very low potency steroids should be used under occlusion.

Antibiotics are needed to treat infected eczema; they may be given topically or systemically. Topical antibiotics used include fusidic acid, silver sulphadiazine, polymyxins, neomycin and mupirocin. Formulations of antibiotics combined with topical steroids are available. It is recommended that topical antibiotics should be used for a maximum of 2 weeks continuously to try to reduce the risk of developing resistance in bacteria. Systemic antibiotics used include flucloxacillin (amoxycillin, penicillin) erythromycin (clarithromycin, azithromycin) and ciprofloxacin (levofloxacin, ofloxacin). Antibacterial emollient washes can be useful in active cutaneous infections as well as prophylactically.

Phototherapy with narrow-band UVB (TL-01) or PUVA (psoralen with UVA) can be highly effective for generalized eczema. Each course of phototherapy lasts 6–8 weeks with patients attending 2–3 times per week. There is, however, a limit to the number of courses (cumulative dose) of phototherapy that any individual patient may receive before there is a significantly increased risk of skin cancer (see Chapter 3).

Severe widespread disease not controlled with topical therapy may require systemic immunosuppressants. Occasionally dermatology specialists may prescribe a rapidly reducing course of oral prednisolone (30 mg for 5 days, then reducing by 5 mg every 5 days) to control very severe generalized acute eczema in adults. However, long-term oral steroids should not be used to control eczema. Rather azathioprine, ciclosporin, mycophenolate mofetil and methotrexate can be used for long-term management. If available, levels of thiopurine methyl transferase (TPMT) should be checked before initiation of azathioprine.

Pruritus

Pruritus is a term used to describe itching of the skin that is an unpleasant sensation triggering rubbing or scratching. The sensation of pruritus can be extremely disturbing, leading to disrupted sleep and even depression. Pruritus may be localized or generalized and may be associated with skin changes or with normal skin.

Pruritus with skin changes
Pruritus may be localized or generalized.

Causes of localized pruritus with skin changes
Causes include eczema, psoriasis, lichen planus (flat topped itchy papules of unknown cause), dermatitis herpetiformis (gluten allergy with rash characteristically on elbows and buttocks), insect bites/stings (nodular prurigo may develop after insect bites and is characterized by persistent itching, lichenified papules and nodules), head lice, contact dermatitis, polymorphic light eruption (an acute allergy to sunlight on sun-exposed skin), urticaria or angio-oedema ('hives' with swelling especially of the face), fungal infections (particularly tinea pedis of the feet), pruritus ani (perianal itching, a common condition that may result from anal leakage, skin tags, haemorrhoids, excessive washing, the use of medicated wipes, allergy to haemorrhoid creams containing Balsam of Peru) and pruritus vulvae (intense itching may result from lichen sclerosus et atrophicus, *Candida* infections or eczema).

Causes of generalized pruritus with skin changes
This occurs in more widespread inflammatory skin diseases such as widespread eczema/psoriasis, scabies, allergic drug eruptions (antibiotics, anticonvulsants), graft versus host disease (following bone marrow transplantation), prebullous pemphigoid (dermatitic eruption before blisters appear), cutaneous lymphoma (may start over the buttocks as more localized disease), parasitophobia (belief that there are parasites under the skin; excoriations are seen), body lice or pubic lice (body lice live in the clothing), viral exanthems (rashes associated with systemic viral illness), urticaria (generalized 'hives'), xerosis (dry skin, especially in the elderly).

Investigation and management of pruritus with skin changes should be directed at the suspected underlying cause.

Pruritus with normal skin
Medical practitioners need to be alert to the patient with generalized pruritus and normal skin as itching may be the first symptom of a systemic disorder such as Hodgkin's disease, chronic renal failure, diabetes etc., or may be a side-effect of medication.

Systemic causes
- Endocrine: diabetes, myxoedema, hyperthyroidism, menopause, pregnancy.
- Metabolic: hepatic failure, biliary obstruction, chronic renal failure.
- Haematological: polycythaemia, iron deficiency anaemia.
- Malignancy: lymphoma, leukaemia, myeloma, carcinomatosis.
- Neurological/psychological: neuropathic pruritus, multiple sclerosis, anxiety.
- Infection: filariasis, hookworm, HIV.
- Drugs: opioids.

Investigations
- Full blood count, erythrocyte sedimentation rate, liver and renal function.
- Serum iron, ferritin, total iron-binding capacity.
- Thyroid function, fasting glucose.
- Serum protein electrophoresis.
- HIV antibody (if risk factors).
- Urine analysis.
- Stools for blood and parasites/ova.
- Chest X-ray.
- Skin biopsy for direct immunofluorescence.

Management of pruritus
Identifying and treating the underlying cause of the pruritus is obviously desirable whenever possible. Patients themselves will find

some short-term relief by scratching the skin, but this ultimately leads to further itching and scratching: the so called 'itch–scratch cycle'. To break this cycle the sensation of itch needs to be suppressed, or the patient's behaviour changed by, for example, habit reversal techniques.

Individuals can purchase simple soothing emollients over the counter and apply these frequently to the pruritic areas. The soothing effect can be enhanced by storing the cream in the fridge and applying it cold. Menthol 1–2% in aqueous cream and calamine possess cooling and antipruritic properties. Camphor-containing preparations and crotamiton (Eurax) and topical doxepin hydrochloride applied thinly 3–4 times daily to localized areas may provide relief from itching.

Topical local anaesthetics (containing benzocaine, lidocaine, tetracaine) on sale to the public may give some temporary relief but intolerance may develop and allergic reactions can occur.

Topical and systemic antihistamines can provide relief from itching. Topical antihistamines (mepyramine, antazoline) are on sale to the public in various formulations which may give temporary relief to localized areas. Generally non-sedating oral antihistamines are given during the day and sedating ones at night. Cutaneous itch responds readily to the histamine H1-receptor blockers cetirizine, levocetirizine, desloratadine and fexofenadine during the day and hydroxyzine at night. H2-receptor blockers (ranitidine, cimetidine) may be used in addition to H1-receptor blockers in resistant cases.

Pruritus ani/vulvae

The affected area should be washed once daily; excessive washing should be avoided. Aqueous cream or emulsifying ointments can be used as a soap substitute. Patients should avoid perfumed, coloured and medicated toilet tissue or wipes. Simple paraffin or zinc cream can be used as a barrier ointment to prevent skin irritation from anal leakage/vaginal discharge. Weak topical steroids can help to reduce inflammation and itching. If symptoms persist patients should see a dermatology specialist who may do patch testing (contact dermatitis) or perform a skin biopsy (neoplasia, lichen sclerosus, lichen planus).

Further reading

Elsner P, Kanervan L, Wahlberg JE, Maibach HI. *Condensed Handbook of Occupational Dermatology*. Springer-Verlag, Berlin and Heidelberg, 2003.

Holden C, Ostlere L. *Pocket Guide to Eczema and Contact Dermatitis*. Blackwell Science Ltd, Oxford, 2000.

Rycroft RJG, Menne T, Frosch PJ, Lepoitterin JP. *Textbook of Contact Dermatitis*, 3rd edn. Springer-Verlag, Berlin and Heidelberg, 2001.

www.bad.org.uk/public/leaflets/other_atopic_-_index.asp

CHAPTER 5

Urticaria and Angio-oedema

OVERVIEW

- Definition and pathophysiology; the role of vasodilators.
- Classification.
- Clinical presentation of different types of urticaria.
- Causes and investigation of non-physical urticarias.
- Management and treatment.

Introduction

Urticaria describes transient pruritic swellings on the skin, often referred to as wheals, hives or nettle rash by the patient. Urticaria is due to oedema in the superficial layers of the skin resulting in well-demarcated erythematous lesions. It may be associated with allergic reactions, infection or physical stimuli, but in most patients no cause can be found. Similar lesions may precede or be associated with vasculitis (urticarial vasculitis), pemphigoid or dermatitis herpetiformis.

Angio-oedema in contrast is usually painful rather than itchy and appears as diffuse swelling that affects the deeper layers of the skin; it can occur rapidly and may involve the mucous membranes. Laryngeal oedema is the most serious complication and can be life-threatening. Hereditary angio-oedema is a rare form with recurrent severe episodes of subcutaneous oedema, swelling of the mucous membranes and systemic symptoms.

Urticaria is a common skin disorder that may occur as a single episode or be chronically recurrent. It is often self-limiting and controlled with over-the-counter antihistamine. The prognosis is varied depending on the underlying cause, but in chronic idiopathic urticaria symptoms may persist for several years.

Pathophysiology

Urticaria results from histamine, bradykinin and proinflammatory mediators being released from basophils and mast-cells in response to various trigger factors. The chemicals released by degranulation cause capillaries and venules to leak causing tissue oedema. Urticaria may be IgE mediated with cross-linking of two adjacent IgE receptors, or complement mediated (causing direct degranulation of mast cells), or mast cells may be directly stimulated by an exogenous or unknown substance. In patients with chronic urticaria histamine can be released spontaneously or in response to non-specific stimuli and their vasculature is more sensitive to histamines.

Clinical history

Careful history-taking is of great importance in diagnosing patients with urticaria and/or angio-oedema because frequently there are no clinical signs for the medical practitioner to see. Ask about the onset, duration and course of lesions, rashes and swelling. Urticaria is very itchy and angio-oedema usually painful. Patients with urticaria complain of itchy spots or rashes lasting minutes or hours (usually less than 24 hours) that resolve leaving no marks on the skin. Patients may complain of swelling (angio-oedema) of their face, particularly eyelids, lips, and tongue, which may last hours or days.

Box 5.1 **Causes of non-physical urticaria**

- Food allergies: fish, eggs, dairy products, nuts, strawberries
- Food additives: tartrazine dyes, sodium benzoates
- Salicylates: medication, foods
- Infections: viral, bacterial, protozoal
- Systemic disorders: autoimmune disorders, connective tissue disease, carcinoma
- Contact urticaria: meat, fish, vegetables, plants
- Papular urticaria: persistent urticaria often secondary to insect bites
- Aeroallergens: pollens, house dust mite, animal dander

Box 5.2 **Causes of physical urticaria**

- Heat
- Sunlight
- Cold
- Pressure
- Water

ABC of Dermatology, 5th edition. Edited by P. K. Buxton and R. Morris-Jones.
© 2009 Blackwell Publishing, ISBN: 978-1-4051-7065-9.

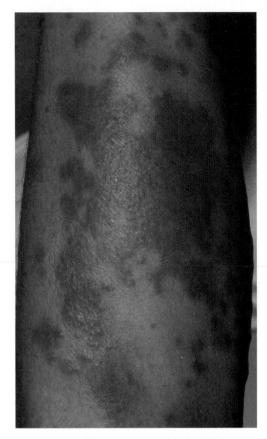

Figure 5.1 Urticarial vasculitis on the arm with area of bruising.

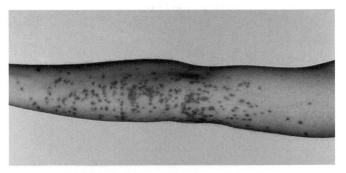

Figure 5.2 Urticaria from contact with brown caterpillar moths.

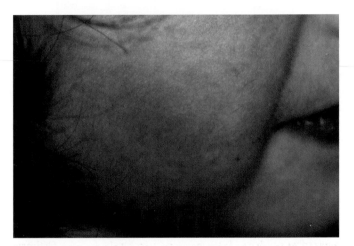

Figure 5.3 Cold-induced urticaria on the cheeks.

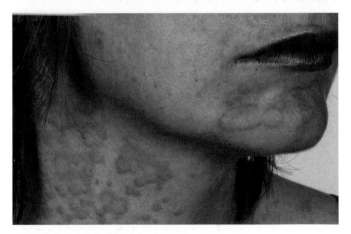

Figure 5.4 Ordinary urticaria on the neck.

If the skin eruption lasts for more than 24 hours, is painful and resolves with bruising then urticarial vasculitis is more likely than ordinary urticaria (Figure 5.1).

Patients may feel unwell before the onset of the rash or swelling and rarely in severe reactions anaphylaxis can occur. You should always ask about any associated respiratory distress.

An attempt to identify possible triggers before the onset of symptoms is important. In particular ask about any food eaten (nausea/vomiting), exercise, heat/cold, sun, medications/infusions, latex exposure, insect stings, animal contact, physical stimuli, infections, family history and any known medical conditions (Figures 5.2 & 5.3).

Classification of urticaria

Urticaria is traditionally classified as acute or chronic depending on whether symptoms last for less or more than 6 weeks. Another approach is to classify urticaria according to the underlying cause, but in 50% of cases no cause is identified (idiopathic). Urticaria can therefore broadly be divided into ordinary/idiopathic (acute/chronic), contact allergic, cholinergic, physical or urticarial vasculitis. See Boxes 5.1 and 5.2.

Ordinary urticaria

This is the most common form of urticaria characterized by intermittent fleeting wheals at any skin site, with or without angio-oedema (Figures 5.4 & 5.5). Lesions may be papular, annular and even serpiginous (Figure 5.6). The urticarial lesions themselves last minutes to hours only and may recur over <6 weeks – acute urticaria, or attacks may become chronic (>6 weeks). In 50% of patients with ordinary urticaria no underlying cause is found. Possible triggers of acute urticaria include infections, vaccinations, medications and food. Generally the more persistent the attacks of urticaria, the less likely an underlying cause is identified; this is termed chronic idiopathic urticaria.

Cholinergic urticaria

Patients are usually aged 10–30 years and typically report urticaria following a warm shower/bath, or after exercise. Patients report

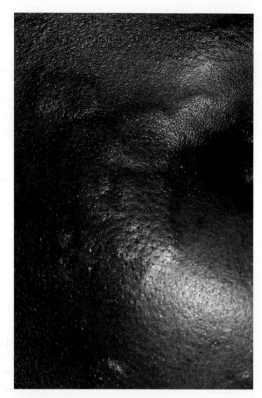

Figure 5.5 Ordinary urticaria on the face.

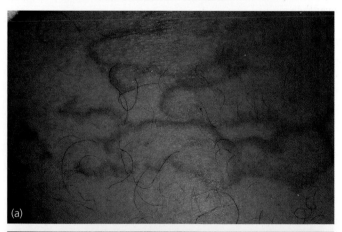

(a)

(b)

Figure 5.6 (a) Serpiginous and (b) annular lesions of urticaria.

erythema and burning pruritus followed by extensive urticaria. The lesions consist of pinhead-sized wheals with a red flare around them. The underlying trigger is not fully understood, but deficiency in α_1-antitrypsin may predispose to urticaria in which sweat has been show to play a role and where serum histamine levels are raised following exertion. Avoidance of heat usually helps to reduce the frequency and severity of symptoms.

A rarer form of cholinergic urticaria can result from exposure to the cold. Patients report urticaria on exposed skin during cold weather, lip/tongue/hand swelling following the holding and ingestion of cold beverages and a more generalized reaction following swimming in an outdoor pool. Affected individuals should avoid swimming in cold water and ingestion of ice-cold drinks as anaphylaxis and death have been reported.

Solar urticaria

Solar urticaria is a rare condition in which sunlight causes an acute urticarial eruption. Patients complain of stinging, burning and itching at exposed skin sites within 30 minutes of ultraviolet or artificial light source exposure. Lesions resolve rapidly (minutes to hours) when light exposure ceases. Photosensitive drug eruptions can present in a similar fashion so a detailed drug history is important. The differential diagnosis may include porphyria (lesions resolve with scarring) and polymorphic light eruption (lesions take days to weeks to resolve). The pathophysiology is poorly understood but is thought to be mediated by antigen production as serum transfer can induce similar symptoms in asymptomatic controls. Light-testing confirms the diagnosis. Management can be difficult but avoidance of sunlight is helpful.

Pressure urticaria

Urticarial wheals occur at the site of pressure on the skin, characteristically around the waistband area (from clothing), shoulders (from carrying a backpack), soles of feet (from walking), hands (using tools), buttocks (from sitting), genitals (sexual intercourse). The urticarial rash may occur immediately but a delay of up to 6 hours can occur (delayed pressure urticaria), and lesions resolve over several days. Symptoms are usually recurrent over many years. The cause is unknown and although histamine is thought to play a role patients are less likely to respond to antihistamines than in other forms of urticaria. Eosinophils and interleukin are thought to play a role. Investigation can include pressure challenge testing. Patients may respond to dapsone or montelukast.

Angio-oedema

Patients present with swelling with or without urticaria that develops over hours and resolves over days. Angio-oedema causes well-demarcated swelling of the subcutaneous tissues (Figure 5.7) and/or mucous membranes, from increased vascular permeability. A detailed drug history should be taken because allergy to medication (ACE inhibitors) may be the cause. Laryngeal swelling is the most serious complication and should ideally be managed by emergency medicine specialists.

A hereditary form of angio-oedema presents in young persons as recurrent severe attacks affecting the skin and mucous membranes.

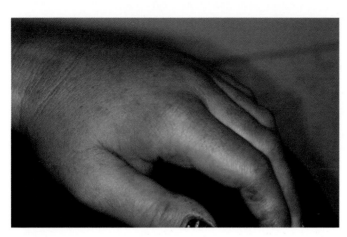

Figure 5.7 Angio-oedema of the hand.

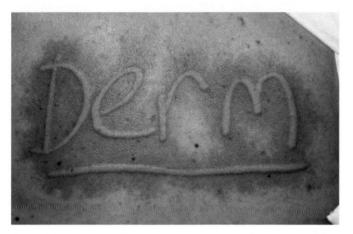

Figure 5.8 Dermatographism.

Tingling, tightness and pain are the main symptoms associated with the oedema. Patients may suffer associated gastrointestinal symptoms and life-threatening laryngeal oedema. Hereditary angio-oedema is caused by a deficiency in C1 (esterase) inhibitor. Serum complement C4 levels are low following attacks. Danazol can be used to reduce the frequency and severity of attacks and fresh frozen plasma can be used before elective surgery.

General investigations

Apart from a detailed history and examination most patients need no further investigations. If food allergy is suspected patients can be asked to keep a food diary, particularly if their urticaria is recurrent and episodic. An attempt to elicit dermatographism (exaggerated release of histamine causing wheal and flare) should be made by firmly stroking the skin with a hard object such as the end of a pen; this is usually positive in physical urticaria (Figure 5.8).

A skin biopsy can be useful if urticarial vasculitis is suspected; plain lidocaine should be used for the local anaesthetic (as adrenaline causes release of histamine from mast cells). Histology from urticaria may show dermal oedema and vasodilatation. In urticarial vasculitis, there is a cellular infiltrate of lymphocytes, polymorphs and histiocytes.

In patients with more severe reactions a RAST (radio-allergosorbent test) or skin prick testing (although not in patients with anaphylaxis) may help to identify specific allergies. In addition, patch testing to identify contact urticaria can be undertaken in specialist centres.

If you suspect hereditary angio-oedema check the complement C3 level and C1 esterase which are usually low.

If heat or cold are the possible precipitants then exercise for 5 minutes or placing an ice-cube on the skin for 20 minutes may be diagnostic. Physical urticaria can be elicited by firm pressure on the skin. Solar urticaria can be assessed in specialist centres using a solar simulator.

General management

Patients often make their own observations concerning trigger factors, especially food, medication and insect stings, and know what they should try to avoid. Treatment of any underlying medical condition identified should help to settle the urticaria. Oral antihistamines are the mainstay of treatment/prevention of urticaria and angio-oedema. Patients can manage their own symptoms by purchasing antihistamines (cetirizine, loratadine, chlorphenamine) over the counter.

In severe recalcitrant cases physicians may need to prescribe synergistic combinations of H1-receptor blockers (as above plus desloratadine, levocetirizine, terfenadine, hydroxyzine) plus H2 blockade (ranitidine, cimetidine) and leukotriene receptor antagonists (montelukast, zafirlukast) to control symptoms. Depending on the frequency of symptoms antihistamines may be taken daily prophylactically or intermittently to treat symptoms.

Oral corticosteroids may be indicated in very severe eruptions, particularly those associated with urticarial vasculitis.

For emergency management of urticaria/angio-oedema with respiratory distress the use of a pre-assembled syringe and needle (EpiPen®, Anapen®) to inject adrenaline intramuscularly (300–500 mcg) may be life-saving. Oxygen and intramuscular/intravenous adrenaline can then be administered.

Further reading

Kaplan AP, Greaves MW. *Urticaria and Angioedema*. Marcel Dekker Ltd, New York, 2004.

Wanderer AA. *Hives: the Road to Diagnosis and Treatment of Urticaria*. Anson Publishing, Montana, 2003.

www.allergyclinic.co.uk/urticaria

CHAPTER 6

Skin and Photosensitivity

OVERVIEW

- Definition of photosensitivity.
- Nature of ultraviolet radiation.
- Skin types and photosensitivity.
- Genetic disorders: albinism, xeroderma pigmentosum.
- Metabolic disorders: porphyria.
- Idiopathic photosensitivity: polymorphic light eruption, solar urticaria and chronic actinic dermatitis.
- Sunscreens: types and indications.

Introduction

The term photosensitive is used to describe patients with cutaneous disorders that result from exposure to normal levels of ultraviolet (UV) light. Sun-exposed skin is predominantly affected in acquired photosensitivity: particularly the face, neck, dorsi of the arms/hands and lower legs. There is marked sparing of sun-protected sites particularly the buttocks, behind the ears and under the chin, which can provide useful diagnostic clues.

Skin tolerance of UV light will depend on a number of factors including the intensity of UV light, skin type (Fitzpatrick skin types classified according to inherited levels of skin pigmentation – see below), genetic disorders (sun-damage repair mechanisms may be defective), acquired allergic conditions and photosensitizing medications.

Taking a thorough history of sun exposure and reactions to it is important in patients with suspected photosensitivity. Some patients may not develop symptoms unless they are exposed to high-intensity sunlight whereas others will be affected throughout the year with low-intensity UV exposure. The time to onset of symptoms following UV exposure is an important part of the history, the course of any skin eruption (frequency, duration) and whether any scarring or marks are left behind on the skin following

ABC of Dermatology, 5th edition. Edited by P. K. Buxton and R. Morris-Jones.
© 2009 Blackwell Publishing, ISBN: 978-1-4051-7065-9.

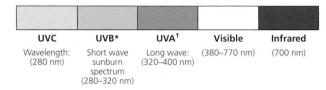

UVC	UVB*	UVA†	Visible	Infrared
Wavelength: (280 nm)	Short wave sunburn spectrum (280–320 nm)	Long wave: (320–400 nm)	(380–770 nm)	(700 nm)

* The UVB band (280–320 nm) is responsible for erythema, sunburn, tanning and skin malignancy
† UVA light (320–400 nm) has the greatest penetration into the dermis and augments UVB erythema and skin malignancy

Figure 6.1 Light spectrum.

the acute phase. Symptoms of itching, burning and even pain can be reported.

This chapter considers cutaneous disorders related to UV light. Precancerous and cancerous skin lesions are discussed elsewhere (see Chapters 21 & 22).

Ultraviolet radiation

Ultraviolet A and B radiation penetrate the earth's atmosphere and are known to play a role in sun-induced skin damage (Figure 6.1). UV intensity is greatest near the equator and at high altitudes. Environmental factors can influence the intensity of UV light such as the season, time of day and reflective surfaces (water, snow, sand). There is evidence that holes in the ozone layer have led to pockets of high-intensity UV.

UVB has a short wavelength and varies according to the season. UVB levels are at their highest in the summer months and during the middle of the day. UVB is important in both sunburn and the development of skin cancer. UVA has a longer wavelength and is present all year round and throughout the day at fairly constant levels. UVA can pass through glass; it is known to play a role in skin ageing and tanning, and there is increasing evidence that it plays a role in skin cancer development.

UV light can cause immediate effects on the skin in the form of photosensitivity and sunburn, and long-term effects such as skin ageing (wrinkling, solar keratoses) and skin cancer.

Fitzpatrick skin type classification

Natural skin pigmentation is formed by melanin which is synthesized by melanocytes. The quantity of melanin in the skin determines its ability to withstand UV radiation. In healthy skin the number of melanocytes remains constant, but the amount of melanin they synthesize is genetically determined, leading to different levels of skin pigmentation. Fitzpatrick devised a classification based on skin type according to inherited pigmentation and the skin's response to UV light. Patients with type I skin are likely to burn even if the UV intensity is low, whereas patients with type VI skin will not usually suffer sun damage. An assessment of a patient's skin type will help the physician determine the patient's susceptibility to UV as well as guiding certain therapies, such as phototherapy and laser treatments. Fitzpatrick skin type can be used to determine the starting doses and increments of UVA/TL-01 during phototherapy.

- Type I (very fair skin/freckled/red hair): always burns, never tans.
- Type II (fair skin): usually burns, tans eventually.
- Type III (fair to olive skin): occasionally burns, tans easily.
- Type IV (brown skin): very rarely burns, tans easily.
- Type V (dark brown skin): tans easily.
- Type VI (black skin): never burns, tans easily.

Genetic disorders causing photosensitivity

Oculocutaneous albinism

Genetic mutations that control melanin synthesis, distribution and degradation result in a group of inherited disorders that lead to loss of skin/hair/eye pigment. Oculocutaneous albinism is an autosomal recessive condition characterized by little or absent melanin pigment at birth (Figure 6.2). Oculocutaneous albinism affects skin, hair and ocular pigmentation resulting in sun-induced skin changes, photophobia, nystagmus and reduced visual acuity.

Oculocutaneous albinism is traditionally classified into two groups – tyrosinase positive or negative – depending on whether the enzyme is absent or dysfunctional, but there are numerous subtypes depending on the specific genetic mutation.

Affected individuals should be assessed in the neonatal period by a dermatologist and an ophthalmologist. The family may wish to consult a geneticist. A sunscreen blocking UVA and UVB light (broad spectrum) should be applied to the skin on a daily basis and reapplied as necessary. Protective clothing and sun avoidance behaviour should be encouraged. Skin checks for any evidence of sun damage or skin cancer should be undertaken regularly. Corrective spectacles may improve visual acuity.

Other genetic conditions associated with loss of skin pigment include piebaldism, phenylketonuria, tuberous sclerosis, and Waardenburg and Apert syndromes.

Xeroderma pigmentosum

This term covers a group of autosomal recessive conditions resulting from deficient cutaneous DNA repair mechanisms. Patients have accelerated UV-associated changes in the skin characterized by photosensitivity, pigmentary changes, premature skin ageing and tumour formation during the first decade of life. Ocular damage also results from photosensitivity. Early signs of the disorder include excessive sunburn, freckling, mottled pigmentation, telangiectasia and skin thinning. Later patients develop multiple skin cancers. Strict sun avoidance (skin and eyes) is paramount for these patients.

Metabolic disorders of photosensitivity

Porphyrias are a group of disorders associated with the accumulation of intermediate metabolites in the metabolic pathway of haem biosynthesis. Most porphyrias are inherited but some may be triggered by alcohol, oestrogens or hepatitis on a background of hereditary predisposition.

The most common form is porphyria cutanea tarda which results in photosensitivity (Figure 6.3). Patients develop cutaneous fragility and blisters that heal with scarring, pigment changes and milia at sun-exposed sites particularly on the face and dorsi of the hands. Patients may have scarring alopecia, facial hypertrichosis and onycholysis. Men with excessive alcohol intake are most frequently affected.

Hepatic porphyrias lead to skin fragility and blistering from exposure to sunlight or minor trauma. Patients with erythropoietic

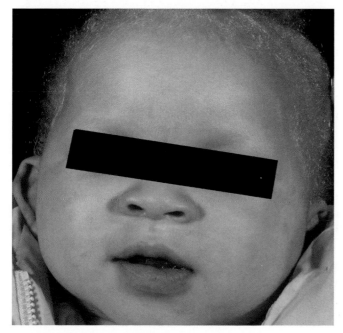

Figure 6.2 Oculocutaneous albinism.

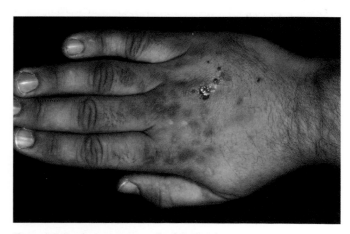

Figure 6.3 Porphyria cutanea tarda of the hand.

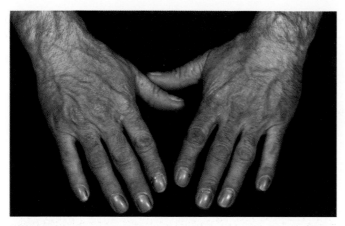

Figure 6.4 Erythropoietic porphyria.

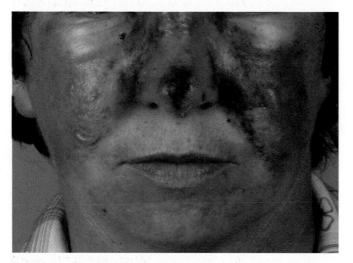

Figure 6.5 Variegate porphyria on face.

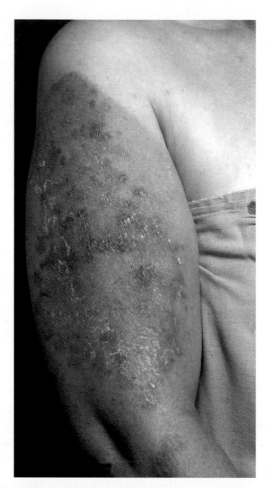

Figure 6.6 Photosensitive drug eruption.

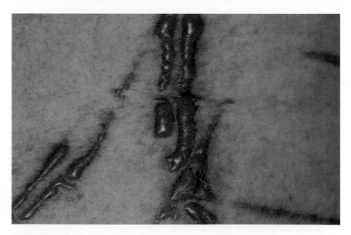

Figure 6.7 Phytophotodermatitis.

and erythrohepatic photoporphyrias are highly photosensitive (Figures 6.4 & 6.5), even to UVA that can pass through glass. Patients with acute intermittent porphyria do not have cutaneous involvement.

Patients need to be given sun avoidance advice including keeping out of midday sun, wearing protective tight-weave clothing (long sleeves, gloves, hat), the use of high-factor broad-spectrum sunscreen (Dundee cream), and tinted film that can be applied to windows, β-carotene and avoidance of precipitants.

Exogenous substances causing photosensitivity

Both topical and systemic medications can lead to localized and generalized photosensitive eruptions (see Chapter 7) (Figure 6.6). In addition, vegetables, fruit, fragrances, dyes and certain chemicals can lead to exogenous localized skin reactions in combination with sunlight. Phytophotodermatitis is a blistering skin rash resulting from photosensitizing plant material in contact with the skin plus UVA light (Figure 6.7). This is a phototoxic skin reaction not requiring any previous exposure to the plant. Outdoor activities in children and agricultural work, particularly in the spring, are usually present in the history. Implicated plant materials include

meadow grass, common rue, poison ivy/oak, celery and limes. The cutaneous rashes usually blister and look exogenous with bizarre linear streaks on the legs and 'drip marks' down the arms.

Idiopathic disorders causing photosensitivity

Polymorphic light eruption (PLE)

The underlying cause of PLE is not fully understood but there is evidence that it is an allergic type IV hypersensitivity reaction to

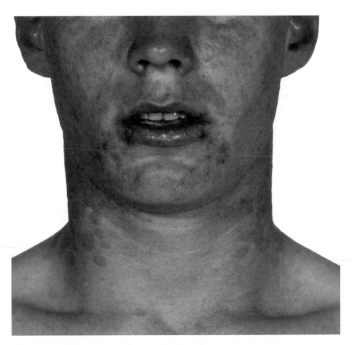

Figure 6.8 Polymorphic light eruption.

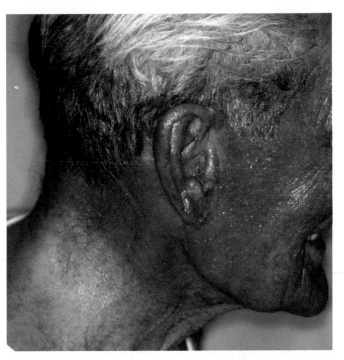

Figure 6.9 Chronic actinic dermatitis.

sunlight. PLE is most common in women and usually occurs in the spring; any skin type can be affected. PLE is triggered after a few hours of sunlight exposure or occasionally an artificial UV source. The rash is usually papular – but as its name suggests this disorder can have a varied morphology, including blisters and widespread inflamed oedematous lesions (Figure 6.8). The eruption of PLE usually takes several weeks to resolve and heals without scarring, although post-inflammatory pigment changes can result. Management includes sun avoidance, seeking shade, protective clothing and sunscreens. Topical or even oral corticosteroids may be needed in severe cases. Desensitization using TL-01 (narrow-band UVB) before sun exposure can be effective.

Solar urticaria

This relatively rare photoallergic condition presents with rapid onset of an itchy, erythematous and urticated eruption following less than 30 minutes of sun exposure (or an artificial light source). Careful history-taking is the key to making the diagnosis as the rash is transient resolving within minutes or hours after retreating from the light. A wide range of UV wavelengths can reportedly trigger the reaction which is thought to be antigen mediated. Studies have shown that injection of serum from those affected into the dermis of healthy individuals can passively transfer the condition. The diagnosis can be confirmed by solar simulator or TL-01 light tests. Solar urticaria can be very debilitating and difficult to manage. Patients quickly learn to avoid sunlight and often become reclusive. Oral antihistamines, high factor broad-spectrum sunscreen and paradoxically phototherapy may prevent or control symptoms.

Chronic actinic dermatitis (CAD)

Middle-aged or elderly men are most commonly affected by this itchy photosensitive eruption that affects the face, posterior and 'V' of the neck, and dorsi of the hands (Figure 6.9). Sunlight all year round can trigger CAD and consequently the rash usually resembles chronic lichenified eczema. UVB, UVA, visible and artificial light sources have all been implicated. Therefore sunscreen should be used daily all year round, even if patients remain indoors. Patch and photopatch testing can be very useful in identifying compounding contact allergies especially to compositae plants (daisy family), perfumes, sunscreen and colophony (pine trees, elastoplast). As well as sun-protective measures patients should be managed in a similar way to those with eczema, with topical steroids and emollients. Patients may, however, require short courses of systemic corticosteroids and in recalcitrant cases, azathioprine.

Photoprotective behaviour

The benefits versus the dangers of UV exposure are hotly debated. Some experts suggest the only safe tan is an artificial one, whilst others argue vitamin D levels may be inadequate and the frequency of some systemic cancers may increase if the sun is avoided.

Although not universal, current fashions in many societies view a tanned skin as desirable and 'healthy'. Fifty years ago a tanned skin was mainly a consequence of outdoor work. Nowadays a tanned skin is associated with increased leisure time, relative ease of travel to sunny climates and deliberate tanning through sun-bed use.

A sensible approach to sun protection is advisable according to each individual's susceptibility to burning and ability to tan. Simple measures to avoid excessive UV exposure include avoidance of midday sun (between 11 am and 3 pm), sitting in the shade (equivalent SPF 9, i.e. not 'out of the sun'), protective clothing (tighter weaves give greater protection), regular application of sunscreen and sun-protective eyewear.

Suncreens

There is a confusing array of sunscreens available to buy over the counter. Sunscreens are formulated to protect the skin from UV radiation. However, some experts believe that when people apply sunscreen they stay out in higher-intensity UV light for longer than they would without the sunscreen, and therefore its use may in fact increase their sun-seeking behaviour.

There are two main types of sunscreen: physical and chemical. As a general rule physical sunscreens look opaque when applied to the skin and are therefore viewed as less cosmetically acceptable. Chemical sunscreens are more likely to cause skin irritation or allergy.

Physical sunscreens contain minute particles of titanium dioxide or zinc/ferric oxide that reflect and scatter UV radiation. Chemical sunscreens contain combinations of para-amino benzoic acid (PABA), cinnamates and benzophenones that absorb UV radiation.

The degree of protection provided by each sunscreen is formally measured in terms of its UVB (SPF number) and UVA (number or star rating) blocking activity. SPF is the ratio of the minimum UV radiation required to cause minimal skin erythema, with and without sunscreen. The level of protection is calculated by using a specific number of grams of cream applied to a specific surface area of skin and irradiated with a known dose of UV. Unfortunately there is evidence that in reality individuals do not apply their sunscreen in similar quantities and therefore tend to achieve only one-third to a half of the predicted SPF/star rating specified on the bottle.

The apparent failure of sunscreens to protect the skin from sun damage usually results from not using high protection sunscreen, inadequate application (not put on before going outside, insufficient amounts, infrequent reapplication), washing off by water/sweat and breakdown of photoprotective chemicals by UV light itself.

Further reading

Ferguson J. *Photodermatology*. Blackwell Publishing, Oxford, 2006.

Lim HW, Honigsmann H, Hawk JLM. *Photodermatology (Basic and Clinical Dermatology)*. Informa Healthcare, New York, 2007.

CHAPTER 7

Inflammatory Dermatoses: Drug Rashes

Introduction

Skin reactions to medications can present in a number of ways. A 'reactive' skin rash is usually generalized and may result from an allergic reaction to a systemic drug. A more localized patch of inflammation may also result from a systemic drug (a 'fixed drug eruption') but may be a reaction to a topical application or transdermal medication. However, these types of rashes may have nothing to do with medication at all, and therefore knowledge concerning the clinical presentations of drug reactions will help to clarify whether drugs are to blame.

Skin disorders as a result of medications are very common indeed; they account for approximately 3% of all adverse drug reactions. The majority of drug rashes are mild and self-limiting and can be managed by patients themselves using simple emollients. However, at the other end of the spectrum, drug rashes can be very severe,

requiring management by dermatology specialists in the intensive care unit. The most severe reactions such as Stevens–Johnson syndrome and toxic epidermal necrolysis have associated mortality rates of 5% and 30%, respectively. Predicting which patients will develop cutaneous reactions to medications is currently not possible although it is known that females and the elderly seem to be the most commonly affected. In addition, patients with the human immunodeficiency virus (HIV) are more susceptible to drug rashes in both frequency and severity.

Pathophysiology

Cutaneous reactions to medications are extremely varied, but they may be divided into two groups according to their pathophysiology: immune and non-immune mediated reactions. On a more practical level they can be divided into localized and generalized.

Immune-mediated rashes are the most common and include hypersensitivity reactions from types I to IV. Type I immediate reactions (IgE) tend to manifest in the skin as urticaria or angio-oedema. Type II cytotoxic reactions result in cutaneous purpura. Type III immune complex-mediated reactions lead to cutaneous vasculitis. Type IV delayed hypersensitivity reactions are by far the most common group of drug rashes resulting in generalized exanthems, phototoxic rashes and contact dermatitis to topical medicaments.

Non-immune-mediated rashes include accumulation of medications in the skin (causing pigment changes), instability of mast cells (histamine released), slow acetylators (metabolism of drugs affected) and photosensitivity reactions (increased susceptibility to UV light).

Localized drug reactions include contact dermatitis to topical medicament creams/ointments/drops and transdermal drug delivery through medicated 'patches', cutaneous reactions to injections given via the skin, contact urticaria, fixed drug eruptions, phototoxic/photosensitive eruptions, lupus-like rash, pigment deposition in the skin and erythema nodosum.

Generalized drug reactions include toxic erythema, urticaria, vasculitis (may be limited to limbs), acute generalized exanthematous

ABC of Dermatology, 5th edition. Edited by P. K. Buxton and R. Morris-Jones.
© 2009 Blackwell Publishing, ISBN: 978-1-4051-7065-9.

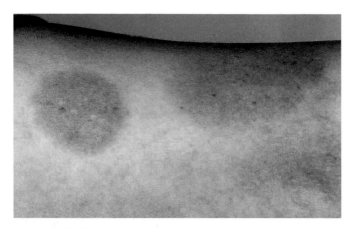

Figure 7.2 Fixed drug eruption.

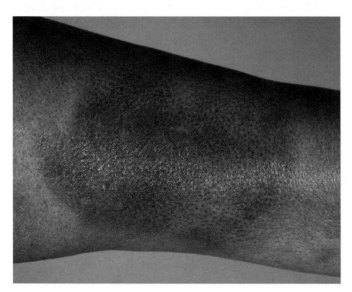

Figure 7.3 Fixed drug eruption.

The most common sites affected include the genitals, hands/feet and mouth. The skin eruption itself is usually an annular plaque which may be a purplish colour; bullae formation is not uncommon (Figures 7.2 & 7.3). The eruption usually fades leaving post-inflammatory pigment changes. Management includes identifying the offending medication and avoiding it in the future. Skin reactions can be treated with a potent topical steroid (betamethasone).

Photosensitive drug eruption

The skin eruption appears on sun-exposed sites, including the face, neck and dorsi of arms/hands. Lesions may appear in rings (annular) with central clearing, or as confluent erythema (sunburn-like), lichenoid or morbilliform eruptions. Drug-induced lupus causes skin changes typically seen in lupus patients, but the rash tends to settle within weeks of stopping the drug. Patients may develop arthritis and pleurisy. Antihistone antibodies are usually positive in drug-induced lupus. Management includes sunscreen, protective clothing, sunglasses, topical steroids and in severe cases hydroxychloroquine or oral prednisolone.

Drug-induced erythema nodosum

Patients present with tender nodules, usually over the anterior shins. The skin pigment is often discoloured and the area may settle with bruising. A deep skin biopsy for histology classically shows septal panniculitis (inflammation between the fat cells). Infections, inflammatory bowel disease, pregnancy and lymphoma may also cause erythema nodosum. Management is to withdraw the drug or treat the underlying cause. Pain may respond to leg elevation, light compression and non-steroidal anti-inflammatory drugs (NSAIDs).

Drug-induced skin pigmentation

Pigmentation in the skin has been reported with many different medications such as amiodarone and minocycline, and less commonly clofamazine and mepacrine. The mechanisms involved in pigmentary changes include accumulation or deposition of the drug in the skin, stimulation of melanogenesis and formation of drug–melanin complexes. Sun-exposed skin sites are commonly affected. The pigmentation is usually benign but can be disfiguring (Figures 7.4 & 7.5). Pigmentation may fade on stopping the drug; sunscreen and camouflage can be useful.

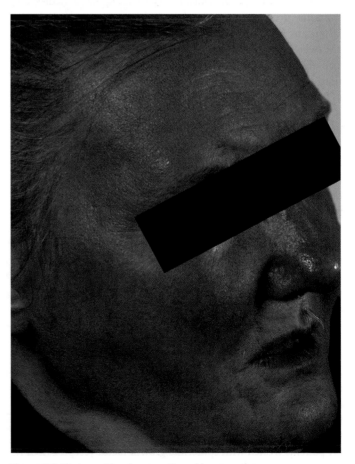

Figure 7.4 Photosensitive drug eruption: chlorpromazine.

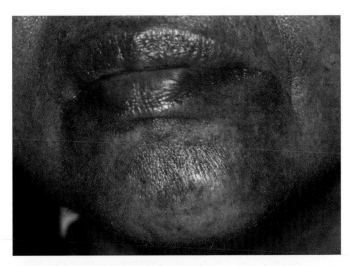

Figure 7.5 Diltiazem pigmentation of the face.

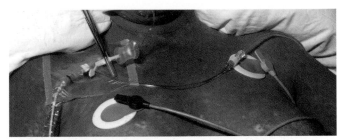

Figure 7.7 Erythrodermic drug rash.

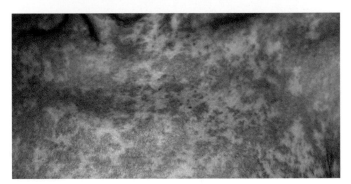

Figure 7.6 Toxic erythema.

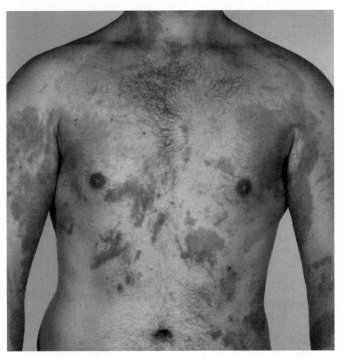

Figure 7.8 Widespread urticaria.

Generalized drug rashes

Toxic erythema

Toxic erythema typically occurs within 2 weeks of starting a new medication.

This is the most common drug rash, presenting as a symmetrical exanthem with erythematous macules and papules, sparing the palms and soles (Figure 7.6).

The rash commonly spreads in a craniocaudal direction, and is mildly pruritic. If possible, the likely culprit drug should be stopped. Application of a moderately potent topical steroid and emollients usually helps to settle the rash quickly.

Drug-induced erythroderma (red man syndrome)

Drug-induced erythroderma is most common in elderly males; 90% of the skin surface is affected by the rash, usually an exfoliative dermatitis (Figure 7.7). Patients complain of pruritus and feeling cold (they lose heat due to impaired barrier function), they have lymphadenopathy and may develop high-output cardiac failure. Patients usually feel unwell and should be managed in hospital, where they require regular emollients (to prevent heat and fluid loss through their skin), nursing in a warm room, mild/moderate topical steroids, and antihistamines.

Drug-induced widespread urticaria

This is characteristically a widespread very pruritic eruption that starts within hours or days of starting the offending medication (Figure 7.8). The individual wheals are erythematous and palpable and last a few hours at any particular site. The wheals can form annular patterns. Occasionally urticarial vasculitis can result, when individual lesions typically last more than 48 hours and resolve with bruising. Urticaria usually settles rapidly following withdrawal of the drug. Oral antihistamines can help to ease the pruritus.

Lichenoid drug eruption

The mechanism is thought to involve autoreactive cytotoxic T lymphocytes, an immune complex formed by the drug and a class II MHC antigen. This causes the immune system to view the keratinocytes and Langerhans cells as non-self, causing the resultant attack. The lichenoid eruption is usually very itchy and widespread consisting of multiple flat-topped shiny purple papules (Figure 7.9). The eruption may develop weeks to months following the initiation of the offending drug. Lesions only slowly resolve after the drug is stopped, taking many months to settle.

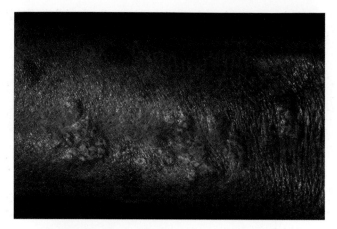

Figure 7.9 Lichenoid drug eruption.

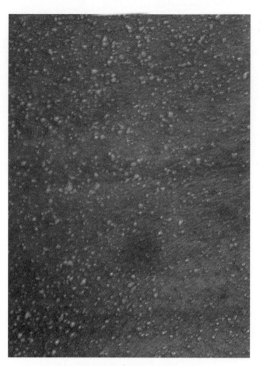

Figure 7.11 Acute generalized exanthematous pustulosis.

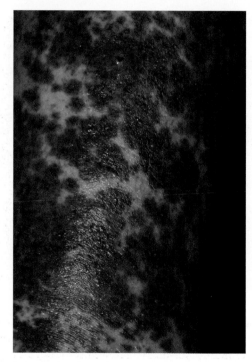

Figure 7.10 Drug-induced vasculitis.

Drug-induced vasculitis

The exact mechanisms involved in drug-induced vasculitis are poorly defined but both humoral and cell-mediated immune mechanisms are thought to play a role. Vasculitis is inflammation of blood vessels that causes them to leak and even occlude. The cutaneous manifestation is a palpable non-blanching purpuric rash scattered mainly on the limbs. In severe cases the purpuric lesions can blister (Figure 7.10) and ulcerate. There are numerous causes of vasculitis so although a particular drug may be suspected screening investigations for other underlying triggers may be indicated, particularly if the patient has any constitutional symptoms (see Chapter 10). Macular purpura may occur if patients are taking warfarin or heparin, or if their platelet count is low. Drug-induced vasculitis may manifest solely in the skin,

but internal organs may also be affected in more severe cases. The offending medication should be withdrawn and the patient may require systemic corticosteroids.

Acute generalized exanthematous pustulosis (AGEP)

Patients present with multiple monomorphic sterile pustules on an erythematous background, particularly on the face and flexures (Figure 7.11). Patients are frequently unwell with a high fever and a raised neutrophil count. Skin biopsy reveals vasculitis with subcorneal (superficial) pustules. The pustules usually resolve over 2 weeks once the drug has been stopped; systemic corticosteroids can help to speed resolution.

Drug rash with eosinophilia and systemic symptoms (DRESS)

DRESS (previously known as drug-induced hypersensitivity syndrome) is a poorly defined condition. It typically occurs 8–12 weeks after initiation of a new medication. Patients are systemically unwell with a high fever, lymphadenopathy, eosinophilia and a pleomorphic skin eruption (Figure 7.12). Secondary hepatitis, arthritis, myocardial involvement and interstitial nephropathy/lung disease may also occur; mortality rates reach 10%. Management involves stopping the drug implicated and giving systemic corticosteroids, often in the form of methyl prednisolone.

Erythema multiforme (EM)

Classically target lesions are seen symmetrically, especially at acral sites (palms, soles, elbows, face). The target lesions are erythematous

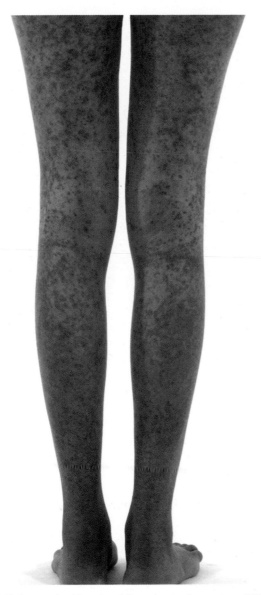

Figure 7.12 Drug rash with eosinophilia and systemic symptoms (DRESS).

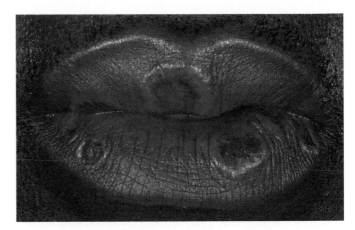

Figure 7.13 Erythema multiforme on the lips.

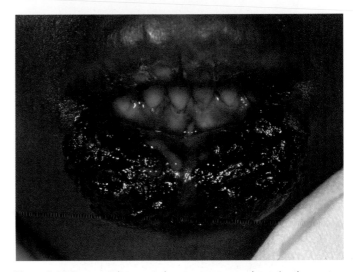

Figure 7.14 Stevens–Johnson syndrome: mucous membrane involvement.

often with a central vesicle (Figure 7.13). Patients are usually well, but may have a fever and mild involvement of mucous membranes. The cause of EM is poorly defined but it is thought to be a hypersensitivity reaction. In addition to medication EM may be triggered by infections including herpes simplex, *Mycoplasma*, hepatitis and tuberculosis. EM is thought to be the mild end of the spectrum of conditions including Stevens–Johnson syndrome and toxic epidermal necrolysis. If the diagnosis is in doubt then a skin biopsy for histology can be helpful, generally showing an extensive lymphocytic infiltrate, necrotic keratinocytes and blister formation. Moderate topical steroids and regular emollients can be used to settle the eruption over 2–4 weeks.

Stevens–Johnson syndrome (SJS)

Stevens–Johnson syndrome (SJS) is the more severe end of the spectrum of immune-complex mediated drug hypersensitivity.

Reactions usually occur within the first 2 months of taking a new medication. Patients are unwell (fever, headache, malaise) and have severe mucous membrane involvement (oral, eyes, genitals, gastrointestinal and respiratory) (Figure 7.14). The rash may be localized to the limbs but is usually widespread (10–30% skin surface involved) and may be Nikolsky positive (skin sloughing off with lateral pressure). The morphology of the cutaneous eruption is variable with confluent erythema, papules, pustules, blisters and erosions. Histology shows skin necrosis as a split between the epidermis and dermis. The offending drug should be stopped and patients should be managed on a high-dependency unit. Treatment is supportive: fluid balance, pain relief, airway maintenance, topical paraffin and body suit, mouthwashes and ophthalmic care.

Toxic epidermal necrolysis (TEN)

Toxic epidermal necrolysis (TEN) is a very severe and life-threatening mucocutaneous drug-induced disorder. More than 30% of the skin surface area becomes necrotic following blistering and sloughs off leaving denuded areas (Figure 7.15). Patients are unwell

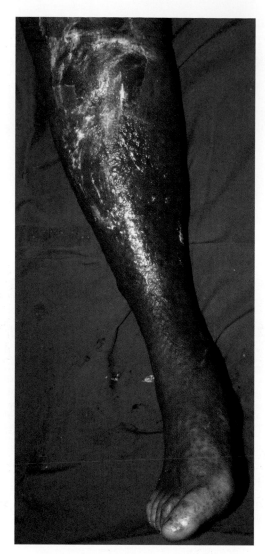

Figure 7.15 Toxic epidermal necrolysis secondary to penicillin.

and their skin is painful. Involvement of the mucous membranes is rapid; mouth, eyes and genitals are affected but in addition the oesophagus, alveolar membranes and urethra may be involved. Patients should be managed in intensive care units by a specialist team including an experienced dermatologist. Management includes immediate withdrawal of the suspected drug and intensive topical emollients. Patients should ideally be nursed in Lyofoam covered with white soft paraffin and receive high-dose intravenous immunoglobulin. There is a 30% mortality rate.

Further reading

Goldstein S, Wintroub BV. *Adverse Cutaneous Reactions to Medication.* Lippincott Williams and Wilkins, Philadelphia, 1996.

Nigen S, Knowles SR, Shear NH. Drug eruptions: approaching the diagnosis of drug-induced skin diseases. *J Drugs Dermatol* 2003; **2**(3): 278–99.

CHAPTER 8

Inflammatory Dermatoses: Immunobullous and Other Blistering Disorders

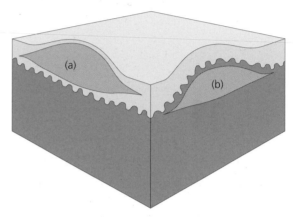

Figure 8.1 Section through the skin with (a) intraepidermal blister, (b) subepidermal blister.

Introduction

Blisters, whether large bullae or small vesicles, can arise in a variety of conditions. There may be *destruction* of epidermal cells in a burn or by a virus such as herpes. *Loss of adhesion* between the cells may occur within the epidermis in pemphigus or at the basement membrane in pemphigoid. In eczema there is *oedema* between the epidermal cells. Sometimes there are associated *inflammatory* changes in the dermis as in erythema multiforme/vasculitis or a metabolic defect as in porphyria.

The integrity of normal skin depends on intricate connecting structures between cells (Figure 8.1). In autoimmune blistering conditions autoantibodies attack these superficial or deep adhesion structures and this is reflected in the clinical changes. The level of the separation of epidermal cells within the epidermis is determined by the specific structure that is the target antigen. Clinically these splits are visualized as superficial blisters which may be fragile and flaccid (intraepidermal split) or deep mainly intact blisters (subepidermal split). Therefore the clinical features can be used to predict the level of the underlying target antigen in the skin.

Pathophysiology

A susceptibility to develop autoimmune disorders may be inherited, but the triggers for the production of these skin-damaging autoantibodies remains unknown. In some patients possible triggers have been identified including drugs (rifampicin, captopril, D-penicillamine), certain foods (garlic, onions, leeks), viral infections, hormones, UV radiation and X-rays.

Bullous pemphigoid results from IgG autoantibodies that target the basement membrane cells (hemidesmosome proteins BP180 and BP230). Complement activates an inflammatory cascade, leading to disruption of skin cell adhesion and blister formation. The subepidermal split leads to tense bullae formation.

Pemphigus vulgaris results from autoantibodies that attack adhesion proteins (desmogleins) between epidermal cells in mucous membranes and skin. This causes the epidermal cells to separate, resulting in intraepidermal blister formation. This relatively superficial split leads to flaccid blisters and erosions (where the blister roof has sloughed off).

Differential diagnosis

Many cutaneous disorders present with blister formation. Presentations include large single bullae through to multiple

ABC of Dermatology, 5th edition. Edited by P. K. Buxton and R. Morris-Jones.
© 2009 Blackwell Publishing, ISBN: 978-1-4051-7065-9.

Other causes of cutaneous blistering	Key clinical features	Diagnostic tests	Further reading
Erythema multiforme	Target lesions with a central blister, acral sites	Skin biopsy for histology	Chapter 7
Stevens–Johnson syndrome/ toxic epidermal necrolysis	Mucous membrane involvement, Nikolsky-positive, eroded areas of skin	Skin biopsy for histology	Chapter 7
Chicken pox	Scattered blisters in crops appear over days	No tests usually required; serology	Chapter 14
Herpes simplex/varicella zoster virus	Localized blistering of mucous membranes or dermatomal	Vesicle fluid for viral analysis	Chapter 14
Staphylococcus impetigo	Golden crusting associated with blisters	Bacterial swab for culture	Chapter 13
Insect bite reactions	Linear or clusters of blisters, very itchy	Clinical diagnosis	Chapter 17
Contact dermatitis	Exogenous pattern of blisters	Patch testing	Chapter 4
Phytophotodermatitis	Blisters where plants/extracts touched the skin with sunlight	Clinical diagnosis	Chapter 6
Porphyria	Fragile skin with scarring at sun-exposed skin sites	Urine, blood, faecal analysis for porphyrins	Chapter 6
Fixed drug eruption	Blistering purplish lesion/s at a fixed site each time drug taken	Skin biopsy for histology	Chapter 7

Table 8.1 Differential diagnosis of immunobullous disorders – i.e. other causes of cutaneous blistering.

small vesicles, and differentiating the underlying cause can be a clinical challenge (Table 8.1). The history of the blister formation can give important clues to the diagnosis, in particular the development, duration, durability and distribution of the lesions – the 'four Ds'.

Development

If erosions or blisters are present at birth then genodermatoses must be considered in addition to cutaneous infections.

Preceding systemic symptoms suggest there may be a viral infection such as chicken pox or hand, foot, and mouth disease. If the lesions are pruritic then consider dermatitis herpetiformis or pompholyx eczema.

A tingling sensation may herald herpes simplex, and pain, herpes zoster. Eczema may precede bullous pemphigoid.

Duration

Some types of blistering arise rapidly (allergic reactions, impetigo, erythema multiforme, pemphigus), whilst others have a more gradual onset and follow a chronic course (dermatitis herpetiformis, pityriasis lichenoides, porphyria cutanea tarda, bullous pemphigoid). The rare genetic disorder epidermolysis bullosa is present from, or soon after, birth and has a chronic course.

Durability

The blisters themselves may remain intact or rupture easily and this sign can help elude the underlying diagnosis. Superficial

---

Box 8.1 Widespread blistering eruptions

- Bullous pemphigoid
- Pemphigus vulgaris
- Dermatitis herpetiformis (or localized)
- Erythema multiforme
- Drug rashes: Stevens–Johnson syndrome, toxic epidermal necrolysis
- Chicken pox

---

blisters in the epidermis have a fragile roof that sloughs off easily. Clinically this results in superficial eroded areas and deflated blisters typically seen in pemphigus vulgaris, porphyria, Stevens–Johnson syndrome, toxic epidermal necrolysis, staphylococcal scalded skin, and herpes viruses. Subepidermal blisters have a stronger roof and usually remain intact and are classically seen in bullous pemphigoid, linear IgA and erythema multiforme. Scratching can result in traumatic removal of blister roofs which may confuse the clinical picture.

Distribution

The distribution of blistering rashes helps considerably in making a clinical diagnosis (Boxes 8.1 & 8.2). In general, immunobullous diseases present with widespread eruptions with frequent mucous membrane involvement. Herpes infections usually remain localized to lips, genitals or dermatomes. Photosensitive blistering disorders involve sun-exposed skin.

Clinical features of immunobullous disorders (Table 8.2)

Bullous pemphigoid

This usually presents in the elderly with tense blisters on a background of either erythema or normal skin (Figure 8.2). The condition may present acutely or be insidious in onset, but usually enters a chronic intermittent phase before remitting after approximately 5 years. Some patients have a prolonged prebullous period in which persistent pruritic urticated plaques (Figure 8.3), or eczema, precede the blisters. Characteristically blisters have a predilection for flexural sites on the limbs and truck. Mucous membrane involvement is rare (Figure 8.4). Blisters heal without scarring.

Potential triggers include vaccinations, drugs (NSAIDs, furosemide, ACE inhibitors, antibiotics), UV radiation and X-rays. In children bullous pemphigoid usually follows vaccination, where the condition characteristically affects the face, palms and soles.

Pemphigoid gestationis

This rare autoimmune disorder usually occurs in the second/third trimester of pregnancy. Mothers may have other associated autoimmune conditions. Acute-onset intensely pruritic papules, plaques and blisters spread from the periumbilical area outwards (Figure 8.5). Mucous membrane involvement can occur. Babies may be born prematurely or small for dates and can have a transient blistering eruption that rapidly resolves. The maternal

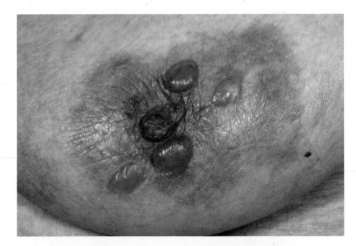

Figure 8.2 Bullous pemphigoid: close-up of blisters on the breast.

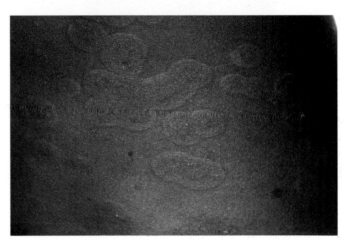

Figure 8.3 Urticated plaques of bullous pemphigoid.

Box 8.2 Localized blistering eruptions

- Dermatitis herpetiformis (knees, elbows, buttocks)
- Pemphigus gestationis (abdomen)
- Porphyria (sun-exposed sites)
- Pompholyx eczema (hands, feet)
- Contact dermatitis
- Fixed drug eruption
- Insect bite reactions (often in clusters or linear patterns)
- Infections: herpes simplex, herpes zoster, staphylococcus (impetigo)

Table 8.2 Clinical features of immunobullous disorders.

Immunobullous disorder	Typical patient	Distribution of rash	Morphology of lesions	Mucous membrane involvement	Associated conditions
Bullous pemphigoid	Elderly	Generalized	Intact blisters	Common	None
Mucous membrane pemphigoid	Middle aged or older	Varied	Erosions, flaccid blisters, scarring	Severe and extensive	Autoimmune disease
Pemphigoid gestationis	Pregnant	Periumbilical	Intact blisters, urticated lesions	Rare	Thyroid disease
Pemphigus vulgaris	Middle aged	Flexures, head	Flaccid blisters, erosions	Common	Autoimmune disease
Dermatitis herpetiformis	Young adults	Elbows, knees, buttocks	Vesicles, papules, excoriations	Rare	Small bowel enteropathy (gluten-sensitive), lymphoma
Linear IgA	Children and adults	Face and perineum (children) Trunk and limbs (adults)	Annular urticated plaques with peripheral vesicles	Common	Lymphoproliferative disorders

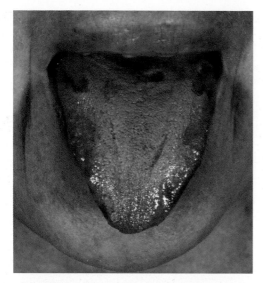

Figure 8.4 Bullous pemphigoid: mouth erosions.

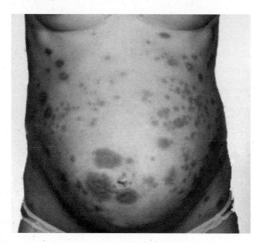

Figure 8.5 Pemphigoid gestationis on the abdomen.

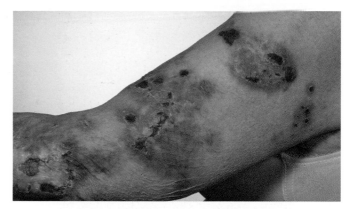

Figure 8.6 Mucous membrane pemphigoid: scarring skin eruption.

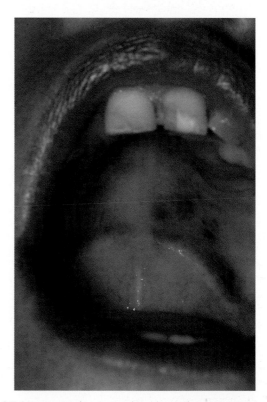

Figure 8.7 Mucous membrane pemphigoid: mouth.

cutaneous eruption usually resolves within weeks after birth, but may flare immediately postpartum.

Mucous membrane pemphigoid (cicatricial pemphigoid)

Patients usually present with painful sores in their mouth, nasal and genital mucosae, and may complain of a gritty feeling in their eyes. Cutaneous lesions occur in around 30% of patients; tense blisters may be haemorrhagic and heal with scarring (Figure 8.6). Scalp involvement can lead to scarring alopecia. Symptoms from mucous membrane sites can be very severe with chronic painful erosions and ulceration that heals with scarring (Figure 8.7).

Ocular damage can include symblepharon (tethering of conjunctival epithelium), synechiae (adhesion of iris to cornea) and fibrosis of the lacrimal duct (dry eyes) resulting in opacification, fixed globe and eventually blindness (Figure 8.8).

Pemphigus vulgaris

Seventy per cent of patients develop oral lesions in chronic progressive pemphigus vulgaris. Mucous membrane involvement

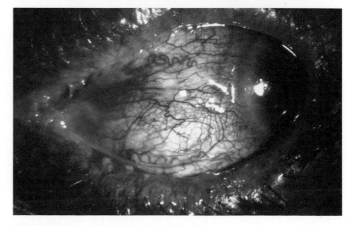

Figure 8.8 Mucous membrane pemphigoid: eyes.

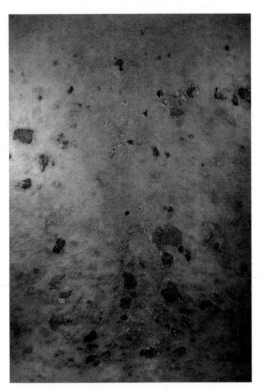

Figure 8.9 Pemphigus vulgaris on the trunk.

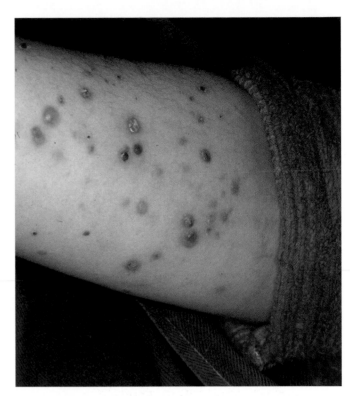

Figure 8.11 Dermatitis herpetiformis.

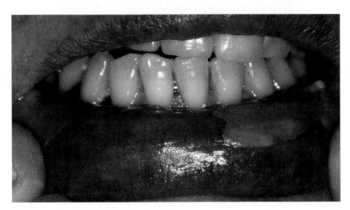

Figure 8.10 Pemphigus vulgaris of the lips.

may precede cutaneous signs by several months. Skin lesions do, however, occur in most patients and are characterized by painful flaccid blisters and erosions arising on normal skin (Figure 8.9). The bullae are easily broken, and even rubbing apparently normal skin causes the superficial epidermis to slough off (Nikolsky sign positive).

Slow healing painful erosions occur in the mouth, particularly on the soft/hard palate and buccal mucosae, but the larynx may also be affected. The oral cavity lesions may be so severe that patients have difficulty eating, drinking and brushing their teeth (Figure 8.10).

Recognized drug triggers of pemphigus vulgaris include rifampicin, ACE inhibitors and penicillamine. Paraneoplastic pemphigus is clinically similar to pemphigus vulgaris but with an associated underlying malignancy such as non-Hodgkin's lymphoma or chronic lymphocytic leukaemia. Pemphigus foliaceus and pemphigus erythematosus are less common variants.

Dermatitis herpetiformis (DH)

This is an intensely pruritic autoimmune blistering disorder that affects young/middle-aged adults and is associated with an underlying gluten-sensitive enteropathy. Several HLA types have been identified in patients with DH (HLA-DQ2, -DR3, -B8) and 10% of patients report an affected relative. Cutaneous lesions are characteristically intermittent and mainly affect the buttocks, knees and elbows (Figure 8.11). The intense pruritus leads to excoriation of the small vesicles which are therefore rarely seen by clinicians.

Most patients do not report any bowel symptoms unless prompted, but may experience bloating and diarrhoea. Low ferritin and folate can result from malabsorption. Interestingly, small bowel investigation reveals abnormalities (villous atrophy, raised lymphocyte count) in 90% of patients. There is an increased frequency of small bowel lymphoma in patients with enteropathy.

DH patients should be encouraged to follow a strict gluten-free diet, as this may control the cutaneous and gastrointestinal symptoms and is thought to reduce the risk of small bowel lymphoma. Patients should avoid wheat, rye and barley. Dapsone and sulphapyridine can be used to control symptoms if dietary manipulation is unsuccessful. DH is a chronic condition and therefore lifelong management is needed.

Linear IgA

Children and adults can be affected by this autoimmune subepidermal blistering disorder. The clinical picture is heterogeneous

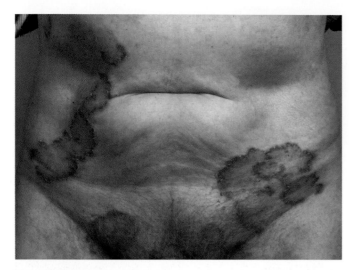

Figure 8.12 Linear IgA on the trunk.

ranging from acute onset of blistering to insidious pruritus before chronic tense bullae. In children the blisters tend to affect the lower abdomen and perineum, whereas in adults the limbs and trunk are most commonly affected (Figure 8.12). Blisters are usually intact and are classically seen around the periphery of annular lesions ('string of beads sign') or in clusters ('jewel sign'). Mucous membrane involvement is common.

Reported drug triggers include vancomycin, ampicillin and amiodarone. Management is similar to that for dermatitis herpetiformis, with patients responding to dapsone and sulphapyridine.

Investigation of immunobullous disease

The gold standard for diagnosing immunobullous disease is direct immunofluorescent analysis of perilesional skin. Skin biopsies are taken across a blister/erosion; the lesional part is sent for histopathology and the adjacent skin sent for direct immunofluorescence (Table 8.3). The histological features can be diagnostic or supportive of the diagnosis. The level and pattern of immunoglobulin staining on direct immunofluorescence is usually diagnostic. Blood may be sent for indirect immunofluorescence to detect autoantibodies in the serum which is positive in the majority of patients (Figures 8.13–8.16).

Management of immunobullous disease

Tense intact blisters can be deflated using a sterile needle (the roof of the blister should be preserved as this provides a 'natural wound covering'). Use of non-adherent dressings or a bodysuit can be used to cover painful cutaneous erosions. Liquid paraffin should be applied regularly to eroded areas to help retain fluid and prevent secondary infection.

In most cases of immunobullous disease immunosuppressive treatments are required. Bullous pemphigoid presenting in an elderly patient may respond to intensive potent topical steroids to affected skin. Reducing courses of systemic corticosteroids can

Table 8.3 Skin biopsy findings in immunobullous disorders.

Immunobullous disorder	Histology features	Immunofluorescence features
Bullous pemphigoid	Subepidermal blister containing mainly eosinophils	Linear band of IgG at the basement membrane zone
Pemphigoid gestationis	Subepidermal blister containing mainly eosinophils	Linear band of C3 at the basement membrane zone
Mucous membrane pemphigoid	Subepidermal blister with variable cellular infiltrate	Linear band of IgG/ C3 at the basement membrane zone
Pemphigus vulgaris	Suprabasal split (basal cells remain attached to basement membrane, looking like 'tombstones')	IgG deposited on surface of keratinocytes in a 'chicken-wire' pattern
Dermatitis herpetiformis	Small vesicles containing neutrophils and eosinophils in the upper dermis	Granular deposits of IgA in the upper dermis (dermal papillae)
Linear IgA	Subepidermal blisters with neutrophils or eosinophils	Linear deposition of IgA at the basement membrane zone

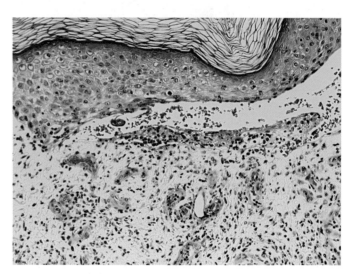

Figure 8.13 Histopathology of bullous pemphigoid.

be helpful in the short term, but most patients are maintained on azathioprine or minocycline (anti-inflammatory properties).

Severe forms of pemphigoid gestationis may require high doses of systemic corticosteroids which can usually be rapidly reduced during the postpartum period. Care should be taken if mothers are breastfeeding as most drugs pass into breast milk.

Mucous membrane pemphigoid is chronic and resistant to most treatments, making management difficult. Oral disease lesions may respond to topical steroids and tetracycline mouthwashes. Ophthalmic disease should be managed carefully as scarring can result in blindness. Topical steroid drops and mitomycin may be useful, but usually systemic immunosuppression is required.

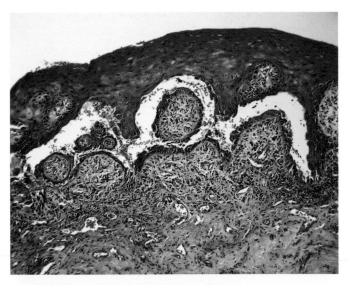

Figure 8.14 Histopathology of pemphigus vulgaris.

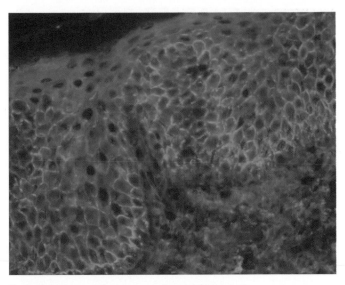

Figure 8.16 Immunofluorescence of pemphigus vulgaris.

Pemphigus vulgaris is a chronic disease that usually requires high doses of systemic corticosteroids to control the disease with steroid-sparing agents as maintenance. Mycophenolate mofetil, azathioprine, immunoglobulin, cyclophosphamide and rituximab have all been shown to be useful.

Further reading

Fassihi H, Wong T, Wessagowit V, McGrath JA, Mellerio JE. Target proteins in inherited and acquired blistering skin disorders. *Clin Exp Dermatol* 2006; **31**(2): 252–9.

Humbert P, Pelletier F, Dreno B, Puzenat E, Aubin F. Gluten intolerance and skin diseases. *Eur J Dermatol* 2006; **16**(1): 4–11.

McCuin JB, Hanlon T, Mutasim DF. Autoimmune bullous diseases: diagnosis and management. *Dermatol Nurs* 2006; **18**(1): 20–5.

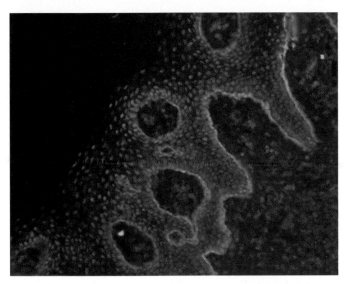

Figure 8.15 Immunofluorescence of bullous pemphigoid.

A gluten-free diet is an effective way of controlling the cutaneous eruption of dermatitis herpetiformis as well as relieving gastrointestinal symptoms and reducing the risk of developing small bowel lymphoma. Dapsone or sulphapyridine are both helpful in controlling the disease.

CHAPTER 9

Inflammatory Dermatoses: Connective Tissue Disease, Vasculitis and Related Disorders

OVERVIEW

- Skin lesions commonly occur in many connective tissue diseases, which involve an autoimmune reaction.

- Vasculitis causes various types of lesions as a result of changes in the cutaneous capillaries and arterioles and may involve internal organs. Raynaud's phenomenon may be associated.

- Other vascular lesions include Henoch–Schönlein purpura and polyarteritis nodosa.

- The causes of cutaneous vasculitis include inflammatory, viral and haematological conditions. A wide range of investigations may be indicated.

- Fibrosis of connective tissue is a feature of a systemic sclerosis, morphoea, CREST syndrome and lichen sclerosus.

- Dermatomyositis, in which there is involvement of skin and muscle tissue, is a marker of internal malignancy.

- Lichen planus is a chronic inflammatory condition of the skin of unknown cause.

- Lupus erythematosus can be a severe systemic illness or occur as a localized, discoid form.

Introduction

The skin is a dynamic interface of trafficking immune cells that may remain localized and respond to nearby stimuli, or migrate through the skin in response to more distant triggers. The skin has been called 'the immunological battle ground of the body' and immune cells involved in inflammatory reactions may be part of a local immune reaction or migrate to the skin as a result of antigenic stimuli at distant sites.

Malfunction of the sophisticated human immune system may result in the body attacking its own tissues, i.e. failure to distinguish 'self' from 'non-self'. These autoimmune responses may develop against a tissue in a specific organ such as the thyroid gland, or to tissues within and between organs resulting in connective tissue diseases.

ABC of Dermatology, 5th edition. Edited by P. K. Buxton and R. Morris-Jones.
© 2009 Blackwell Publishing, ISBN: 978-1-4051-7065-9.

Connective tissue disease

Connective tissue disease can be difficult to define but encompass disorders that involve tissues connecting and surrounding organs.

Connective tissues include the extracellular matrix and support proteins such as collagen and elastin. Acquired disorders of connective tissue are thought to have an autoimmune basis, many of which have distinctive clinical features and patterns in laboratory investigations. However, at times classification may not be easy.

What triggers the production of autoantibodies in the first place is unknown; however some possible factors are sunlight, infections or drugs. There is thought to be an underlying hereditary susceptibility to autoimmune diseases, marked by specific HLA (human lymphocyte antigen) types in some cases.

In autoimmune disorders immune cells may be attracted to particular targets within the skin locally (pemphigus, pemphigoid) or accumulate at sites of connective tissues in multiple organs (systemic lupus erythematosus, dermatomyositis). Once at their destination these immune cells trigger a cascade of chemical messages leading to inflammation.

The possibility of an underlying connective tissue disorder should be considered if a patient complains of any combination of symptoms including the following: cutaneous lesions (particularly photosensitive sites, dorsi of fingers and vasculitic lesions), joint pains, muscle aches, malaise, weakness, photosensitivity, Raynaud's phenomenon and alopecia.

Linking the clinical symptoms and signs with the most appropriate investigations in order to arrive at a unifying diagnosis is a challenge to even the most experienced medical practitioner (Box 9.1).

Vasculitis

Complex reactions occurring specifically in the capillaries and arterioles of the skin may lead to cutaneous erythema (redness). The erythema may be macular or papular and may be transient or last for weeks. Blood vessels can become leaky leading to pouring out (extravasation) of red blood cells into the tissue with or without inflammation of the blood vessel walls. Inflammation of blood vessel walls is called vasculitis and may involve arteries and/or veins.

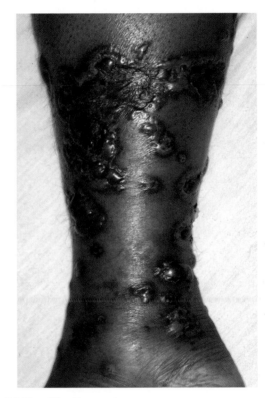

Figure 9.2 Vasculitis with necrosis.

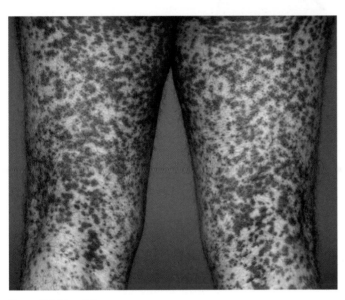

Figure 9.1 Vasculitis.

Symptoms can include pain in the skin, general malaise, fever, abdominal pain and arthropathy. Clinically patients have a non-blanching skin eruption that is most commonly seen on the lower limbs (Figure 9.1). Individual skin lesions may be macular or palpable purpura, blistering, ulcerated and necrotic (Figure 9.2). Vasculitis confined to the skin can be painful and unpleasant, but systemic vasculitis may be life-threatening.

There are numerous possible underlying causes of vasculitis including infections, medications, connective tissue disease, underlying malignancy, vascular/coagulopathy disorders, inflammatory bowel disease and sarcoidosis.

The pathophysiology of vasculitis is complex and poorly characterized but is thought to be antibody or immune complex mediated. Blood vessel endothelial lining cells become damaged as a result of immune complex deposition, antibody targeting and consequent inflammatory cascades. Inflammation involves activation of complement and the release of inflammatory mediators resulting in vasodilatation and polymorph accumulation.

Confirmation of cutaneous vasculitis from a skin biopsy for histology and immunofluorescence (IMF) can be helpful but is not usually diagnostic of the underlying cause (Box 9.2). However, in Henoch-Schönlein purpura the IMF from the skin biopsy usually shows IgA deposition.

Polyarteritis nodosa

This is a disease of small to medium-sized blood vessels that can affect any organ but most commonly affects the skin and joints. Immune complexes mediate the disease activating the complement cascade leading to inflammatory damage to vessels. Antineutrophil cytoplasmic antibodies (ANCA) may be positive.

Patients present with general malaise, fever, weight loss, weakness, neuropathies and skin lesions. Cutaneous manifestations may include a subtle mottled pattern (livedo reticularis), purpura, tender subcutaneous nodules, ulceration and necrosis, particularly on the lower limbs.

Henoch-Schönlein purpura

This usually occurs in children or young adults, the aetiology is unknown but up to 50% of patients have preceding upper respiratory tract symptoms and a positive antistreptolysin O titre (ASOT). The skin, kidneys (IgA nephropathy), GI tract and joints are mainly affected. IgA, complement and immune complexes are deposited in small vessels leading to systemic vasculitis. The diagnosis is made on clinical grounds, although deposition of IgA in the skin/kidneys on immunofluorescence can be supportive. The treatment is mainly supportive and most patients recover within weeks. Occasionally the condition can persist and systemic corticosteroids may be needed.

Management of cutaneous vasculitis

Treat any underlying cause. For mild to moderate cutaneous involvement a potent topical steroid can be applied to the affected skin. If the lower legs are affected then support hosiery should be used and the legs elevated on sitting.

In more severe cases systemic corticosteroids (30–60 mg) are usually required. Anticoagulation with heparin or warfarin may be needed. If the vasculitis persists then an alternative immunosuppressant may be needed in the long term such as azathioprine or methotrexate.

Raynaud's phenomenon

This is reversible vasospasm of peripheral arterioles leading to transient ischaemia of the digits associated with an underlying autoimmune disease. The most common associations are with systemic sclerosis, mixed connective tissue disease, systemic lupus erythematosus and cryoglobulinemia. In the cold the affected digits characteristically turn white (vasospasm) then blue (cyanosis) and finally red (hyperemia); these colour changes may be associated with pain or numbness.

Systemic sclerosis

This is a condition in which there is extensive sclerosis of the subcutaneous tissues in the fingers and toes as well as around the mouth (scleroderma), with similar changes affecting the internal organs, particularly the lung and kidneys. There are vascular changes producing Raynaud's phenomenon and telangiectasia around the mouth and fingers (Figure 9.3). It is associated with antinuclear antibodies (speckled or nucleolar), and in about 50% of cases circulating immune complexes may be present. Endothelial cell damage in the capillaries results in fibrosis and sclerosis of the organs concerned. There is considerable tethering of the skin on the fingers and toes, which becomes very tight with a waxy appearance and considerable limitation of movement. A variant is the CREST syndrome (Box 9.3).

Morphoea is a benign form of localized systemic sclerosis in which there is localized sclerosis with very slight inflammation. There is atrophy of the overlying epidermis. In the early stages the skin may have a dusky appearance, but as the disease progresses the skin becomes a whitish colour and feels very firm (Figure 9.4). Localized

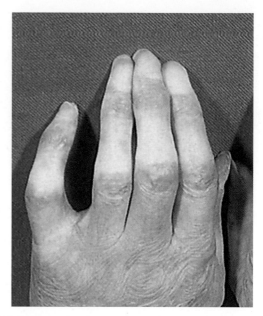

Figure 9.3 Systemic sclerosis.

Box 9.3 **CREST syndrome**

C Calcinosis cutis
R Raynaud's phenomenon
E Esophageal dysmotility
S Sclerodactyly
T Telangiectasia

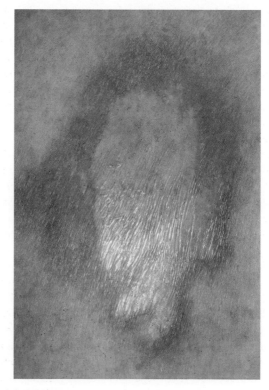

Figure 9.4 Morphoea.

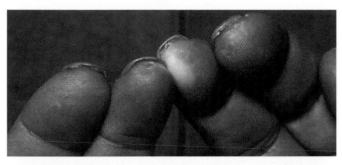

Figure 9.5 Calcinosis cutis.

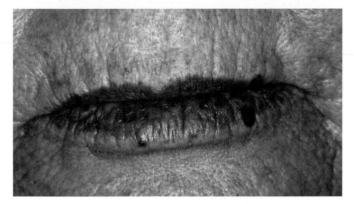

Figure 9.6 CREST syndrome.

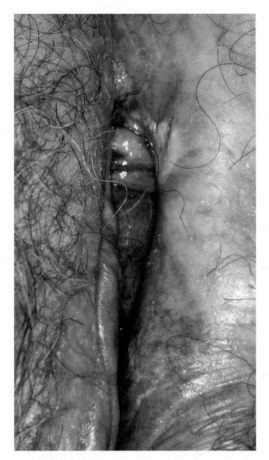

Figure 9.7 Lichen sclerosus.

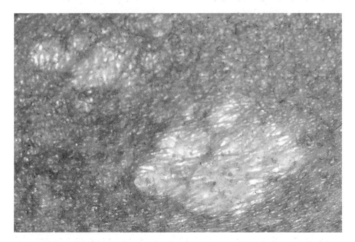

Figure 9.8 Extragenital lichen sclerosus.

morphoea in the frontoparietal area ('en coup de sabre') is associated with alopecia and a sunken groove of firm sclerotic skin.

Patients who develop CREST usually first complain of Raynaud's phenomenon, followed by thickening of the skin of the digits due to scleroderma (progressive fibrosis) leading to sclerodactyly. Calcium deposits in the skin are seen as chalky-white material which can be painful (Figure 9.5). Patients then develop multiple telangiectasia usually first seen on the face (Figure 9.6) but mucous membranes and the gastrointestinal tract may also be affected. Dysmotility of the oesophagus is usually a late development.

Investigations should include an FBC, antinuclear antibody (ANA), anticentromere antibody and anti-Scl-70.

A multidisciplinary team approach to management is usually needed, including psychological support. Patients should keep themselves warm, especially their hands. Calcium-channel blockers and prostagandins/protacyclin may help prevent and treat Raynaud's phenomenon. Calcitriol may soften the sclerodactyly and pulsed dye laser may treat facial telangiectasia.

Lichen sclerosus

This is an itchy eruption which has many features in common with lichen planus. Lichen sclerosis is, however, less common and mainly affects the genital and perineal regions in women. The disorder is characterized by well-demarcated atrophic patches and plaques with a distinctive ivory white colour. There is fibrosis of the underlying tissues with associated loss of normal genital architecture. It frequently affects the vulva (Figure 9.7) and perineum, but may also affect the penis. Extragenital lesions may occur anywhere on the skin (Figure 9.8). A more acute form can affect children, which tends to resolve but in adults it is a chronic condition. There is an increased incidence of squamous cell carcinoma.

The cause of the hyalinized collagen and epidermal atrophy is unknown, but in early lesions there is an infiltrate of lymphocytes with CD3, CD4, CD8 and CD68 markers. An immunological basis for the disease has been suggested because patients have an increased incidence of autoimmune disease. Treatment is with potent topical steroids and excision of any neoplasms.

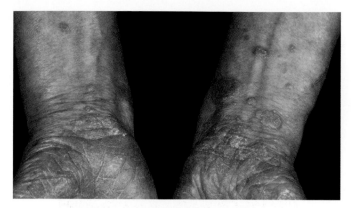

Figure 9.9 Lichen planus: wrist.

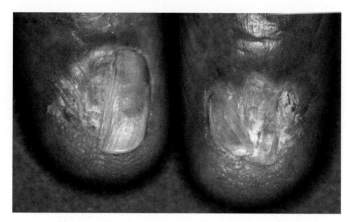

Figure 9.11 Lichen planus: nails.

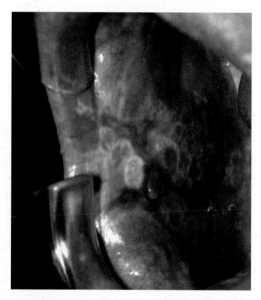

Figure 9.10 Lichen planus: oral mucosa.

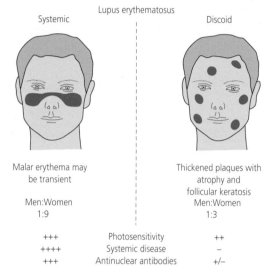

Figure 9.12 Characteristics of systemic and discoid lupus erythematosus.

Lichen planus

The underlying cause is unknown, but the condition is thought to have an immunological aetiology. The histological features are characterized by a band of lymphocytes attacking the basal keratinocytes which results in oedema, subepidermal clefts and death of some keratinocytes. Clinically patients have an itchy eruption consisting of shiny purple-coloured flat-topped papules that characteristically appear on the wrists (Figure 9.9) and ankles. White lines called Wickham's striae may appear on the surface of the lesions at any site. Lesions may appear in clusters or in linear scratches/surgical scars (Koebner phenomenon).

In black skin lichen planus (LP) lesions may be very hypertrophic and heal with marked post-inflammatory hyperpigmentation. The mouth (Figure 9.10) and genitals may also be involved, and distinctive linear ridges and dystrophy may affect the nails (Figure 9.11). Scalp lesions are often scaly with marked follicular plugging that may result in scarring alopecia.

Most cases resolve over 1–2 years. Hypertrophic LP may, however, persist for decades. Potent topical steroid applied to the itchy active lesions is usually effective. Occlusion of the steroid for treatment of hypertrophic lesions is usually more effective than steroid alone.

Lichenoid drug eruptions are clinically similar to LP but lesions are usually more extensive and oral involvement is rare (see Chapter 7). Lesions only resolve very slowly after the drug is stopped, generally taking 1–4 months to settle and usually leaving pigmentation on the skin.

Lupus erythematosus

There are four main clinical variants of lupus erythematosus: systematic, subacute, discoid and neonatal (Figure 9.12, Box 9.4).

Systemic lupus erythematosus (SLE) is an autoimmune disorder characterized by the presence of antibodies against various components of the cell nucleus. SLE has been triggered by drugs including chlorpromazine, quinine and isoniazid. SLE is a multisystem disease; 75% of patients have skin involvement, most commonly an erythematous 'butterfly' distribution rash on the face (Figure 9.13). Photosensitivity, hair loss and areas of cutaneous vasculitis may occur. The systemic changes include fever, arthritis and renal involvement, but there may be involvement of a wide range of organs.

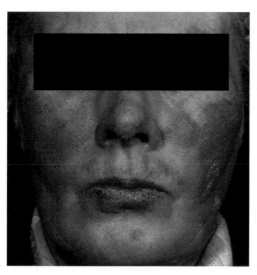

Figure 9.13 Systemic lupus erythematosus: butterfly rash.

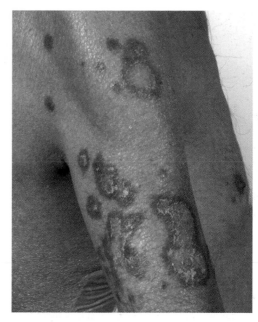

Figure 9.14 Subacute lupus erythematosus.

Box 9.4 **Clinical variants of lupus erythematosus**

- Systemic
- Subacute cutaneous
- Discoid
- Neonatal

Diagnostic criteria for SLE include four of the following at any given time:
- malar rash
- serositis
- discoid plaques
- neurological disorders
- photosensitivity
- haematological changes
- arthritis
- immunological changes
- mouth ulcers
- antinuclear antibodies
- renal changes.

Subacute lupus erythematosus is a variant that presents with an erythematous annular and serpiginous eruption on the skin (Figure 9.14). Systemic involvement is less common and severe than in SLE. It is associated with a high incidence of neonatal lupus erythematosus in children born to mothers with the condition. The extractable nuclear-antibodies (ENA) test is positive in 60% and anticytoplasmic antibodies are present in 80% of patients.

Discoid lupus erythematosus is a photosensitive disorder in which well-defined erythematous lesions with atrophy, scaling and scarring occur on the face (Figure 9.15), scalp (alopecia) and occasionally arms. This is a condition in which circulating antinuclear antibodies are very rare and only 5% of patients go on to develop SLE.

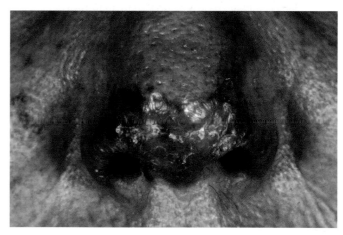

Figure 9.15 Discoid lupus erythematosus.

Neonatal lupus erythematosus is caused by transplacental passage of maternal lupus antibodies (particularly Ro/La) to the neonate who may suffer skin lesions and congenital heart block (which may require pacing).

Treatment of SLE with threatened or actual involvement of organs is important. Prednisolone is usually required and sometimes immunosuppressant drugs such as azathioprine as well. Treatment of DLE is generally with topical steroids and sunscreen. Hydroxychloroquine 200 mg daily can be effective. Hydroxychloroquine can cause ocular toxicity and therefore patients should be told to report any visual disturbance.

Dermatomyositis

A rare disorder that affects the skin, muscle and blood vessels. The cause is unknown but derangement of normal immune responses is observed. Evidence suggests dermatomyositis may be

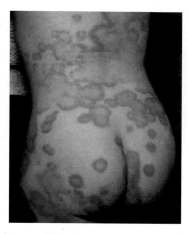

Figure 10.1 Erythema multiforme.

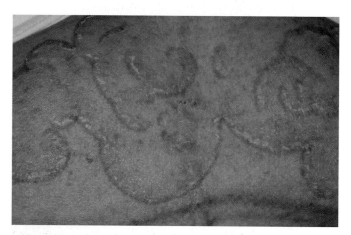

Figure 10.2 Annular erythema.

connective tissue disease, sarcoidosis and reactions to drugs such as sulphonamides.

The lesions consist of erythematous macules that become raised and typically develop into 'target lesions' in which there is a dusky red or purpuric centre with a pale indurated zone surrounded by an outer ring of erythema. The lesions may be few or multiple and diffuse, often involving the hands, feet, elbows and knees. Blisters may develop.

In the more severe forms there may be dermal changes and blister formation with involvement of the mucous membranes (*Stevens–Johnson syndrome*). There is often pyrexia with gastrointestinal and renal lesions.

Erythema annulare is a specific pattern in the skin with a large number of reported associations, ranging from fungal and viral infections to sarcoidosis and carcinoma. It consists of a small erythematous macule that enlarges to form an expanding ring, usually on the trunk (Figure 10.2).

Erythema chronicum migrans is a migrating erythema that results from a cutaneous inflammatory response to infection caused by *Borrelia burgdorferi* (Lyme disease) (Chapter 17).

There are many other types of 'figurate erythemas'. *Erythema gyratum repens* is associated with underlying carcinoma and *erythema marginatum*, which is now rare, with rheumatic fever.

Erythema of the nailbeds
This may be associated with connective tissue disease, such as lupus erythematosus, scleroderma and dermatomyositis.

Angiomas

Spider naevi, which show a central blood vessel with radiating branches, are frequently seen in women (especially during pregnancy) and children (see Chapter 21). If they occur in large numbers, particularly in men, they may indicate liver failure. Palmar erythema and yellow nails may also be present.

Congenital angiomas
Eruptive angiomas may be associated with systemic angiomas of the liver, lung and brain. Port wine stain due to abnormality of the dermal capillaries commonly develops on the head and neck. It may be associated with congenital vascular abnormalities of the meninges and epilepsy. Vascular abnormalities of the eye, and also glaucoma, occur with lesions on the face.

Changes in pigmentation

Hypopigmentation

Hormonal
A widespread partial loss of melanocyte functions with loss of skin colour is seen in hypopituitarism and is caused by an absence of melanocyte-stimulating hormone.

Genetic
In albinism, an autorecessive condition, there is little or no production of melanin, with loss of pigment from the skin, hair and eyes (see Chapter 6). Other genetic conditions with loss of skin pigment include piebaldism (Figure 10.3), phenylketonuria and tuberous sclerosis.

Localized depigmentation is most commonly seen in vitiligo; a family history of the condition is found in one-third of the patients. In the sharply demarcated, symmetrical macular lesions there is loss of melanocytes and melanin (Figure 10.4). There is an increased incidence of organ-specific antibodies and their associated diseases (Box 10.3).

Other causes of hypopigmented macules include: post-inflammatory conditions such as psoriasis, eczema, lichen planus and lupus erythematosus; infections, for example pityriasis versicolor and leprosy; chemicals, such as hydroquinones, hydroxychloroquine and arsenicals, reactions to pigmented naevi, seen in halo naevi (when the mole develops a pale ring around it); and genetic diseases, such as tuberous sclerosis ('ash leaf' macules).

Hyperpigmentation
There is wide variation in the pattern of normal pigmentation as a result of heredity factors and exposure to the sun. Darkening of

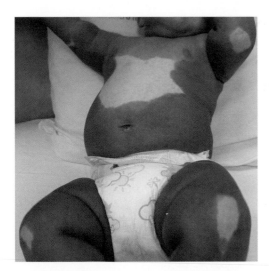

Figure 10.3 Piebaldism.

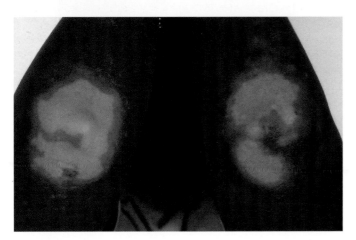

Figure 10.4 Vitiligo.

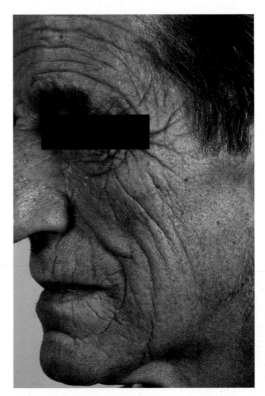

Figure 10.5 Haemochromatosis.

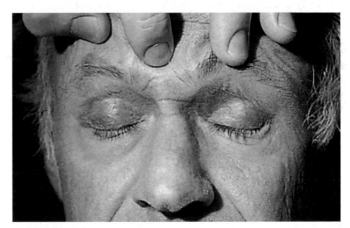

Figure 10.6 Agyria.

Box 10.3 **Autoimmune associations with vitiligo**

- Thyroid disease
- Myasthenia gravis
- Pernicious anaemia
- Alopecia areata
- Hypoparathyroidism
- Halo naevus
- Addison's disease
- Morphoea and lichen sclerosus
- Diabetes

the skin may be due to an increase in the normal pigment melanin or to the deposition of bile salts from liver disease, iron salts (haemochromatosis) (Figure 10.5), drugs or metallic salts from ingestion. In agyria ingested silver salts are deposited in the skin (Figure 10.6).

Causes of hyperpigmentation include the following factors.

Hormonal

An increase in circulating hormones that have melanocyte-stimulating activity occurs in hyperthyroidism, Addison's disease and acromegaly. In pregnant women or those taking oral contraceptives there may be a localized increase in melanocytic pigmentation of the forehead and cheeks known as melasma (or chloasma) (Figure 10.7). It may fade slowly if ultraviolet light is excluded from the affected skin using daily sunblock.

Increased deposition of haemosiderin is generalized in haemochromatosis. Localized red-brown discolouration of the lower legs is seen with longstanding varicose veins. It also occurs in a specific localized pattern in Schamberg's disease, when there is a 'cayenne pepper' appearance of small pigmented macules on the legs and thighs.

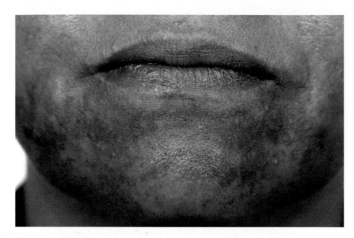

Figure 10.7 Melasma.

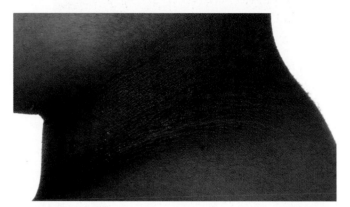

Figure 10.8 Acanthosis nigricans.

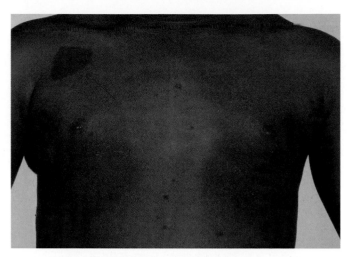

Figure 10.9 Neurofibromatosis: café au lait macules.

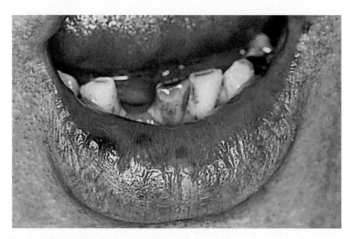

Figure 10.10 Peutz–Jeghers syndrome.

Neoplastic conditions

Lymphomas may be associated with increased pigmentation. Acanthosis nigricans characterized by darkening and thickening of the skin of the axillae (Figure 10.8), neck, nipples, and umbilicus, occurs with internal cancers, usually adenocarcinoma of the stomach. Pseudoacanthosis nigricans is much more common, consisting of simple darkening of the skin in the flexures of obese individuals; it is not associated with malignancy but more with insulin resistance. Increased skin pigmentation may also be observed in patients with acromegaly who have an underlying pituitary tumour.

Drugs

Chlorpromazine, other phenothiazines and minocycline may cause an increased pigmentation in areas exposed to the sun (see Chapter 7). Phenytoin can cause local hyperpigmentation of the face and neck.

Inflammatory reactions

Post-inflammatory pigmentation is common, often after acute eczema, fixed drug eruptions or lichen planus. Areas of lichenification from rubbing the skin are usually darkened.

Malabsorption and deficiency states

In malabsorption syndromes, pellagra and scurvy there is commonly increased skin pigmentation.

Congenital conditions

There is clearly a marked variation in pigmentation and in the number of freckles in normal individuals. There may be localized well-defined pigmented areas in neurofibromatosis with 'cafe au lait' patches (Figure 10.9). Increased pigmentation with a blue tinge occurs over the lumbosacral region in the condition known as Mongolian blue spot.

Peutz–Jeghers syndrome is described in the section 'The gut and the skin' below. There are pigmented macules associated with intestinal polyposis in the oral mucosa, lips and face (Figure 10.10).

Malignant lesions

Malignant lesions may cause skin changes such as acanthosis nigricans and dermatomyositis or produce secondary deposits (Boxes 10.4 & 10.5). Lymphomas can arise in or invade the skin. Pruritus may be associated with Hodgkin's disease.

Mycosis fungoides is a T-cell lymphoma of cutaneous origin. Initially well-demarcated erythematous plaques develop on covered areas with intense itching (Figure 10.11). In many cases there is a gradual progression to infiltrated lesions, nodules and ulceration

Box 10.4 **Skin markers of internal malignancy**

- Acanthosis nigricans: gastric adenocarcinoma
- Erythematous rashes, 'figurate erythema' bronchial/oesophageal/breast carcinoma
- Pruritus: lymphoma
- Dermatomyositis (elderly): lung/breast/ovarian/testicular carcinomas
- Acquired ichthyosis: Hodgkin's disease, sarcoma, lymphoma

Box 10.5 **Non-specific skin changes associated with malignant disease**

- Secondary deposits
- Secondary hormonal effects
- Acne (adrenal tumours)
- Flushing (carcinoid)
- Pigmentation (pituitary tumours)
- Generalized pruritus (particularly lymphoma)
- Figurate erythema
- Superficial thrombophlebitis

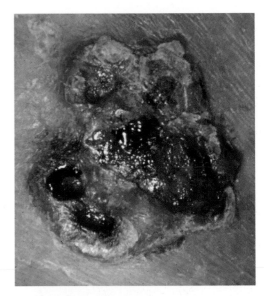

Figure 10.12 Cutaneous T-cell lymphoma.

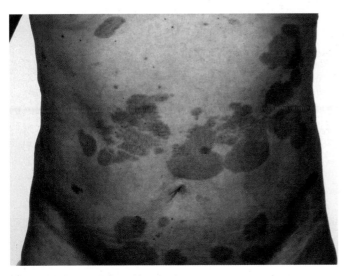

Figure 10.11 Mycosis fungoides: trunk.

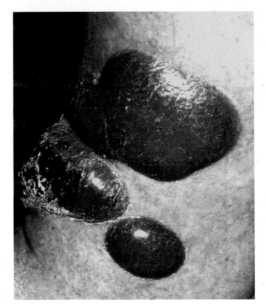

Figure 10.13 B-cell lymphoma of the leg.

(Figure 10.12). In others the tumour may occur *de novo* or be preceded by generalized erythema. Primary cutaneous B-cell lymphoma can also rarely occur (Figure 10.13).

Poikiloderma, in which there is telangiectasia, reticulate pigmentation (Figure 10.14), atrophy and loss of pigment, may precede mycosis fungoides, but it is also seen after radiotherapy and in connective tissue diseases.

Parapsoriasis is a term used for well-defined maculopapular erythematous lesions that occur in middle and old age. Some cases undoubtedly develop into mycosis fungoides and a biopsy specimen should be taken of any such fixed plaques that do not clear with topical steroids.

The gut and the skin

Vasculitis of various kinds, polyarteritis nodosa, connective tissue diseases such as scleroderma, and many metabolic diseases produce both cutaneous and gastrointestinal lesions. There are, however, some specific associations.

Dry skin, asteatosis and *itching*, with superficial eczematous changes and a 'crazy paving' pattern, occur in malabsorption and cachectic states. Increased pigmentation, brittle hair and nails may also be associated.

Pyoderma gangrenosum gives rise to an area of non-specific inflammation and pustules/blisters break down rapidly to form a necrotic ulcer with hypertrophic undermined purplish margins (Figure 10.15). There is a strong association with ulcerative colitis

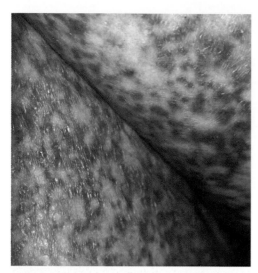

Figure 10.14 Poikiloderma.

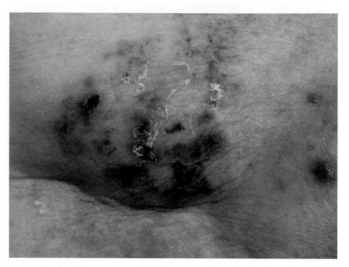

Figure 10.16 Dermatitis herpetiformis.

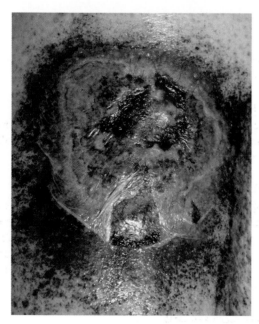

Figure 10.15 Pyoderma gangrenosum.

Box 10.6 **Associations of pyoderma gangrenosum**

- Ulcerative colitis
- Crohn's disease
- Rheumatoid arthritis
- Monoclonal gammopathy
- Leukaemia

---

and Crohn's disease, rheumatoid arthritis, abnormal gamma globulins and leukaemia (Box 10.6).

Dermatitis herpetiformis is an intensely itchy, chronic disorder with erythematous and blistering papules particularly on the elbows, knees and buttocks (Figure 10.16). It is more common in men than women. Most patients have a gluten-sensitive enteropathy with some degree of villous atrophy. There is an associated risk of small bowel lymphoma.

Peutz–Jeghers syndrome is an autosomal dominantly inherited condition characterized by the appearance in infancy of pigmented macules on the oral mucosal membranes, lips and face. Benign intestinal polyps, mainly in the ileum and jejunum, which rarely become malignant, are associated with the condition.

Other conditions include congenital disorders with connective tissue and vascular abnormalities that affect the gut, such as Ehlers–Danlos syndrome and pseudoxanthoma elasticum (arterial gastrointestinal bleeding), purpuric vasculitis (bleeding from gastrointestinal lesions) and neurofibromatosis (intestinal neurofibromas).

In *Crohn's disease* (regional ileitis) perianal erosions/ulceration and sinus formation in the abdominal wall may occur. Glossitis and thickening of the lips and oral mucosa and vasculitis may also be associated.

Liver disease may affect the skin, hair and nails to a variable degree (Box 10.7). Obstructive jaundice is often associated with itching which is thought to be due to the deposition of bile salts in the skin. Evidence of this is the fact that drugs that combine with bile salts such as cholestyramine improve pruritus in some patients. Jaundice is the physical manifestation of bile salts in the skin.

Liver failure is characterized by a number of skin signs, particularly vascular changes causing multiple spider naevi and palmar erythema due to diffuse telangiectasia. It is not unusual to see spider naevi on the trunk in women but large numbers in men should raise suspicion of underlying hepatic disease.

Porphyria cutanea tarda as a result of chronic liver disease produces bullae, scarring and hyperpigmentation in sun-exposed areas of the skin (Figure 10.17). Xanthomas may be associated with primary

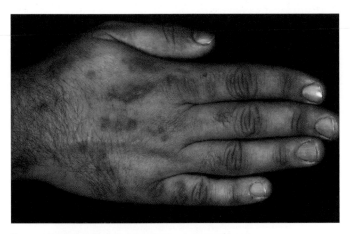

Figure 10.17 Porphyria cutanea tarda: dorsum of hand.

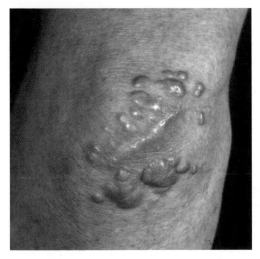

Figure 10.18 Xanthomas.

biliary cirrhosis (Figure 10.18) and in chronic liver disease asteotosis, with dry skin producing a 'crazy paving' pattern.

Diabetes and the skin

In diabetes the disturbances of carbohydrate–lipid metabolism, small blood vessel lesions and neural involvement may be

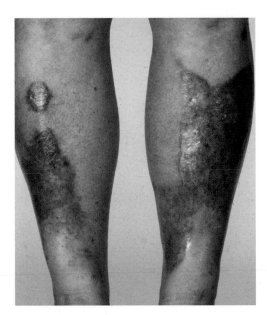

Figure 10.19 Necrobiosis lipoidica.

associated with skin lesions. The more common of these include the following.

Infection

Diabetic patients have an increased susceptibility to cutaneous infections including staphylococcal, streptococcal, coliforms, *Pseudomonas* and *Candida albicans*.

Vascular lesions

'Diabetic dermopathy', due to a microangiopathy, consists of erythematous papules which slowly resolve to leave a scaling macule on the limbs. Atherosclerosis with impaired peripheral circulation is often associated with diabetes. Ulceration due to neuropathy (trophic ulcers) or impaired blood supply may occur, particularly on the feet.

Specific skin lesions

Necrobiosis lipoidica

Between 40% and 60% of patients with this condition may develop diabetes, but it is uncommon in diabetic patients (0.3%). As the name indicates, there is necrosis of the connective tissue with lymphocytic and granulomatous infiltrate. There is replacement of degenerating collagen fibres with lipid material. It usually occurs over the shin but may appear at any site (Figure 10.19).

Granuloma annulare

This usually presents with localized papular lesions on the hands (Figure 10.20) and feet, but may occur elsewhere. The lesions may be partly or wholly annular and may be single or multiple. There is some degree of necrobiosis, with histiocytes forming 'palisades' as well as giant cells and lymphocytes. It is seen more commonly in women under the age of 30. There is an association with insulin-dependent diabetes. It may be pruritic or asymptomatic and is usually self-limiting but may recur.

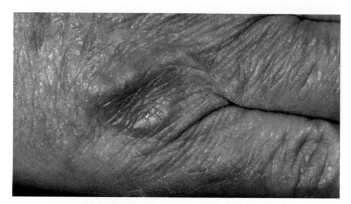

Figure 10.20 Granuloma annulare.

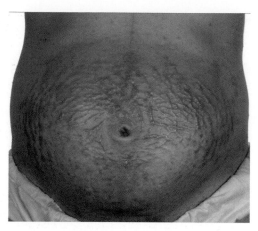

Figure 10.21 Pruritic urticarial papules and plaques of pregnancy (PUPPP).

Other diseases

Porphyrias are due to the accumulation of intermediate metabolites in the metabolic pathway of haem synthesis. There are several types. In hepatic porphyrias there is skin fragility leading to blisters from exposure to the sun or minor trauma. In erythropoietic and erythrohepatic photoporphyrias there is intense photosensitivity including sensitivity to long-wavelength ultraviolet light that penetrates window glass.

Porphyria cutanea tarda usually occurs in men, with a genetic predisposition, who have liver damage as a result of an excessive intake of alcohol. There is impaired porphyria metabolism leading to skin fragility and photosensitivity, with blisters and erosions, photosensitivity on the face and the dorsal surface of the hands.

Xanthomas are lipid-laden macrophages deposited in the skin. They are commonly associated with hyperlipidaemia – either primary or secondary to diabetes, the nephrotic syndrome, hypothyroidism or primary biliary cirrhosis. Diabetes may be associated with the eruptive type.

Necrotizing fasciitis is a rapidly (hours to days) progressive infection of the deep fascia. The infection is often mixed (anaerobic and aerobic bacteria) with gas formation in the subcutaneous tissues. Patients often have a history of recent trauma or surgery. Pain initially at the site followed by anaesthesia is common. Patients appear very unwell – often disproportionately to the clinical picture. Dusky erythema associated with necrosis at the skin surface is usually the tip of the iceberg with much more extensive life-threatening necrosis of the deeper tissues. Urgent surgical debridement is indicated.

Amyloid deposits in the skin occur in primary systemic amyloidosis and myeloma.

Pregnancy

Pregnancy may be associated with pruritus, in which the skin appears normal in 15–20% of women (prurigo gestationis). It is generally more severe in the first trimester.

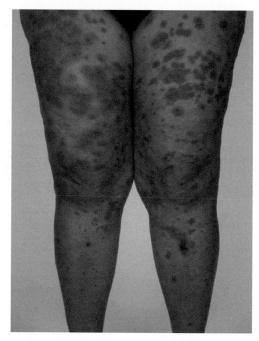

Figure 10.22 Pemphigoid gestationis.

Pruritic urticarial papules and plaques of pregnancy (PUPPP) (Figure 10.21). This polymorphic eruption usually starts on the abdomen in the striae during the third trimester and then becomes widespread. The condition does not affect the baby. It usually resolves post-partum and rarely recurs in subsequent pregnancies with the same partner. Topical steroids may provide symptomatic relief.

Pemphigoid gestationis (PG) is a rare disorder that may initially resemble PUPPP but develops pemphigoid-like vesicles, spreading over the abdomen and thighs (Figure 10.22). PG is an autoimmune disorder, in which cross-reactivity between placental tissues and the skin is thought to be important. It is strongly associated with HLA-DR3/4 and most patients develop anti-HLA antibodies. There is a greater prevalence of premature and small-for-dates babies but no increase in mortality rates.

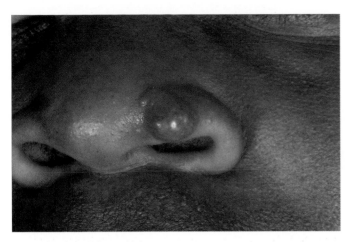

Figure 10.23 Nodular sarcoid.

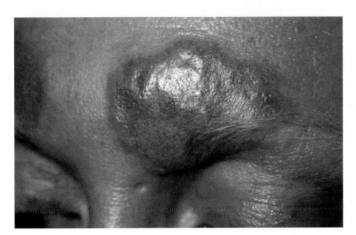

Figure 10.24 Sarcoid plaque.

Sarcoidosis

Pulmonary and other systemic manifestations of sarcoidosis may occur without involvement of the skin. The most common changes are:

- erythema nodosa, which is often a feature of early pulmonary disease
- papules, nodules, and plaques, which are associated with acute and subacute forms of the disease (Figures 10.23 & 10.24)
- scar sarcoidosis, with papules.
- lupus pernio with dusky red infiltrated lesions on the nose and fingers.

Thyroid disease

Thyroid disease is associated with changes in the skin, which may sometimes be the first clinical signs, including changes in texture and hair growth (Table 10.1). Associated increases in thyroid-stimulating hormone concentration may lead to pretibial myxoedema (Figure 10.25). In autoimmune thyroid disease vitiligo and other autoimmune conditions may be present.

Table 10.1 Clinical signs of thyroid disease.

Hypothyroidism	Hyperthyroidism
Dry skin	Soft, thickened skin
Oedema of eyelids and hands	Pretibial myxoedema
Absence of sweating	Increased sweating (palms and soles)
Coarse, thin hair; loss of pubic, axillary, and eyebrow hair	Thinning of scalp hair
	Diffuse pigmentation
Pale 'ivory' skin	Rapidly growing nails
Brittle poorly growing nails	Palmar erythema
Purpura, bruising, and telangiectasia	Facial flushing

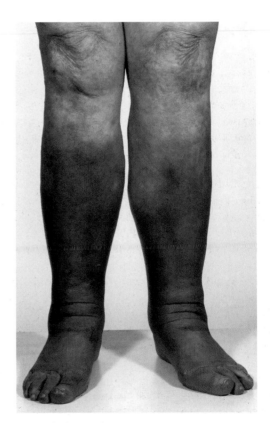

Figure 10.25 Pretibial myxoedema.

Genetics and skin disease

The international project to sequence the human genome (3 billion base pairs) was completed in 2003. This human genome database will allow genetic researchers the opportunity to examine closely the specific genes that are of interest in relation to specific diseases. For example, those working in the field of genodermatoses can look at the structure, function, any detrimental mutations, interaction with other genes and other diseases mapped to that gene's location when undertaking research on a particular cutaneous disorder.

Cutaneous disorders that were originally classified according to clinical manifestations are now being more logically classified according to molecular defects at a genetic level (Table 10.2).

Table 10.2 The abnormality underlying some inherited skin disorders.

Skin disorder	Abnormality
Ehlers–Danlos syndrome	Collagen and the extracellular matrix
Dystrophic epidermolysis bullosa	Type VII collagen
Pseudoxanthoma elasticum	Elastic tissue
Xeroderma pigmentosum	DNA repair
Simple epidermolysis bullosa	Keratins 5 and 14
Epidermolytic hyperkeratosis	Keratins 1 and 10
Palmoplantar keratoderma	Keratins 9 and 16
Junctional epidermolysis bullosa	Laminins
X-linked recessive ichthyosis	Steroid sulphatase
Ichthyosis vulgaris	Filaggrin in stratum corneum
Darier's disease	Epidermal cell adhesion
Albinism (tyrosinase negative type)	Tyrosinase

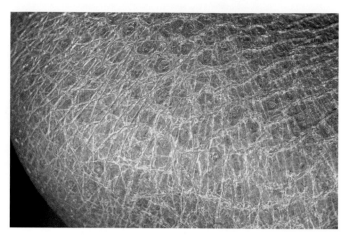

Figure 10.26 Ichthyosis.

Currently around 500 single inheritance gene disorders with a significant cutaneous component have been identified at the molecular level. Although these disorders tend to be rare they can provide valuable information into the function of the particular protein or adhesion molecule etc. that is affected by the gene defect. In addition this has led to a deeper understanding of inheritance patterns, more accurate diagnoses for neonates, where applicable prenatal diagnosis, and the hope for future treatments in the form of gene therapy.

As a general rule common cutaneous disorders that run in families (familial) such as psoriasis, atopic eczema and acne have more complex patterns of inheritance and are therefore more difficult to define genetically. These disorders are referred to as multifactorial as several genes are involved in the expression of the disease in addition to environmental modification (aeroallergens, food allergy, medication, infections).

Recent advances include the identification of the gene defect that is responsible for *ichthyosis vulgaris (IV)* (which affects 1 in 250 individuals) (Figure 10.26), an inherited condition that affects skin barrier function. The pathogenic mutations were identified in the gene encoding *filaggrin* which is an essential structure in the stratum corneum. Abnormalities of filaggrin lead to increased levels of transepidermal water loss. Many patients with IV also suffer from atopic dermatitis (AD) and therefore researchers hypothesized that filaggrin abnormalities may underpin the molecular pathology of AD. However loss of filaggrin expression is not the whole story in AD which is a very heterogeneous disorder. Some patients with AD may possess filaggrin gene mutations whilst others have primary immunological defects or susceptibilities to infections and/or inflammation in the skin or more likely a combination of all these factors.

In the future we may be able to develop therapies, for example, that restore filaggrin expression and function in the skin, resulting in significant clinical benefits to many patients with atopic dermatitis.

Gene therapy is an exciting potential new strategy in the management of genetic abnormalities. The accessibility of the skin as a therapeutic target for gene therapy is being exploited in developing novel treatments for delivery of corrected genes into skin tissues and beyond. Inherited blistering disorders such as epidermolysis bullosa could in theory be corrected by the delivery of corrective gene transfer using retroviral vectors. In the delivery of gene therapy the skin's barrier function needs to be overcome and effects need to persist. Stem cells may therefore prove to be the ideal targets. However gene therapy targeted at keratinocytes and fibroblasts are also being evaluated with the hope of providing a range of novel genetic therapy tools for treatments in the future.

Single gene disorders

These tend to be rare disorders that are inherited in a Mendelian pattern: autosomal recessive, autosomal dominant and X-linked recessive/dominant. Most of these disorders result from a single gene mutation that affects its protein product which may in turn be increased, lost or modified. Not all these genetic disorders are evident at birth: many may present in later life such as neurofibromatosis type 2. The 'two-hit' principle is thought to be responsible for later presentations of genetic disorders when patients possess one mutant gene but its counterpart is normal until a second event occurs later in life. When the second gene mutates the disease is expressed.

Single gene mutations may affect particular molecular structures in the skin such as the hemidesmosome (BP180) leading to one of the inherited types of junctional epidermolysis bullosa. However, the same BP180 protein may be targeted by acquired disorders such as bullous pemphigoid. Clinically both conditions are characterized by skin fragility due to subepidermal splits.

Mosaicism refers to two or more cell populations that are genotypically different from each other but occur in the same individual. Cutaneous mosaicism may result from a mutation during development that is restricted to a few particular skin cells. This frequently results in linear abnormalities in the skin, usually present at birth. The mosaic defects often follow Blashko's lines (Figure 10.27), a bizarre pattern of lines and whorls which are thought to represent the developmental growth patterns in the skin (Figure 10.28). The genetic abnormalities found in localized mosaic cells may be identical to those found in generalized

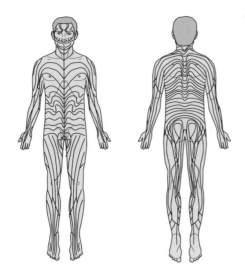

Figure 10.27 Blashko's lines.

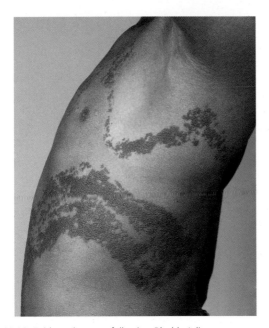

Figure 10.28 Epidermal naevus following Blashko's lines.

genodermatoses. For example, the same abnormalities in the genes controlling the production of keratins 1 and 10 can be responsible both for a generalized epidermolytic hyperkeratosis and for localized warty linear naevi.

Genetically complex disorders

Psoriasis is an example of a familial disorder that clusters in families but does not follow classical Mendelian inheritance. However, in many families the inheritance appears to be autosomal dominant with decreased penetrance. Environmental triggers are thought to be important as there is not 100% concordance amongst monozygotic twins. Several HLA associations have now been identified for psoriasis including B13, B17 and Cw6. Several genes have also been identified that confer susceptibility to psoriasis including *PSOR1* on chromosome 6 (lies within the major histocompatibility complex, MHC) which is found in 50% of patients with psoriasis. In addition, six other psoriasis susceptibility loci (*PSOR2, PSOR3, PSOR4, PSOR5, PSOR6, PSOR7*) have been identified, as well as the transcription factor *RUNX1*.

Atopic eczema is a genetically complex familiarly transmitted disease. Extrinsic environmental factors are thought to play a significant role in the increased lifetime prevalence of the disease in children, which is currently estimated to be between 10–20%. Several chromosomal regions have been identified via genetic linkage analyses in patients with atopic eczema including 5q31 (T helper cell (Th2) gene region), 1q21 (shared with psoriasis), 3q21 (encoding co-stimulatory T-cells) and FcεRI (encodes for the β subunit of the high affinity IgE receptor) that lies on chromosome 11q13 as well as multiple other regions as yet uncharacterized. Children of parents with atopic eczema have a 50% chance of being affected, but 20–30% of affected children have unaffected parents. The inheritance of atopic eczema probably involves genes that predispose to the state of atopy (genotype) and others that determine the expression (phenotype): asthma, eczema or hay fever.

Further reading

Lebwohl MG. *The Skin and Systemic Disease. A Colour Atlas and Text*, 2nd edn. Churchill Livingstone, Oxford, 2003.

Sarzi-Puttini P, Doria A, Girolomoni G, Kuhn A. *The Skin In Systemic Autoimmune Disease.* Elsevier Science, Amsterdam, 2006.

Spitz JL. *Genodermatoses: a Clinical Guide to Genetic Skin Disorders*, 2nd edn. Lippincott Williams and Wilkins, Philadelphia, 2004.

Leg Ulcers

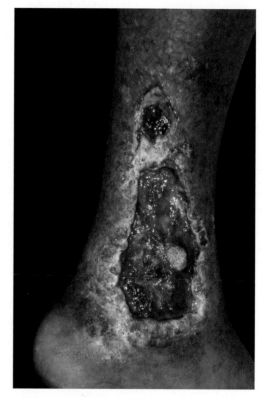

Figure 11.1 Venous leg ulcer.

Introduction

The prevalence of leg ulceration is estimated to be 0.3% of the general population rising to 2% of those over the age of 80 years. Leg ulcers cause significant morbidity for those affected and the cost to the National Health Service in the UK is estimated to be £300–600 million per annum. Many patients have recurrent ulceration requiring repeated courses of bandages and dressings; 80% of patients are treated in the community. The management of leg ulcers usually requires a multidisciplinary approach. If the underlying cause of ulceration cannot be relieved by an operation or medical intervention then the key worker will often be the specialist nurse who has considerable experience of assessing and facilitating the healing of difficult chronic ulcers.

Assessment of any ulcer should include consideration of the following parameters: site, size, edge, base, surrounding skin, leg shape, duration, symptoms, underlying systemic/cutaneous diseases, peripheral pulses/sensation, medication, and current and past ulcer treatments. Investigations may include ankle:brachial pressure indices,

venous and/or arterial duplex scanning, microbiology swabs, ulcer biopsy (usually through the edge) and patch testing.

A basic understanding of the underlying principles of ulceration is essential in reaching a clinical diagnosis and appreciating the different approaches to management. Most (95%) of ulcers are 'venous' (stasis) in nature and therefore these will be considered first in some detail (Figure 11.1).

Venous ulcers

Pathology

The skin

Ulcers arise because the skin (epidermis and dermis) dies from inadequate provision of nutrients and oxygen. This occurs as a consequence of (a) oedema in the subcutaneous tissues with poor lymphatic and capillary drainage and (b) the extravascular accumulation of fibrinous material that has leaked from the blood vessels. The result is a rigid cuff around the capillaries which

ABC of Dermatology, 5th edition. Edited by P. K. Buxton and R. Morris-Jones.
© 2009 Blackwell Publishing, ISBN: 978-1-4051-7065-9.

prevents diffusion of oxygen and nutrients through the vessel wall into the surrounding tissues with consequent fibrosis.

The blood vessels

Arterial perfusion of the leg is usually normal or increased, but stasis occurs in the venules. The lack of venous drainage is a consequence of incompetent valves between the superficial veins and the deeper large veins on which the calf muscle 'pump' acts. In the normal leg there is a superficial low-pressure venous system and deep high-pressure veins (Figures 11.2 & 11.3). If the blood flow from superficial to deep veins is reversed then the pressure in the superficial veins may increase to a level that prevents venous drainage (Figure 11.4). The resulting back pressure leads to varicose veins with stasis and oedema, consequently there is diminished blood flow to the skin causing ulceration (Figure 11.5). Chronic venous insufficiency and the resulting venous hypertension cause venous ulcers.

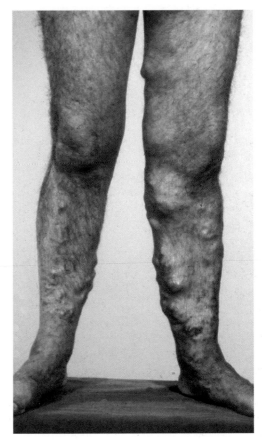

Figure 11.4 Varicose veins.

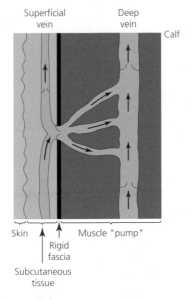

Figure 11.2 Healthy valves in legs.

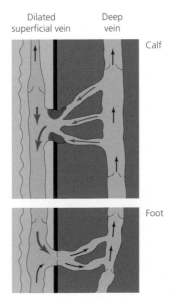

Figure 11.3 Incompetent valves in legs.

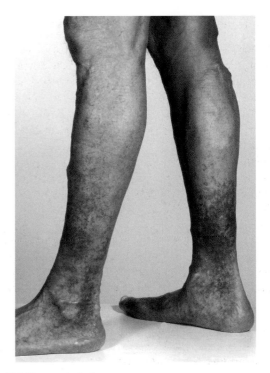

Figure 11.5 Venous stasis changes.

Incompetent valves

Incompetent valves leading to gravitational ulcers may be preceded by:

1 deep vein thrombosis (DVT) associated with pregnancy, injury, immobilization, or infarction
2 primary long saphenous vein insufficiency
3 familial venous valve incompetence that presents at an earlier age (approx 50% of patients)
4 deep venous obstruction.

Risk factors for venous ulceration

Women are more at risk than men. Other factors are a family history of venous disease, increasing age, immobility, obesity, lower leg trauma, peripheral oedema, DVT, varicose veins and a previous history of venous leg ulceration.

Clinical features

Venous ulcers occur around the ankle (gaiter area), most commonly over the medial malleolus. Patients frequently have swollen lower legs with marked pitting oedema. Chronic pitting oedema and fibrinous exudate often lead to fibrosis of the subcutaneous tissues, which may be associated with localized loss of pigment and dilated capillary loops, an appearance known as 'atrophie blanche' (Figure 11.6). This occurs around the ankle with oedema and dilated tortuous superficial veins proximally and can lead to 'inverted champagne bottle'-shaped legs. Lymphoedema results from obliteration of the superficial lymphatics, with associated fibrosis (Figure 11.7). There is often hypertrophy of the overlying epidermis known as lipodermatosclerosis which is a scleroderma-like hardening of the legs in patients with venous insufficiency characterized by induration, hyperpigmentation and depression of the skin (Figure 11.8).

Ulceration often occurs for the first time after a trivial injury. The ulcer margin is usually well defined with a shelving edge and central slough. The surrounding skin may be eczematous (erythematous, inflamed and itchy): so-called varicose eczema. Venous ulcers may be mildly painful, may exude serous fluid and may become odorous from secondary infection.

It is important to check the pulses in the leg and foot as compression bandaging of a leg with impaired blood flow can cause

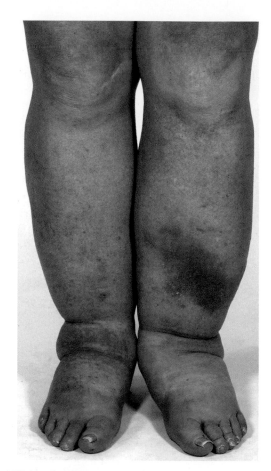

Figure 11.7 Lymphoedema.

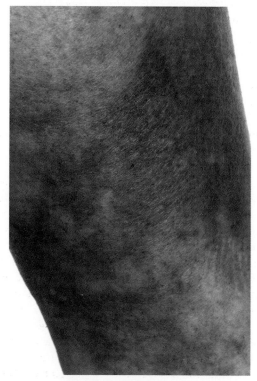

Figure 11.8 Lipodermatosclerosis.

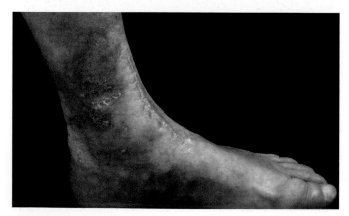

Figure 11.6 Atrophie blanche.

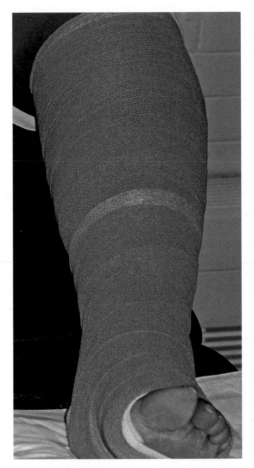

Figure 11.9 Compression bandaging

ischaemia and necrosis. Longstanding ulcers can rarely undergo malignant change (Marjolin's ulcer) when the edge becomes heaped up and atypical due to transformation to squamous cell carcinoma.

Treatment

When new epidermis can grow across an ulcer it will, and the aim is to produce an environment in which this can take place. To this end several measures can be taken (Box 11.1).

1 Oedema may be reduced by means of: (a) diuretics; (b) keeping the legs elevated when sitting; (c) avoiding standing as far as possible; (d) raising the heels slightly from time to time to help venous return by the 'calf muscle pump'; (e) applying compression bandages with greater pressure at the ankle than the thigh (see Chapter 25) (Figure 11.9).

2 Exudate and slough should be removed. Lotions can be used to clean the ulcer, such as 0.9% saline solution, sodium hypochlorite solution or 5% hydrogen peroxide (Figure 11.10). Modern dressings such as alginate, hydrocolloid and Hydrofiber® can efficiently absorb exudate.

There is some evidence that antiseptic solutions and chlorinated solutions delay collagen production and cause inflammation. Enzyme preparations may help by 'digesting' the slough. To prevent the formation of granulation tissue use silver nitrate 0.25% compresses, a silver nitrate 'stick' for more exuberant tissue, and curettage, if necessary.

1 The dressings applied to the ulcer can consist of: (a) simple non-stick, paraffin gauze dressings (an allergy may develop to those with an antibiotic); (b) wet compresses with saline or silver nitrate solutions for exudative lesions; (c) silver sulphadiazine (Flamazine) or hydrogen peroxide creams (Hioxyl, Crystacide); and (d) absorbent dressings, consisting of hydrocolloid patches or powder, which are helpful for smaller ulcers (see Chapter 25).

2 Paste bandages, impregnated with zinc oxide and antiseptics or ichthammol, help to keep dressings in place and provide protection. They may, however, traumatize the skin, and allergic reactions to their constituents are not uncommon.

3 Treatment of infection is less often necessary than is commonly supposed. All ulcers are colonized by bacteria to some extent, usually coincidental staphylococci. A purulent exudate is an indication for a broad-spectrum antibiotic and a swab for

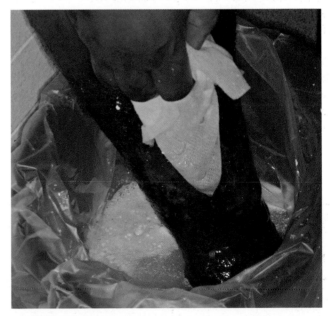

Figure 11.10 Cleaning leg ulcers.

bacteriology. Erythema, oedema and tenderness around the ulcers suggest a β-haemolytic streptococcal infection, which will require long-term antibiotic treatment. Dyes can be painted on the edge of the ulcer, where they fix to the bacterial wall as well as the patient's skin. These may be bright red eosin or blue gentian violet. Soaking the leg in a bucket containing potassium permanganate can be a very effective antiseptic and can help to reduce exudate and slough. Systemic antibiotics have little effect on ulcers but are indicated if there is surrounding cellulitis. A swab for culture and sensitivity helps to keep track of organisms colonizing the area.

4 Surrounding eczematous changes should be treated with moderate-strength topical steroids avoiding the ulcer itself. Ichthammol 1% in 15% zinc oxide and white soft paraffin or Ichthopaste bandages can be used as a protective layer, and topical antibiotics can be used if necessary. It is important to remember that any of the commonly used topical preparations can cause an allergic reaction: neomycin, lanolin, formaldehyde, tars, clioquinol (the 'C' of many proprietary steroids).

5 Skin grafting can be very effective. There must be a healthy viable base for the graft, with an adequate blood supply; natural re-epithelialization from the edges of the ulcer is a good indication that a graft will be supported. Pinch grafts or partial-thickness grafts can be used.

6 Maintaining general health, with adequate nutrition and weight reduction, is important.

7 Corrective surgery for associated venous abnormalities.

Arterial ulcers

Ulcers on the leg also occur as a result of: (a) atherosclerosis with poor peripheral circulation, particularly in older patients; (b) vasculitis affecting the larger subcutaneous arteries; and (c) arterial obstruction in macroglobulinaemia, cryoglobulinaemia, polycythaemia, and 'collagen' disease, particularly rheumatoid arthritis.

Arterial ulcers are sharply defined and accompanied by pain, which may be very severe, especially at night. The pretibial area of the lower leg, dorsal foot and toes are most commonly affected. In patients with hypertension a very tender ulcer can develop posteriorly (Martorelli's ulcer). The legs may be hairless and pale with poor peripheral pulses (Figure 11.11).

Simple or magnetic resonance angiography may be needed to map the arterial tree and look for obstructions and narrowing.

As mentioned above, compression bandaging will make arterial ulcers worse and may lead to ischaemia of the leg.

Neuropathic ulcers

These are usually painless and occur on pressure points of the feet and toes. Diabetic patients may be affected. The ulcers are usually well-defined and 'punched-out', occasionally with deep sinus tracts that can be explored in the clinic with a sterile probe (Figure 11.12).

Inflammatory conditions

Ulcers of the lower legs may occur in polyarteritis nodosa and vasculitis. Pyoderma gangrenosum, a rapidly developing necrotic ulcer with surrounding induration, may occur in association with ulcerative colitis or rheumatoid vasculitis (Figures 11.13 & 11.14).

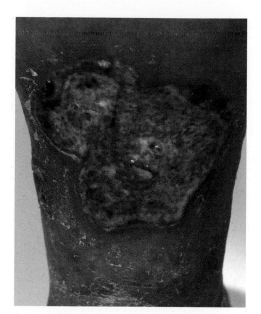

Figure 11.11 Arterial ulcer.

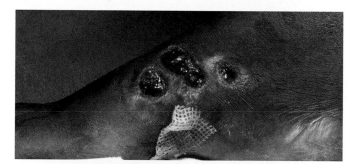

Figure 11.12 Ulcer in diabetic foot.

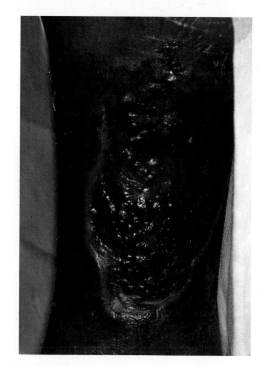

Figure 11.13 Vasculitic ulcer.

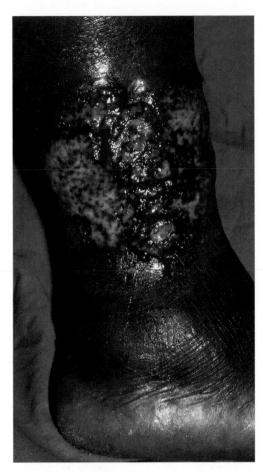

Figure 11.14 Pyoderma gangrenosum.

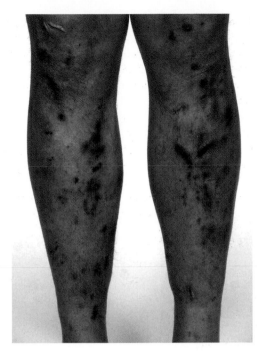

Figure 11.16 Dermatitis artefacta.

Infectious ulcers

Infections that cause ulcers include staphylococcal or streptococcal infections, tuberculosis (which is rare in the UK but may be seen in recent immigrants), and anthrax. Leishmaniasis may present with an ulcer at the cutaneous site of a sandfly bite (see Chapter 18).

Malignant diseases

Squamous cell carcinoma may present as an ulcer or, rarely, develop in a pre-existing ulcer (Marjolin's ulcer) (Figure 11.15). Basal cell carcinoma and melanoma may develop into ulcers, as may Kaposi's sarcoma.

Trauma

Patients with diabetic or other types of neuropathy are at risk of developing trophic ulcers. Rarely, they may be self-induced: 'dermatitis artefacta' (Figure 11.16).

Further reading

Moffatt C, Martin R, Smithdale R. *Leg Ulcer Management (Essential Clinical Skills for Nurses)*. Blackwell Publishing, Oxford, 2007.

Morison M, Moffatt C, Franks P. *Leg Ulcers: a Problem-Based Learning Approach*. Elsevier Health Sciences, Edinburgh, 2006.

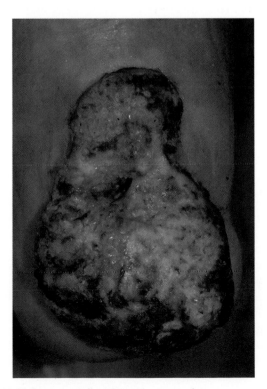

Figure 11.15 Squamous cell carcinoma in venous ulcer.

Acne and Rosacea

Introduction

In Westernized societies acne affects 80–100% of individuals at some point in their lives leading many to conclude that acne is a 'normal' part of life. However, the significant morbidity associated with it means it frequently has a negative impact on people's lives. Acne from the Greek 'acme' meaning 'prime of life' suggests a disorder mainly during adolescence; however, this is somewhat misleading as acne can affect young infants through to individuals in their 40s. Indeed over the past two decades the number of individuals who suffer from acne in later life has been increasing. Estimates show that 5% of the population over the age of 45 years still suffer from acne. Acne can have a significant psychological impact on patients regardless of its severity. Nonetheless severe acne may in addition also be very painful, may cause irreversible scarring and may be associated with systemic symptoms including fever, joint pains and malaise.

What is acne?

Acne lesions develop from the sebaceous glands associated with hair follicles: face, back, chest, and anogenital area (Figure 12.1). (Sebaceous glands are also found on the eyelids and mucosa, prepuce and cervix; however they are not associated with hair follicles.) The sebaceous gland contains holocrine cells that secrete triglycerides, fatty acids, wax esters, and sterols as 'sebum'. The main changes in acne include:

- thickening of the keratin lining and subsequent obstruction of the sebaceous duct resulting in the closed comedones ('whiteheads') (Figure 12.2) or open comedones ('blackheads' whose colour is due to melanin, not dirt) (Figure 12.3)
- an increase in sebum secretion
- an increase in *Propionibacterium acnes* bacteria within the duct
- inflammation around the sebaceous gland, probably as a result of the release of bacterial enzymes.

Underlying causes

There are various underlying causes of these changes (Box 12.1).

Hormones

Androgenic hormones increase the size of sebaceous glands and the amount of sebum in both male and female adolescents. Although androgen levels may be normal there is thought to be an increased sensitivity of the glands to androgen hormones. In some women with acne there is a lowered sex hormone-binding globulin concentration with a consequent increase in free testosterone levels. This change in the hormone balance is mimicked by many combined oral contraceptive pills resulting in increased acne. Oral contraceptives containing more than 50 micrograms ethinyloestradiol

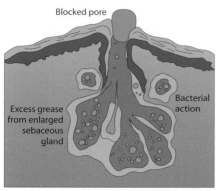

(a)

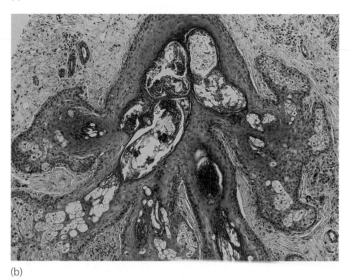

(b)

Figure 12.1 (a) Sebaceous gland: pathology in acne. (b) Histology of acne.

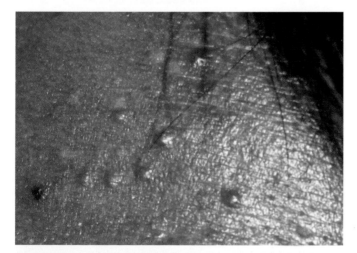

Figure 12.2 Acne with comedones.

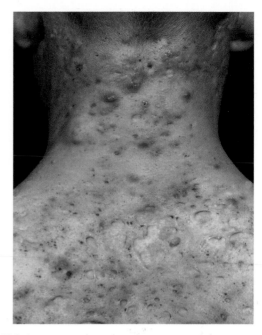

Figure 12.3 Acne cysts and scars.

Box 12.1 **Factors causing acne**

Intrinsic factors
Hormones
- Polycystic ovary syndrome
- Virilizing tumours
- Congenital adrenal hyperplasia
- Increased cortisol (Cushing's syndrome)
- Increased growth hormone (acromegaly)

Medications
- Topical and systemic steroids
- Oral contraceptive pill (higher androgen content)
- Phenytoin
- Barbiturates
- Isoniazid
- Ciclosporin
- Lithium

Extrinsic factors
- Oils/pomades
- Coal and tar
- Chlorinated phenols
- DDT and weed killers

Fluid retention

The premenstrual exacerbation of acne is thought to be due to fluid retention leading to increased hydration of and swelling of the sebaceous duct. Sweating also makes acne worse, possibly by the same mechanism.

Diet

Many patients believe their acne is exacerbated by eating certain foods. Most commonly implicated foods include dairy products, chocolate, nuts, coffee and fizzy drinks. Some epidemiological

can also make acne worse. Oestrogens have the opposite effect in prepubertal boys and eunuchs. Infantile acne occurs in the first few months of life. It can rarely be caused by congenital adrenal hyperplasia or virilizing tumours, but is most commonly due to transplacental stimulation of the adrenal gland by maternal hormones causing increased adrenal androgens.

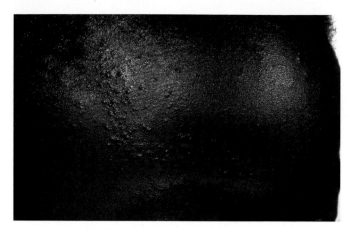

Figure 12.4 Oil-induced acne.

Box 12.2 **Types of acne**

Acne vulgaris
- Affects comedogenic areas
- Occurs mainly in puberty, boys more than girls
- Familial tendency

Infantile acne
- Face only
- Clears spontaneously
- May require treatment

Severe acne
- Acne conglobata/fulminans
- Pyoderma faciale
- Gram-negative folliculitis

studies have suggested that a Westernized diet of high levels of refined sugars and starch may explain striking differences in the prevalence of acne amongst different populations that are not thought to be explained by genetic factors or weight differences.

Seasons

Acne often improves with natural sunlight. Phototherapy with artificial light sources using visible blue light alone or in combination with red light has been shown in several clinical trials to be an effective treatment for acne in a proportion of patients.

External factors

Oils, whether vegetable oils in the case of cooks in hot kitchens or mineral oils in engineering, can cause 'oil folliculitis', leading to acne-like lesions through contact with the skin (Figure 12.4). Other acnegenic substances include coal tar, dicophane (DDT), cutting oils and halogenated hydrocarbons. Cosmetic acne is seen in adult women who have used cosmetics containing comedogenic oils over many years. Individuals who use rich oils in the scalp can suffer from 'pomade acne' which occurs close to the hairline.

Iatrogenic factors

Corticosteroids, both topical and systemic, can cause increased keratinization of the pilosebaceous duct resulting in acne. Androgens, gonadotrophins and corticotrophin can induce acne in adolescence. Oral contraceptive pills (OCP) of the combined type and antiepileptic drugs may also cause acne. However an OCP with a high oestrogen combined with low androgen can actually be used to treat acne in women.

Types of acne (Box 12.2)

Acne vulgaris

Acne vulgaris, the common type of acne, occurs during puberty and affects the comedogenic areas of the face, back and chest. There may be a familial tendency to acne. Acne vulgaris is more common in boys, 30–40% of whom develop acne between the ages of 18 and 19 (Figure 12.5). In girls the peak incidence is between 16 and 18 years. Adult acne is a variant affecting 3% of men and

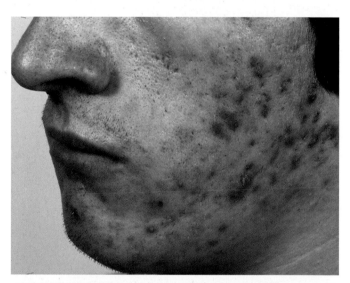

Figure 12.5 Acne vulgaris.

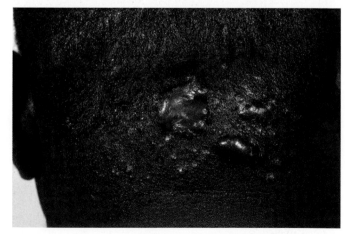

Figure 12.6 Acne keloidalis nuchae.

5% of women over the age of 40. Acne keloidalis is a type of scarring acne seen particularly on the neck in men (Figure 12.6).

Patients with acne often complain of excessive greasiness of the skin, with 'spots', 'zits', 'blackheads' or 'pimples'. These may be associated with inflammatory papules and pustules developing into larger cysts and nodules. Resolving lesions leave post-inflammatory

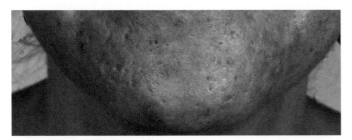

Figure 12.7 'Ice-pick' scars.

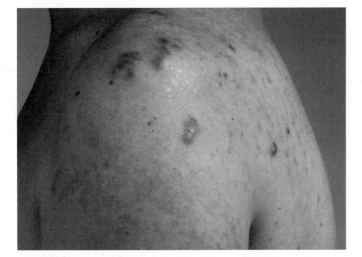

Figure 12.8 Keloid scars.

Figure 12.9 Keloid scars.

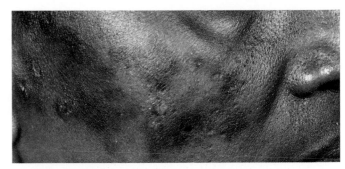

Figure 12.10 Acne excoriée.

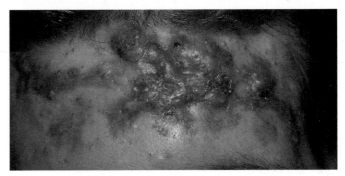

Figure 12.11 Acne conglobata.

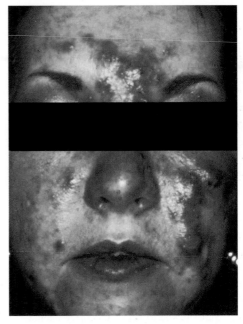

Figure 12.12 Acne fulminans.

pigment changes and scarring. Scars may be atrophic, so-called 'ice pick' (Figure 12.7) lesions or keloid formation. Keloids consist of hypertrophic scar tissue and occur predominantly on the neck (Figures 12.8 & 12.9), upper back, shoulders and sternum.

Acne excoriée

In this variant of acne the patient picks at the skin producing disfiguring erosions (Figure 12.10). The acne itself is usually mild but tends to be persistent as it is often very difficult to help the patient break this habit.

Infantile acne

Localized acne lesions occur on the face in the first few months of life. Infantile acne may require topical or systemic therapy as although it will resolve spontaneously it may last up to 5 years and can cause scarring. There is an association with severe adolescent acne.

Acne conglobata/fulminans

This is a severe form of acne, more common in boys and in tropical climates. There is extensive, nodulocystic acne and abscess formation affecting particularly the trunk, face and limbs (Figure 12.11). Acne fulminans is similarly severe but is associated with systemic symptoms of malaise, fever and joint pains (Figure 12.12).

It appears to be associated with a hypersensitivity to *P. acnes*. Another variant is pyoderma faciale, which produces erythematous and necrotic lesions and occurs mainly in adult women (Figure 12.13).

Gram negative folliculitis occurs with a proliferation of organisms such as *Klebsiella*, *Proteus*, *Pseudomonas* and *Escherichia coli*.

Treatment of acne (Table 12.1)

Although acne can be very painful and may result in pigment change and scarring it is the psychological impact of the condition that is often the most debilitating for those affected. In the past some medical practitioners have underestimated the effect acne has on patients' lives and consequently patients were often dismissed with no treatment on the assumption they would 'grow out of it'. Although most acne will settle with time early intervention for those seeking medical advice results in a significant improvement in their quality of life scores as determined by DLQI (dermatology life quality index which is a validated questionnaire to assess the impact of skin disease on quality of life). DLQI scores for acne are similar to those for psoriasis. Early intervention can also help reduce the likelihood of permanent scars and post-inflammatory pigment changes (Figure 12.14).

When choosing a topical formulation to prescribe for a patient with acne it is worth bearing in mind the patient's skin type: for dry/sensitive skin prescribe creams; for oily skin use solutions or gels; and for combination skin and hair-bearing sites lotions are well tolerated.

When treating patients with acne it is important to warn them they may not see any improvement in their acne for several months and treatment may need to continue for months or years.

Cleansers

Mild acne may respond well to simple measures such as cleansing the skin with proprietary keratolytics; these dissolve the keratin plug of the comedones. Cleansers need to be used with care as they can cause considerable dryness and scaling of the skin.

Topical treatments

Benzoyl peroxide has been available for the treatment of acne for many years; it has bacteriostatic effects against *P. acnes* and is mildly comedolytic. It is available with or without prescription at concentrations ranging from 1 to 10% in numerous formulations including lotions, creams, gels and washes. Mild irritant dermatitis may result, particularly if the patient is using additional anti-acne treatments. Bleaching of clothing and bedding may occur.

Salicylic acid promotes desquamation of follicular epithelium and therefore inhibits the formation of comedones. It is available over the counter at concentrations between 0.5 and 2% in cream and lotion formulations to be used twice daily.

Azelaic acid appears to be effective through its antikeratinizing and antibacterial effects. Twenty per cent azelaic acid cream is available on prescription and can be used twice daily for up to 6 months. Mild skin irritation can result in approximately 5% of patients. Azelaic acid can cause depigmentation of the skin and therefore should be used with care.

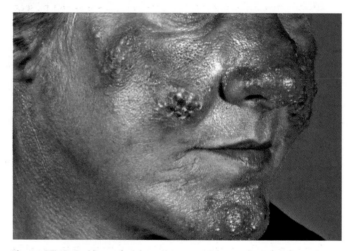

Figure 12.13 Pyoderma faciale.

Table 12.1 Treatment of acne.

Treatment	Comedones	Inflammatory papules/ pustules	Mixed picture	Nodulocystic
First line	Topical retinoid Azelaic acid Salicylic acid	Benzoyl peroxide	Topical retinoid ± topical antibiotic ± benzoyl peroxide Combination of all three	Oral antibiotic + topical retinoid
Second line	Physical comedone extraction	Oral antibiotic Oral contraceptive pill (high oestrogen, low androgen, e.g. Yasmin®)	Azelaic acid + benzoyl peroxide ± topical antibiotic	Oral isotretinoin A short course of systemic steroids may be given initially with the isotretinoin
Third line		Antiandrogens e.g. co-cypindiol (Dianette®) Different oral antibiotic	Hormone therapy Oral antibiotic Oral isotretinoin	Triamcinolone injections to unresponsive lesions

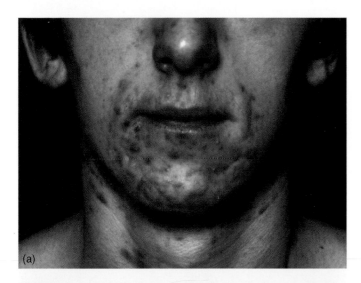

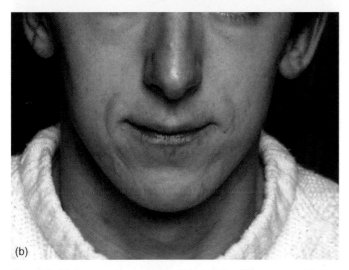

Figure 12.14 Severe cystic acne before (a) and after (b) treatment with tetracycline.

Topical retinoids are vitamin A derivatives that are anti-inflammatory and comedolytic. Treatments currently available include tretinoin, adapalene and tazarotene. Topical retinoids are available in cream and gel formulations and are usually applied once daily at night (as they can cause photosensitivity). The main side-effect is skin irritation that results in erythema and desquamation; if this occurs patients may be able to tolerate alternate night applications. Tolerance to the irritation usually appears with continued use. Occasionally an initial acne flare may occur with the use of topical retinoids; this is not, however, an indication to stop treatment as it usually heralds accelerated resolution of the acne.

Topical antibiotics are effective through their bactericidal activity against *P. acnes* and consequent anti-inflammatory effects. The most commonly prescribed antibiotics include erythromycin and clindamycin either alone or in combination with other agents such as zinc or benzoyl peroxide. Preparations are usually applied twice daily. Antibiotic resistance has been reported more commonly with antibiotics used alone than in combination.

Phototherapy with ultraviolet or visible light is an alternative therapy that may be helpful in those unresponsive to or unable to tolerate conventional treatments.

Systemic treatments

Hormone therapies. These include certain types of oral contraceptive pill (OCP) that increase sex hormone-binding globulin and consequently reduce free testosterone levels. These generally are OCPs that have higher oestrogen and lower androgen potential (such as Yasmin®). *Antiandrogen* treatment alone can be teratogenic and therefore is given women in the form of a contraceptive which contains cyproterone acetate with ethinyloestradiol (Dianette®). Long-term safety data are available up to 5 years. Dianette® may also help to diminish mild hirsutism.

Oral antibiotics. Tetracyclines remain the mainstay of treatment in those over the age of 12 years (below this age they may cause dental hypoplasia and staining of teeth). Once-daily preparations (lymecycline, minocycline (MR)) are more convenient to use than twice-daily preparations (tetracycline, doxycycline, oxytetracycline) and are equally well tolerated. Tetracyclines should be avoided in pregnancy and breastfeeding. Erythromycin and trimethoprim are alternatives. Treatment benefits may not be seen for the first 6–8 weeks of therapy. An adequate treatment course should last approximately 6–12 months depending on severity and response.

Oral retinoids. Isotretinoin has revolutionized the treatment of severe acne, but it is usually reserved for resistant disease unresponsive to other oral therapies. This is because of its side-effect profile including teratogenesis (90% risk of birth defects) and its ability to cause a rise in liver enzymes and lipids. Blood testing before initiation is essential and during therapy as indicated clinically. Female patients of child-bearing age will need to use a robust form of contraception whilst taking isotretinoin and for 1 month following its cessation. Pregnancy testing is usually undertaken before release of prescriptions for females.

All patients will experience some drying of the lips and skin and it is this side-effect that may limit the dose of isotretinoin tolerated, at least initially. Mood change and depression has been suggested as a possible side-effect of isotretinoin and consequently some practitioners preclude its use in those with a history of mental illness. All patients and their carers should be warned that there is a potential risk of mood swings and depression and to stop the medication immediately if they experience problems. A modern approach to isotretinoin dosing is to begin patients on a low dose for the first 1–2 months (20–40 mg daily) and then increase to 1 mg/kg/day to minimize initial xerosis. The cumulative target dosage for isotretinoin is 120–150 mg/kg based on studies showing that acne is likely to be 'cured' if a full treatment course is taken.

Residual lesions, keloid scars, cysts and persistent nodules can be treated by injection with triamcinolone, topical retinoids, chemical dermabrasion, carbon dioxide laser resurfacing and collagen injections. For severe atrophic 'ice-pick' scarring punch biopsies can be used to remove scars from the face and pinch grafts applied to the areas (harvested from behind the ear). When healing is

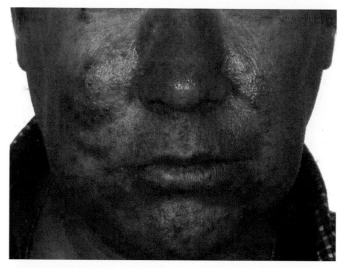

Figure 12.15 Rosacea.

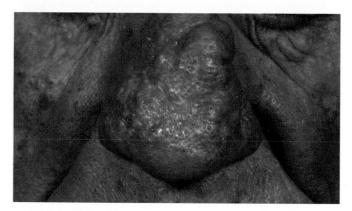

Figure 12.16 Rhinophyma.

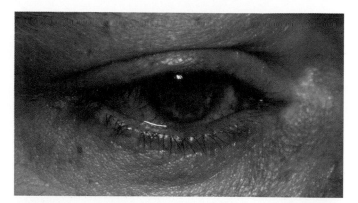

Figure 12.17 Blepharitis.

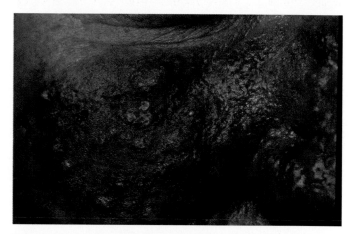

Figure 12.18 Rosacea.

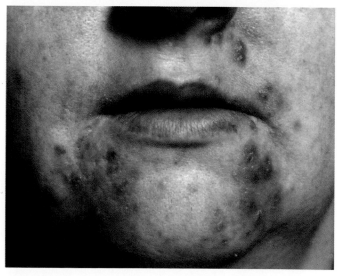

Figure 12.19 Perioral dermatitis on treatment with cyproterone acetate.

complete dermabrasion can then be used for resurfacing with good cosmetic results.

Rosacea

Rosacea is characterized by facial flushing, persistent erythema, telangiectasia, inflammatory papules, pustules and oedema (Figure 12.15). In some individuals with chronic rosacea the nasal skin can become coarse in texture eventually resulting in gross thickening and hypertrophy – known as rhinophyma (Figure 12.16) (from the Greek, 'rhis' nose, 'phyma' growth). Conjunctivitis, blepharitis (Figure 12.17) and eyelid oedema may be associated. Facial flushing and erythema is frequently exacerbated by heat, exercise, hot food/drinks, spicy food, emotion, alcohol and sunlight (Figure 12.18). Eventually facial erythema can become permanent due to multiple dilated blood vessels – telangiectasia.

Differential diagnosis of rosacea

- Acne, in which there are comedones, a wider distribution and improvement with sunlight. (Acne may however coexist with rosacea – hence the older term 'acne rosacea'.)
- Seborrhoeic eczema, in which there are no pustules and eczematous changes are present. (However an overlap syndrome is now recognized.)
- Lupus erythematosus, which shows light sensitivity, erythema and scarring, but no pustules.
- Perioral dermatitis, which occurs in women with pustules and erythema around the mouth and chin (Figure 12.19). This

may be precipitated by the use of potent topical steroids; some patients experience a premenstrual exacerbation. Treatment is to stop the topical steroids and prescribe oral tetracyclines.

Management

Trigger factors should be identified and ideally avoided. All patients should be encouraged to avoid using skin irritants such as soaps or astringent cleansers. There is evidence that regular use of a broad-spectrum sunscreen can be helpful.

Topical metronidazole can be helpful in the treatment of mild disease; however benefits may not be apparent for several months. Gel and cream formulations of metronidazole 0.75–1% should be used twice daily to the affected skin. Fifteen per cent azelaic acid in a gel formulation is now also available for the treatment of rosacea. Topical preparations seem to be more effective at treating the papules and pustules than the erythema and flushing.

Oral antibiotics including tetracycline, doxycycline, erythromycin and minocycline have all been used to effectively treat rosacea. Patients should be warned that there may be no visible clinical improvement for several weeks and treatment courses may need to continue for many months.

The use of low-dose oral isotretinoin has been shown to be effective in those with refractory disease.

Laser ablation of dilated telangiectatic vessels can be undertaken once the inflammatory component has been treated. Carbon dioxide laser or shave removal of excess skin from the nose can significantly improve the appearance of rhinophyma.

Further reading

Cunliffe WJ, Strauss J, Gollnick H, Lucky AW. *Acne Diagnosis and Management.* Taylor and Francis Ltd, Oxford, 2001.
www.bad.org.uk/public/leaflets/rosacea.asp

Bacterial Infections

Introduction

The barrier function of normal skin is highly effective at protecting against invading bacteria. Many micro-organisms come into contact with the skin and many live there as part of the normal skin flora, but they rarely cause disease. Normal skin flora consists of coagulase-negative *Staphylococcus*, *Corynebacterium*, diphtheroids and α-haemolytic *Streptococci* in the epidermis, and *Propionibacterium* in the hair follicles. Normal flora competes with invading pathogenic micro-organisms thereby acting as a 'biological shield'. However, cutaneous bacterial infection from normal flora may result from a weakness in the skin's barrier function (such as a dermatological disease) or a change in the micro-environment which allows the bacteria to become more pathogenic.

Bacterial skin infections may be acquired from the external environment (from plants, soil, fomites, animals or other humans) by implantation, direct contact, aerosols or water-borne transmission.

Bacteria most frequently invade a break in the skin, follicular openings and mucous membranes where host barriers are more vulnerable.

Bacterial skin infections vary from the very minor to life-threatening and overwhelming. It is often tempting to assume a single organism is responsible for any particular cutaneous infection (Occams's razor – the philosophy of assuming the minimum number of factors are involved as possible), but often the contrary is true. Synergistic microbial invasion is frequently present in cutaneous wounds. See Table 13.1 for a summary of the common patterns of bacterial infection in the skin.

Clinical presentation

Patients with a bacterial skin infection may recall an episode of trauma to the skin such as a graze, laceration, insect bite or implantation of foreign material, or they may have a history of ongoing skin disease. A more detailed history may reveal contact with potentially contaminated water via bathing, animal contact, travel abroad, or other family members/close contacts who are similarly affected. However, many patients will not have any obvious source from the history alone.

Acute bacterial infections in the skin generally produce some or all of the classical characteristics of acute inflammation: erythema, swelling/oedema, heat/warmth and pain/discomfort. Patients may develop systemic symptoms such as fever and malaise. Many cutaneous infections start as an isolated lesion that then spreads to involve the surrounding previously uninvolved skin. Multiple lesions may be present in a follicular distribution.

Bacterial investigations

Taking bacterial swabs for microscopy and culture can be very useful in managing patients with probable cutaneous infections. In addition nasal swabs may help to detect those who are *Staphylococcus* carriers who may suffer from recurrent infections if they have a widespread inflammatory skin condition such as eczema. Swabs should be moistened in the transport media before contact with the skin and each surface of the swab should be rotated on the infected skin surface. These manoeuvres will increase the 'pick-up' of micro-organisms. Culture results often report the sensitivities and resistance patterns of the organisms isolated which can help

ABC of Dermatology, 5th edition. Edited by P. K. Buxton and R. Morris-Jones.
© 2009 Blackwell Publishing, ISBN: 978-1-4051-7065-9.

Table 13.1 Common patterns of bacterial infection in the skin.

Infection	Clinical photograph	Clinical presentation	Organisms	Management
Infected eczema		Child with atopic eczema which has flared and is not responding to usual treatments. Marked inflammation, crusting exudate and scratching	*Staphylococcus aureus* *Streptococcus pyogenes*	Antiseptic wash/cream Topical antibiotic/steroid combination cream for maximum 2 weeks Oral flucloxacillin or erythromycin
Impetigo		Children are mainly affected, especially on the face and limbs. Highly contagious. Background erythema with yellow crusting and exudate	*S. aureus* *S. pyogenes*	Antiseptic wash/cream Topical fusidic acid, mupirocin, or polymyxin Oral flucloxacillin or erythromycin
Bullous impetigo		Children and adults. Face, limbs and flexures affected. Erythema with bullae which rupture leaving superficial crusts	*S. aureus* with exfoliative toxins A/B (may become generalized – staphylococcal scalded skin syndrome)	Oral flucloxacillin or erythromycin
Boils (furuncles)		Tender, inflamed pustules or nodules at the hair follicle that may coalesce to form a carbuncle. Heal with scarring	*S. aureus*	Antiseptic wash/cream Oral flucloxacillin or erythromycin
Bacterial folliculitis		Hair-bearing skin sites particularly the legs, beard area and scalp. Adults and children affected. In recurrent infections look for Staph. nasal carriage	*S. aureus* *Pseudomonas aeruginosa* (differential diagnosis *Malassezia* spp)	Topical fusidic acid or mupirocin (acetic acid cream EarCalm® for *P. aeruginosa*) Oral flucloxacillin or erythromycin
Ecthyma		Children, the elderly/debilitated. Mainly on the legs. Initially small bullae that form adherent crusts with underlying ulceration. Heal slowly with scarring	*S. pyogenes* *S. aureus*	Antiseptic wash/cream Oral penicillin V or erythromycin
Erysipelas		Face or lower leg. Portal of entry is broken skin. Well-demarcated bright erythema	*S. pyogenes* (group A *Strep.* but also B, C, G) *S. aureus* (less common)	Intravenous benzyl penicillin or erythromycin

to guide therapy There is an increasing incidence of antibiotic resistant bacteria in the community as well as in the hospital setting. Skin biopsies may also be sent in sterile saline for microbiological analyses including culture and PCR.

General approach to management

The treatment approach depends on the extent and the severity of the cutaneous infection.

Antiseptic skin washes or creams containing chlorhexidine hydrochloride can be helpful in removing superficial bacteria, and many of the novel formulations are suitable to use in patients with sensitive skin such as atopic eczema. Potassium permanganate soaks can be very effective at treating any cutaneous infections, particularly on the lower legs which may be submersed in a solution. The skin should be washed daily whenever possible to remove adherent infected crusts.

Topical antibiotics applied twice daily can be used alone to treat mild localized infections. Fusidic acid, mupirocin, neomycin, polymyxins, retapamulin, silver sulphadiazine and metronidazole are all available in topical formulations. Topical antibiotics should not be used over large areas of skin as systemic toxicity may result. As a general rule any course of topical antibiotic should be limited to a maximum of 2 weeks, as prolonged exposure is more likely to select for resistant organisms. In addition patients may develop allergies to topical antibiotics particularly neomycin which may result in contact dermatitis.

Topical antibiotic/steroid combinations may be used to treat infection and inflammation simultaneously.

Systemic antibiotics may be needed for more extensive cutaneous bacterial infections.

Staphylococcal cover is provided by flucloxacillin, erythromycin, co-fluampicil (contains flucloxacillin and ampicillin), co-amoxiclav, clindamycin, fusidic acid, azithromycin, ciprofloxacin, cefuroxime, dicloxacillin, cloxacillin, linezolid, pristinamycin, roxithromycin. For methicillin-resistant *Staphylococcus aureus* (MRSA) use vancomycin, nafcillin, daptomycin, tigecycline.

Streptococcal cover is provided by penicillin V, amoxicillin, flucloxacillin, erythromycin, clarithromycin, azithromycin, co-amoxiclav, cefuroxime, ceftazidime, clindamycin, pristinamycin, roxithromycin, vancomycin and levofloxacin.

Superficial infections

Impetigo is usually caused by *Staphylococcus aureus* or *Streptococcus pyogenes*. Impetigo is highly contagious between close contacts and develops rapidly into clusters of pustules and vesicles which break down into the classic golden crusts (Figure 13.1). Bullous lesions are more likely to occur with *Staphylococcal* infections which produce epidermolytic toxins A/B. *Streptococcus* is more likely to be

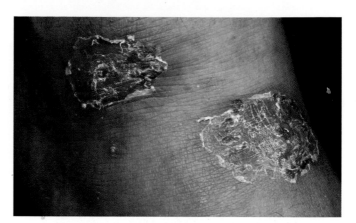

Figure 13.1 Impetigo.

the causative organism if there is associated regional lymphadenopathy, but many patients will have a mixed infection. Several family members may be affected simultaneously particularly in conditions of poor hygiene in hot humid climates. There may be an association with minor trauma such as insect bites. Secondary impetigo may co-exist with any pre-existing skin lesion. Topical treatment includes antiseptic washes, fusidic acid, mupirocin, and polymyxins. Oral antibiotics most frequently used include flucloxacillin and erythromycin.

Bacterial folliculitis is defined as infection in the hair follicles which may be superficial and/or deep and is usually caused by *S. aureus*. The majority of those affected by folliculitis never seek medical advice as these infections are frequently mild and self-limiting. Clinically there is a pustule and erythema around the follicular orifice which may be associated with mild irritation (Figure 13.2). Folliculitis may result from minor trauma such as hair removal by shaving or waxing.

Deeper follicular infections are characterized by abscess formation (which is termed sycosis barbae in the beard area), boils (Figure 13.3) and furunculosis. When several furuncles coalesce they form a carbuncle.

Hot-tub folliculitis caused by *Pseudomonas aeruginosa* appears within 2 days of exposure to contaminated water or water accessories (such as loofahs and wet-suits).

Pseudofolliculitis has a similar clinical appearance but this is caused by occlusion of the follicular openings by heavy emollients rather than bacterial infection. In pseudofolliculitis the lesions are all at the same stage of development and are clinically very monomorphic, and the pustules are sterile (Figure 13.4). *Pseudofolliculitis barbae* in the beard area has a similar clinical appearance but is in fact a perifolliculitis. Coarse curly hair punctures the skin adjacent to the hair follicle (from which it has arisen) resulting in a foreign body reaction with inflammation which can become chronic and lead to scarring.

In the occipital area of the scalp *acne keloidalis nuchae* results from folliculitis and perifolliculitis with resultant alopecia and keloid scarring from chronic inflammation. A similar appearance

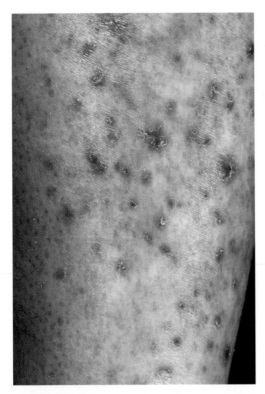

Figure 13.2 Bacterial folliculitis.

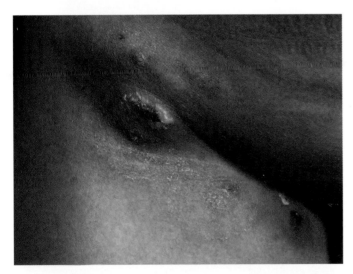

Figure 13.3 Boils.

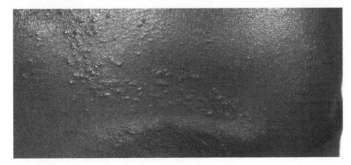

Figure 13.4 Pseudofolliculitis: forehead.

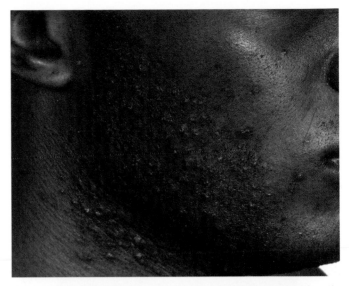

Figure 13.5 Acne keloidalis.

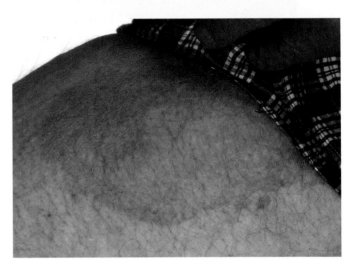

Figure 13.6 Erythrasma.

is seen in the beard area (Figure 13.5). The cause is unknown but it occurs almost exclusively in black males who shave their hair very short.

Erythrasma usually affects the flexural skin sites, particularly the axilla and groin. There is superficial scaling and mild inflammation often with a reddish-brown discolouration (Figure 13.6). It is frequently mistaken for a fungal infection so isolation of the causative bacterium *Corynebacterium minutissimum* from skin scraping can be useful. Under Wood's ultraviolet light the affected skin (bacteria) fluoresces pink. First-line treatment is usually oral erythromycin (250 mg QDS for 7–14 days), but if topical treatment is preferred then clotrimazole, miconazole, fusidic acid or neomycin can be effective.

Deeper infections

Erysipelas is caused by a *Streptococcus* infection. Over approximately 48 hours the inflammation spreads across the skin

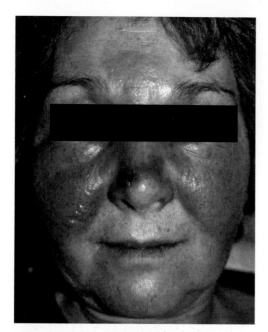

Figure 13.7 Erysipelas.

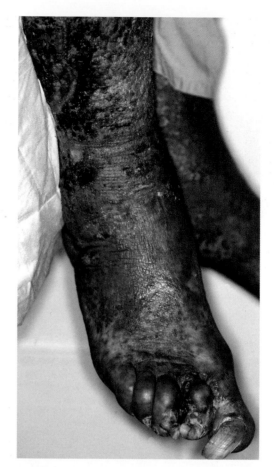

Figure 13.8 Cellulitis.

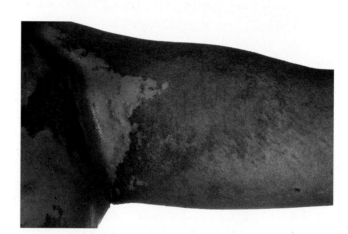

Figure 13.9 *Staphylococcus* scalded skin syndrome.

with a characteristic red, shiny, raised, spreading plaque with a well-demarcated edge (Figure 13.7). Occasionally blistering may occur at the active edge; patients may have fever and malaise. The face (*S. pyogenes* from throat colonization) and lower legs are most frequently affected. Differential diagnosis of erysipelas on the face includes contact dermatitis, photodermatitis, rosacea, systemic lupus erythematosus and fifth disease or 'slapped cheek', which is transient.

The *Streptococcus* organisms invade the dermis and penetrate the lymphatics, which gives the contrasting clinical appearance from cellulitis (infection in the deeper layers) which is poorly demarcated. There may be a minor skin laceration or tinea pedis (look between the toes) as the portal of entry. If the infection is severe treat with intravenous benzylpenicillin or orally with amoxicillin, roxithromycin or pristinamycin for 1–2 weeks. Recurrent attacks are reported in 20% of patients with predisposing conditions; these individuals may require long-term secondary prophylaxis.

Erysipelas is the local manifestation of a group A streptococcal infection; however the same organism through the production of toxins or superantigens can cause other skin lesions such as: (a) the rash of scarlet fever; (b) erythema nodosum; (c) guttate psoriasis; and (d) an acute generalized vasculitis.

Cellulitis develops more slowly than erysipelas and has a poorly-defined margin and marked regional lymphadenopathy. Patients may have a fever and general malaise. In cellulitis *S. pyogenes* (also groups C/G β-haemolytic *Streptococcus*, or rarely *Staphylococcus aureus*) organisms invade deeper tissues than those found in erysipelas. The lower leg is the most common site affected (Figure 13.8). Patients may have underlying dermatoses such as a diabetic foot ulcer, tinea pedis or stasis dermatitis which act as a portal of entry for the streptococcal bacteria. In severe infections intravenous benzylpenicillin may be needed for up to a week as the infection settles slowly.

Staphylococcus scalded skin syndrome (SSSS) is caused by strains of *S. aureus* that produce exfoliative toxins A/B resulting in intraepidermal splitting (the target is desmoglein 1 which is responsible for keratinocyte adhesion). A localized form of the disease is called bullous impetigo. The clinical presentation is usually a child below 5 years of age with conjunctivitis, otitis media or a nasopharyngeal infection with fever, malaise and red tender skin. Generalized cutaneous erythema is followed by widespread superficial blistering (Nikolsky sign positive) and exfoliation which may be most striking in the flexures (Figure 13.9). Although most children are

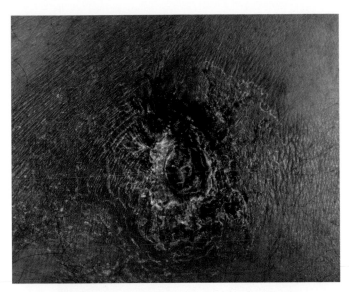

Figure 13.10 Ecthyma.

not unwell there is a 4% mortality rate. Give systemic antibiotics to treat *Staphylococcus*. If patients fail to respond then consider treating for MRSA which has a higher mortality rate.

Ecthyma is often referred to as a deeper form of impetigo as the group A β-haemolytic streptococci (*S. pyogenes*) invade the dermis leading to superficial ulcers. Lesions start as small pustules that have adherent crust and underlying ulceration, and most commonly occur on the lower legs of children and elderly people who live in humid climates. Lesions usually heal slowly with scarring (Figure 13.10).

Mycobacterial disease

Clinical manifestations of mycobacterial infections are largely determined by the ability of the host to mount an immune response. Disease spectrums therefore range from dissemination to mild localized lesions; for example *Mycobacterium tuberculosis* may present with miliary TB or lupus vulgaris, and *Mycobacterium leprae* may present with lepromatous or more tuberculoid phenotypes (see Chapter 18).

Cutaneous *Mycobacterium tuberculosis* (TB) is rare even in endemic areas. TB in the skin usually occurs as a secondary manifestation of disease with its primary focus in the respiratory tract. The most common manifestation is lupus vulgaris which usually presents on the head and neck. Lesions appear as slowly growing well-demarcated red-brown papules that coalesce to form indolent plaques of a gelatinous nature: so-called 'apple-jelly nodules' (Figure 13.11). A number of mechanisms are thought to cause clinical lupus vulgaris, including spread of TB to the skin from lymphatics or blood, and direct extension of TB from underlying tissues, from primary cutaneous inoculation or secondary to BCG vaccination.

Allergic-type hypersensitivity reactions called tuberculids can occur in the skin of patients with underlying TB. Tuberculids are thought to represent hypersensitivity reactions to antigenic

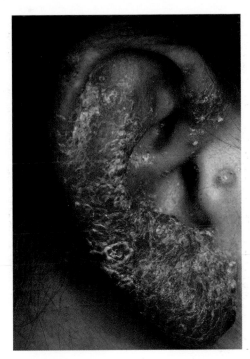

Figure 13.11 Lupus vulgaris.

fragments of dead bacilli deposited in the skin via haematogenous spread. Recent studies have demonstrated TB DNA in the affected skin in 25–75% of cases. Tuberculids include erythema induratum (Bazin's disease) where patients present with tender nodules and plaques that ulcerate and heal with scarring on the lower legs. Papulonecrotic tuberculid (which some authors believe to be a more superficial form of Bazin's disease) (Figure 13.12) and lichen scrofulosorum (very small lichenoid papules over the trunk and limbs in young patients) are also seen.

Atypical mycobacteria (ATM) are often found in the environment in vegetation and water. Immunocompromised patients are most frequently affected or those with underlying systemic diseases such as diabetes, chronic renal failure, connective tissue disease and malignancy. Traumatic implantation of ATM into the skin may cause the initial inoculation.

Mycobacterium marinum or 'fish tank' or 'swimming pool granuloma' usually occurs due to contact with infected tropical fish or contaminated water. The hand or fingers are most frequently affected; initially a single warty nodular lesion appears with subsequent sporotricoid spread along local lymphatics forming a chain of nodules (Figure 13.13).

Injection abscesses may be caused by mycobacteria such as *M. chelonei*. Buruli ulcer, an extensive ulcerating condition due to *M. ulcerans*, is confined to the tropics.

Other infections

Bacillary angiomatosis caused by *Bartonella henselae and B. quintana* infections (previously known as *Rochalimea*) presents

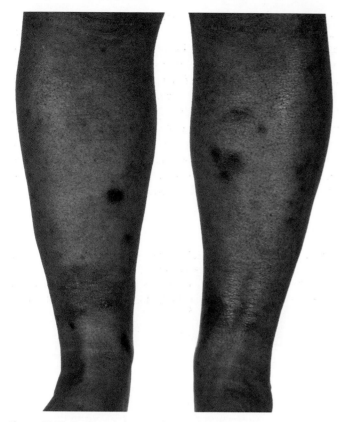

Figure 13.12 Erythema induratum (Bazin's disease).

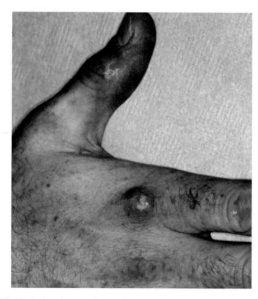

Figure 13.13 Swimming pool granuloma.

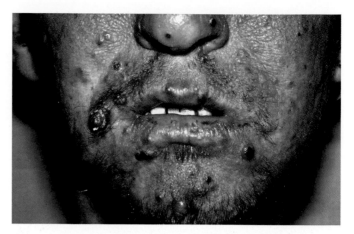

Figure 13.14 Bacillary angiomatosis.

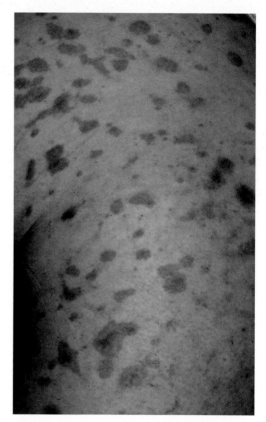

Figure 13.15 Rocky mountain spotted fever.

in AIDS patients with small haemangioma-like papules. Clinical manifestations are most commonly seen in the skin and mucous membranes, but underlying visceral disease (especially liver) may occur simultaneously. Patients usually present with multiple small cherry-like haemangiomas on the skin which appear over weeks to months (Figure 13.14). Erythromycin 500 mg qds for up to 12 weeks is recommended.

Cat-scratch disease is caused by the bacterium *Bartonella hense-lae.* Crusted nodules appear within 3–12 days at the site of a scratch (usually by a kitten) associated with the development of regional painful lymphadenopathy 1 or 2 months later. The disease usually undergoes spontaneous remission within 2–4 months. A 5-day course of azithromycin can speed recovery.

Rickettsial organisms are a diverse group of slow-growing small Gram-negative bacteria that are mainly transmitted by ticks and mites. Rocky Mountain spotted fever (RMSF) is one of the most common rickettsial infections (*Rickettsia rickettsii*) in the USA and has a 4% mortality rate. The most common vector of RMSF

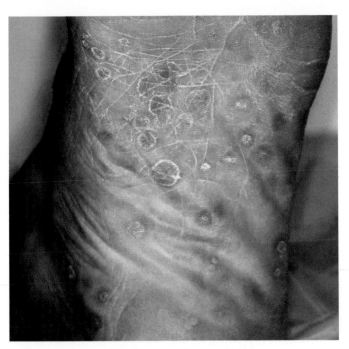

Figure 13.16 Secondary syphilis.

is the dog tick. Within a week of the bite patients present with high fever, headache, myalgia and a petechial rash which characteristically appears on the palms and soles but may spread to the trunk (Figure 13.15). Treat with doxycycline 100 mg twice daily for approximately 1 week.

Syphilis has been termed the 'great impostor' due to its wide range of clinical presentations. It is caused by the spirochete bacterium *Treponema pallidum* which is transmitted through sexual intercourse, by transplacental spread and via unscreened blood transfusions. The incidence of syphilis is steadily increasing due to co-infection with human immunodeficiency virus (HIV) (see Chapter 15 for more details). Primary syphilis manifests as a painless genital ulcer at the site of inoculation. Cutaneous manifestations of secondary syphilis are characterized by a widespread eruption of red-brown scaly macules that affects the trunk and limbs (particularly palms and soles) (Figure 13.16). In patients with AIDS the rash may be florid with marked crusting.

Further reading

Seal DV, Hay RJ, Middleton KR. *Skin and Wound Infection. Investigation and Treatment in Practice.* Blackwell Publishing, Oxford, 2000.

Tan JS, File TM. *Contemporary Diagnosis and Management of Skin and Soft Tissue Infections*, 1st edn. Handbooks in Health Care Company, New York, 2002.

CHAPTER 14

Viral Infections

OVERVIEW

- Because they are intracellular organisms viruses are able to make important changes in cellular function, including alteration in immune response.

- As well as modifying genetic material of the host cell, the viral genome itself undergoes both sudden and gradual change.

- RNA viruses are unstable, undergoing multiple mutations and causing systemic disease whereas DNA viruses are more stable and cause local infections.

- Herpes simplex infections are acquired by local contact: type I affect the mouth and face, type II affect the genitalia.

- Herpes zoster (shingles) is due to reactivation of previously acquired varicella zoster virus (chicken pox).

- The poxviruses are DNA viruses that affect the skin, the most common being molluscum contagiosum.

- Viral warts are due to the human papilloma virus. There are many types, of which 16 and 18 are capable of causing malignant change.

- The majority of viral diseases with rashes are caused by RNA viruses associated with systemic disease of which measles is the most important.

- Specific antiviral vaccines and drugs are increasingly available.

Introduction

The term *virus* comes from the Latin meaning poison or toxin. Most modern medical practitioners think of viruses as micro-organisms rather than toxins, but some experts argue that viruses are not living organisms as they do not fulfil all the necessary criteria. Viruses do not have cell structures and they require host cells to replicate and synthesize new products. This spontaneous self-assembly within the host cells has been likened to the autonomous growth of crystals. Viral self-assembly has also been used to strengthen the hypothesis that the 'origins of life' started from self-assembling organic molecules. Nonetheless, viruses do possess genes, cause disease, trigger immune responses and evolve through

natural selection, so from a practitioner's point of view living or otherwise they have an enormous impact on human health.

The inability of viruses to grow or replicate outside the host cell means they have become masters at persistence within the host. Viruses persist within the host cell because they are often able to replicate without killing the host cells, their gene expression can be restricted, they can mimic host molecules, down-regulate host immunity and directly infect the host's immune cells. Viruses continuously change, either gradually (called 'drift') where they accumulate minor mutations, or suddenly (called 'shift') following major changes during recombination of the viral genome.

RNA viruses such as measles and human immunodeficiency virus (HIV) are unstable, undergoing immense drift and shift with up to 2% of their genome altered each year through multiple mutations. These viruses tend to cause systemic disease in humans leading to generalized cutaneous eruptions such as a 'viral exanthem'. In contrast, DNA viruses such as human papillomavirus (HPV), molluscum contagiosum, herpes simplex virus (HSV), and varicella zoster virus (VZV) are more stable. They are frequently inoculated directly into the skin and replicate in epidermal cells.

Viruses can be transmitted by direct contact skin to skin, through aerosols and via the faecal–oral route. Once inside the host viruses can spread directly from cell to cell, via the blood, or central nervous system by axonal transport. Many viruses demonstrate tropism (in other words a predilection for a certain host cell) via virus attachment protein-specific cell surface receptors. HPV, for example, has tropism for keratinocytes.

The behaviour of different viruses therefore determines the type of disease they cause with resultant either localized or widespread reactive skin disorders. Common viral infections of the skin are usually easily identified by pattern recognition through the characteristic skin or mucous membrane site affected and/or typical lesions.

Herpesviruses

Herpes simplex

Herpes simplex virus (HSV) is spread by direct contact 'shedding' from one host to another. Two viral subtypes exist: type I is associated mainly with facial lesions although the fingers (Figure 14.1) and genitals may be affected. Type II is associated almost entirely with genital infections. HSV remains within the host for life, remaining

ABC of Dermatology, 5th edition. Edited by P. K. Buxton and R. Morris-Jones.
© 2009 Blackwell Publishing, ISBN: 978-1-4051-7065-9.

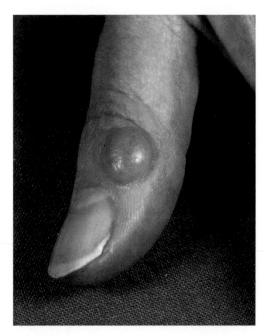

Figure 14.1 Inoculation herpes.

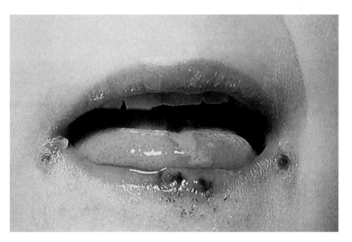

Figure 14.2 Herpes of lips.

Box 14.1 **Herpes simplex – points to note**

- Genital vesicles may not be visualized as they rapidly ulcerate
- Prodrome of itching and tenderness
- Rapid viral detection from scraping the vesicle/ulcer base using electron microscopy, immunofluorescence or PCR
- Genital herpes in pregnancy carries a risk of ophthalmic infection of the infant. Caesarean section may be indicated
- 'Eczema herpeticum' occurs in patients with atopic eczema and can cause severe systemic illness (Figure 14.4). HSV disseminates on the abnormal skin. Treat with oral or parenteral aciclovir.

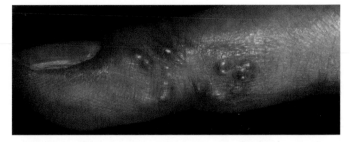

Figure 14.3 Herpes simplex vesicles on finger.

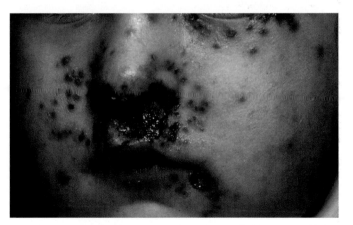

Figure 14.4 Eczema herpeticum.

latent in the sensory nerve ganglia, and therefore reactivation can frequently occur.

Primary herpes simplex (type I) infection usually occurs in or around the mouth, with variable involvement of the face (Figure 14.2). Lesions are small vesicles (Figure 14.3) which crust over and heal but there may be considerable malaise and regional lymphadenopathy. HSV type II infects the external genitalia; the initial vesicle or vesicles rapidly break down into painful ulcers (Box 14.1).

Episodes of reactivation of HSV may be triggered by the cold ('cold sore'), bright sunlight, trauma, immunosuppression or intercurrent illnesses. There is frequently a prodrome of tingling or itching before the appearance of the vesicles, which occur in the distribution of a sensory nerve.

Topical aciclovir/penciclovir/idoxuridine cream can be used to treat mild labial herpes. Severe infections should be treated with oral aciclovir 200–400 mg 5 times daily for 5 days. Secondary prophylaxis for frequent reactivation can be given as 400 mg once or twice daily. Higher doses are needed in immunocompromised patients. Valaciclovir (HSV 500 mg twice daily for 5 days, VZV 1g three times daily for 7 days) and famciclovir (genital HSV 250 mg three times daily for 7 days, VZV 750 mg daily for 7 days) are alternatives that are taken less frequently.

Herpes zoster (shingles)

Varicella zoster virus (VZV) causes chicken pox (the primary illness) and subsequently herpes zoster (reactivation) as the virus remains latent in the sensory nerve ganglia (Box 14.2). The thoracic nerves are most commonly affected. In herpes zoster, pain, fever, and malaise may precede the rash which is characterized by its dermatomal distribution (Figure 14.5). Erythematous papules usually precede vesicles which develop over several days, crusting as they resolve. Secondary bacterial infection is common. Some patients develop severe chronic pain in the affected area – postherpetic

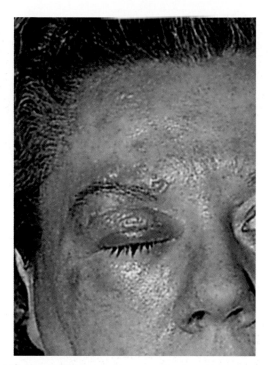

Figure 14.6 Ophthalmic zoster.

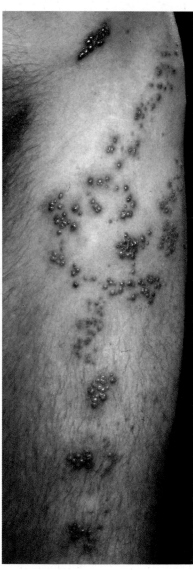

Figure 14.5 Herpes zoster.

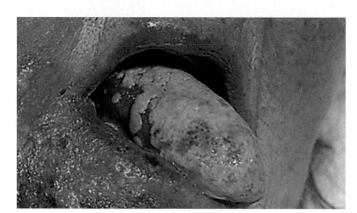

Figure 14.7 Mandibular nerve zoster.

aciclovir (5 mg/kg every 8 hours for 5 days) should be considered and patients may require systemic steroids (prednisolone 40–60 mg daily) to prevent nerve paralysis in severe cases. The skin should be treated directly regularly with emollients (white soft paraffin/liquid paraffin) to prevent cracking and reduce pain from healing lesions. Topical antibiotic ointments can be used to treat secondary bacterial infections (mupirocin, fusidic acid, polymyxin).

Poxviruses

The poxviruses are large DNA viruses, with a predilection for the epidermis. Variola (smallpox), once a disease with high mortality, has been eliminated (last reported case of smallpox occurred in Somalia in 1977) by vaccination with modified vaccinia (cowpox) virus. Vaccination of the general population is no longer required due to the eradication of the virus, but some military and front-line

neuralgia. Skin lesions of herpes zoster and nasopharyngeal secretions can transmit chicken pox.

Patients ideally should receive high-dose aciclovir (800 mg 5 times daily for 7 days) within 72 hours of the onset of the eruption. If the eye is affected or there is nerve compression then intravenous

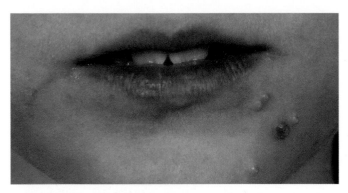

Figure 14.8 Molluscum contagiosum.

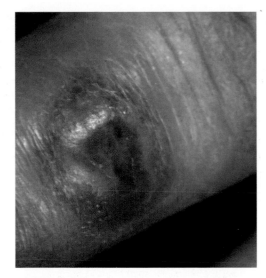

Figure 14.10 Milker's nodule.

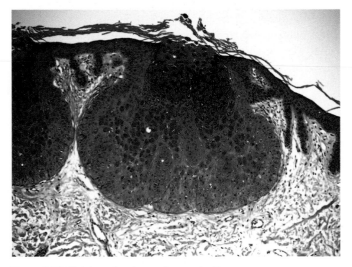

Figure 14.9 Histology showing molluscum bodies.

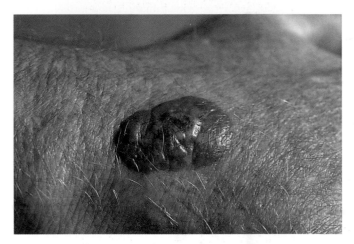

Figure 14.11 Orf.

medical personnel are being vaccinated due to the theoretical threat of biological attack with smallpox.

Molluscum contagiosum

The commonest skin infection due to a poxvirus is molluscum contagiosum, a skin infection usually acquired in childhood. It is spread by direct contact often within families or schools. The incubation period is variable, between 14 days and 6 months. In adults florid molluscum may be an indication of underlying immunodeficiency such as HIV.

The white, umbilicated papules of molluscum contagiosum are characteristic (Figures 14.8 & 14.9). Lesions often itch, particularly in patients with atopy, and may become secondarily infected. Large solitary lesions (giant mollusca) and infected lesions may look atypical. Resolving lesions may be surrounded by a small patch of inflammation.

Parents are often keen for their children with molluscum to be treated. However, most lesions will resolve spontaneously leaving no marks on the skin. Therefore painful treatments that may cause scarring should be actively avoided in children. An antibiotic–hydrocortisone ointment can be used to treat secondary infection/inflammation. More recently topical hydrogen peroxide (Crystacide) has been shown to speed resolution. Cryotherapy can be used to speed resolution but this is often painful and may cause

pigmentary changes or scarring. Other methods include superficial curettage, rotating a sharpened orange stick moistened with phenol in the centre of each lesion and painting on hydrogen peroxide. Gently squeezing a molluscum lesion expels thick white material that can also speed resolution.

Other poxvirus infections

Cowpox only sporadically infects cows from its natural reservoir, probably small mammals, and may affect humans. Papules on the hands enlarge and develop necrosis and crusting.

Milker's nodules are due to a virus that causes superficial ulcers in cows' udders and calves' mouths. In humans papules form on the hands and develop into grey nodules with a necrotic centre, surrounding inflammation, and lymphangitis (Figure 14.10). A more generalized papular eruption can occur.

Orf is often recognized in rural areas. It is seen mainly in early spring as a result of contact with lambs. A single papule or group of lesions develops on the fingers or hands with purple papules developing into bullae (Figure 14.11). These rupture to leave annular lesions 1–3 cm in diameter with a necrotic centre and surrounding inflammation. The incubation period is a few days and the lesions last 2–3 weeks with spontaneous healing. Associated erythema multiforme and widespread rashes are occasionally seen. Lifelong immunity does not result from infections.

Wart viruses

One hundred different DNA subtypes of human papillomavirus (HPV) are currently recognized, 80 of which have undergone gene sequencing. A definite link has been demonstrated between HPV 16 and 18 and the development of carcinoma with the consequent development of a HPV vaccine. It is thought, however, that HPV infection alone does not cause malignant transformation. Identified cofactors include smoking, UV light, folate deficiency and immunosuppression. Women should have regular cervical smears.

Warts are classified as anogenital/mucosal, non-genital cutaneous and epidermodysplasia verruciformis (EV). The latter is a rare condition associated with a defect of specific immunity to wart virus. HPV infections are also described as symptomatic (latent, i.e. viral DNA detected), subclinical (detected with acetic acid under magnification) or clinical (warts easily seen).

HPV only infects humans and is spread by direct contact usually through a small break in the skin/mucous membrane. HPV can remain viable in the environment at low temperatures for prolonged periods and therefore be contracted from contact with inanimate objects. The basal keratinocytes become infected causing epidermal hyperplasia seen clinically as an exophytic warty lesion. Plane warts appear as some papules, and filiform warts have finger-like projections (Figure 14.12). Plantar warts (veruccae) form painful plaques containing black 'dots' that represent thrombosed capillaries.

Cutaneous HPV lesions can undergo malignant transformation particularly in individuals who are immunosuppressed by HIV or secondary to transplantation. If skin lesions suddenly increase in size or are painful then transformation to squamous cell carcinoma should be suspected. Acitretin is given to some transplant patients to try to reduce the rate of cutaneous malignant transformation.

Treatment

Warts commonly occur in children and resolve spontaneously without treatment or with simple topical measures. There are numerous treatment options available indicating that not all warts respond to a particular treatment. Warts are generally slow to clear but studies show 70% will resolve following 4 months of salicylic acid applied once daily. Salicylic and lactic acids in various formulations can be purchased over the counter and high percentages can be prescribed. Gels/ointments/paints/lotions should be applied daily.

Recent studies have demonstrated efficacy of duct tape (used by builders) to treat HPV: 85% of warts resolved following 2 months of treatment with duct tape (which was cut to size, applied to the wart and renewed weekly).

For large or painful warts other measures may be considered.

Liquid nitrogen is effective but has to be stored in special containers and replaced frequently. It can be applied with cotton wool or discharged from a special spray with a focused nozzle. Freezing is continued until a rim of frozen tissue forms around the wart. Cryotherapy is accompanied by a burning sensation or pain and is not usually tolerated in young children. Subsequent pigment changes, blistering and even scarring may occur. Carbon dioxide is more readily available and can be transported in cylinders that produce solid carbon dioxide 'snow'. The temperature (about –64°C) is not as low as liquid nitrogen (–196°C).

Diathermy loop cautery under local anaesthetic is effective for perianal warts. Curettage and cautery for very large warts under local anaesthetic is quick and effective but leaves scars and warts may recur.

Podophyllin derived from the Mayapple is available in various formulations including ointment (Posalfilin®) for plantar warts (daily) and solution/cream (weekly) for genital warts (Warticon®, Condyline®). Podophyllin 15% paint should only be applied to warts by a trained practitioner as it can cause chemical burns. It should not be used on large numbers of warts simultaneously because of toxicity and must never be used in pregnancy.

Immune response modifier Imiquimod® is licensed for the treatment of genital warts. It stimulates cytokine production at the site of application which is carried out 3 times per week. Treatment should continue until the warts resolve or up to a maximum of 16 weeks. Local irritation and inflammation can be severe, especially on mucosal surfaces.

Immunotherapy with the contact sensitizer diphencyprone (DPC) can also be effective. Following sensitization to DPC increasing concentrations are painted onto the warts to cause a local inflammatory response. At 6 months 60% complete cure rates are reported in patients with previously highly recalcitrant warts.

Other treatments include carbon dioxide laser vaporization, cavitron ultrasonic surgical aspiration (vibration causes tissue cavities and heating), 5-fluorouracil, intralesional bleomycin and interferon alpha.

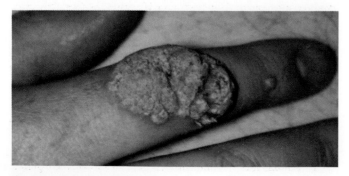

Figure 14.12 Human papillomavirus warts.

Viral diseases with rashes (Box 14.3)

Many childhood viral illnesses have become less common over the past two decades due to increased availability of effective vaccines. However, these vaccines are not universally available or accepted. Approximately 880 000 deaths from measles occur worldwide each year. Recently there has been a resurgence of measles in the UK following a decline in take-up of MMR (measles/mumps/rubella) vaccinations. Measles is probably the best-known example of a viral exanthema – a widespread reactive cutaneous eruption. (In an enanthem the mucous surfaces are affected.) All exanthems, except fifth disease (erythema infectiosum), result from RNA viruses.

Measles

Virus. Measles (Morbillivirus in the Paramyxoviridae family),

Age. Measles usually affects children under the age of 5 years.

Incubation period is 7–14 days. Measles is highly contagious. Prodromal symptoms include fever, malaise, upper respiratory symptoms, conjunctivitis and photophobia. Children are miserable and look unwell.

Initial rash. Koplik's spots (white spots with surrounding erythema) appear on the oral mucosa. After 2 days a macular rash appears, initially behind the ears and on the face and trunk, and then on the limbs (Figure 14.13).

Development and resolution. Papules form and coalesce. There may be haemorrhagic lesions and bullae which fade to leave brown patches.

Complications include encephalitis, otitis media and bronchopneumonia.

Diagnosis. Specific antibodies may be detected; they are at their maximum at 2–4 weeks.

Treatment. Vitamin A supplementation during the acute illness can reduce morbidity/mortality.

Prophylaxis. Two doses of live-attenuated MMR vaccine should be given.

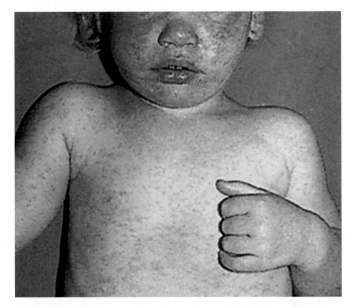

Figure 14.13 Measles.

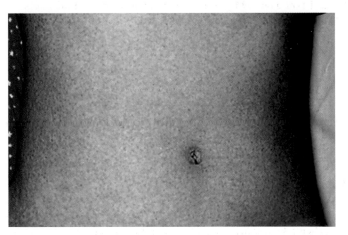

Figure 14.14 Rubella.

Rubella

Virus. Rubella (Rubivirus in the Togaviridae family).

Age. Children and young adults.

Incubation period is 14–21 days.

Prodromal symptoms. There are none in young children. Otherwise fever, malaise, and upper respiratory symptoms occur.

Initial rash. Erythema of the soft palate and lymphadenopathy. Later pink macules appear on the face, spreading to trunk and limbs over 1–2 days (Figure 14.14).

Development and resolution. The rash clears over 1–2 days (occasionally no rash develops).

Complications. Infection during pregnancy can cause congenital defects. The risk is highest in the first trimester.

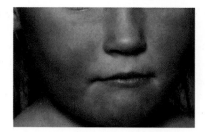

Figure 14.15 Erythema infectiosum.

Diagnosis. Usually clinical. Antibody titres can be measured during the illness and convalescence.

Prophylaxis. Active immunization is routinely available for all schoolgirls.

Erythema infectiosum (fifth disease)
Virus. Parvovirus B19.

Age. Children aged 2–10 years, mainly girls.

Incubation period is 5–20 days.

Prodromal symptoms. Possibly slight fever with the initial rash.

Initial rash. A hot erythematous eruption on the cheeks – hence the 'slapped cheek syndrome'. Over 2–4 days a maculopapular eruption develops on the limbs and trunk (Figure 14.15).

Development and resolution. The rash extends to affect hands, feet, and mucous membranes, and then fades over 1–2 weeks.

Diagnosis. Serology for parvovirus B19-specific IgM antibody.

Complications. There are no reported dermatological complications but haematological disorders such as thrombocytopenia, arthropathy and fetal abnormalities may be associated.

Roseola infantum (sixth disease)
Virus. Human herpesvirus type 6 (HHV6).

Age. Infants below 2 years of age.

Incubation period is 10–15 days.

Prodromal symptoms. Fever for a few days.

Initial rash. A rose pink maculopapular eruption appears on the neck and trunk.

Development and resolution. Rash may affect the face and limbs before clearing over 1–2 days.

Diagnosis. Clinical signs. HHV6 virus can be isolated from the blood or serology to detect antibody responses.

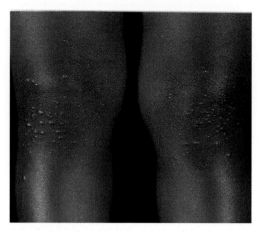

Figure 14.16 Gianotti–Crosti syndrome.

Complications include febrile convulsions.

Gianotti–Crosti syndrome
Virus. Epstein-Barr virus (EBV) and hepatitis B have been implicated.

Age. Children below 14 years of age.

Incubation period is unknown.

Prodromal symptoms. Lymphadenopathy and malaise accompany the acral eruption.

Initial rash. Red papules rapidly develop on the face, neck, limbs, buttocks, palms and soles (Figure 14.16).

Development and resolution. Over 2–6 weeks the lesions become purpuric then slowly fade.

Diagnosis. Clinical diagnosis. Serology for suspected virus.

Complications. Lymphadenopathy and hepatomegaly always occur and may persist for many months. The skin eruption can be very itchy; topical steroids can relieve symptoms.

Hand, foot and mouth disease
Virus. Coxsackievirus A.

Age. Affects both children and adults. More severe in children.

Incubation period is 3–6 days.

Prodromal symptoms. Fever, headache and malaise may accompany the rash.

Initial rash. Initially there may be intense erythema surrounding yellow-grey vesicles 1–1.5 mm in diameter (Figure 14.17). These are mainly distributed on the palms and soles and in the mouth. Sometimes a more generalized eruption may develop.

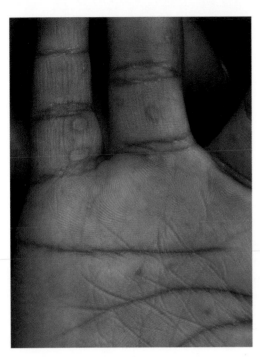

Figure 14.17 Hand, foot and mouth disease.

Development and resolution. Over 3–5 days the rash fades.

Diagnosis. Coxsackie A (usually A16) virus is isolated from lesions and stools. A specific antibody may be found in the serum.

Complications are rare but include widespread vesicular rashes and erythema multiforme.

Further reading

Seal DV, Hay RJ, Middleton KR. *Skin and Wound Infection. Investigation and Treatment in Practice.* Blackwell Publishing, Oxford, 2000.
Straus EG, Strauss JH. *Viruses and Human* Disease, 2nd edn. Academic Press, California, 2007.

HIV and the Skin

Introduction

The human immunodeficiency virus (HIV) is the cause of the acquired immune deficiency syndrome (AIDS). Worldwide 33 million children and adults are currently living with HIV according to current WHO (World Health Organization) statistics (2007).

HIV is an RNA retrovirus that replicates itself by reverse transcriptase to produce a DNA copy; this then becomes incorporated into the host DNA where further replication occurs. HIV persists in the body within the host's immune cells – the CD4 lymphocytes and monocytes, thereby directly weakening the host's immune system. HIV is transmitted by sexual contact, infected blood (transfusions, needle sharing) and transplacental spread; initially the virus remains latent for an average of 10 years before causing profound immunosuppression. The extent to which an individual's immune system is affected by HIV is measured through the CD4

cell count and their HIV viral load. AIDS is defined as a CD4 count of less than 200 cells/μL, or HIV associated with any one of 26 (mainly opportunistic infections) conditions.

Patients with low CD4 counts who are profoundly immunosuppressed tend to have more frequent and more severe skin disorders. Common cutaneous diseases such as psoriasis, eczema, seborrhoeic dermatitis and acne etc. tend to be more severe, have atypical features and are often resistant to conventional treatments. The spectrum of cutaneous manifestations in HIV has changed over the past decade due to the use of highly active antiretroviral therapy (HAART). This treatment, however, is not universally available to patients, and despite treatment for their HIV 70% of patients still suffer from HIV-related skin problems with a high incidence of drug rashes. In addition patients taking HAART can develop problems when their immune system is reconstituted – the so-called immune reconstitution inflammatory syndrome (IRIS).

In general HIV/AIDS should be considered in any patient with a florid or atypical inflammatory skin disease that is resistant to treatment or who has severe and extensive infection of the skin. Because of the atypical nature of cutaneous manifestations in HIV medical practitioners should have a low threshold for performing investigations including a skin biopsy for histology and culture (Box 15.1).

Stages of HIV

Primary HIV infection

Eighty per cent of individuals have acute signs and symptoms associated with their primary HIV infection – the so-called

Box 15.1 **HIV and the skin**

- Skin disorders affect 80% of HIV patients
- Fifty per cent develop a rash during seroconversion
- Severity of skin disorders increases with decreasing CD4 counts
- Cutaneous presentations are frequently atypical
- Consider taking a skin biopsy
- Management of skin diseases can be difficult; HAART is usually beneficial
- Patients have a high risk of developing drug rashes

ABC of Dermatology, 5th edition. Edited by P. K. Buxton and R. Morris-Jones.
© 2009 Blackwell Publishing, ISBN: 978-1-4051-7065-9.

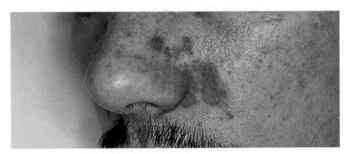

Figure 15.2 Seborrhoeic dermatitis.

Box 15.2 **Skin disorders in HIV/AIDS**

- Seborrhoeic eczema (severe)
- Psoriasis (severe)
- Fungal infections
- Bacterial infections
- Viral infections
- Kaposi's sarcoma
- Frequent drug rashes (often severe)
- Oral hairy leukoplakia

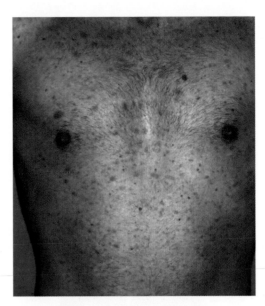

Figure 15.1 Primary HIV infection: seroconversion rash.

'seroconversion illness'. The incubation period is 2–6 weeks. Symptoms include fever, malaise, headache, nausea, vomiting and diarrhoea. Clinical signs include cervical lymphadenopathy, pharyngitis, weight loss and rash. The skin eruption associated with primary HIV infection is present in 50% of patients and consists of a maculopapular rash mainly on the face, neck and trunk lasting 2–3 weeks (Figure 15.1). Some patients develop a papulovesicular eruption or erosions in the mouth rather than a classic viral exanthem. Primary HIV seroconversion illness lasting more than 2 weeks is associated with a poorer long-term prognosis. During seroconversion abnormalities in the full blood count (FBC) may be seen (leukopenia, lymphopenia, thrombocytopenia, low haemoglobin) and diagnostically (after counselling) HIV RNA may be detected in the plasma.

Early stages

Within 1–2 months of the primary infection 50% of patients will have detectable antibodies to HIV. The proportion of CD4 lymphocytes variably decreases and this is associated with an increased frequency and severity of skin disorders. Patients may experience worsening of premorbid skin complaints or present de novo with sudden florid skin disease. Drug rashes associated with any medication are more frequent and often severe.

Late-stage HIV infection

As the patient's immune system becomes increasingly suppressed and their CD4 count falls below 200 cells/μL they are classified as having AIDS. Patients with AIDS are likely to present with severe widespread dermatoses including seborrhoeic dermatitis, crusted scabies, multidermatomal varicella zoster virus, Kaposi's sarcoma, widespread fungal/yeast infections, bacillary angiomatosis and eosinophilic folliculitis. These conditions are described in more detail below.

Skin disorders in HIV (Box 15.2)

Seborrhoeic dermatitis

Fifty per cent of HIV patients develop seborrhoeic dermatitis (SD) compared to 1–3% of the general population. SD may be one of the first indicators of HIV infection. It is interesting to note that as the immune system becomes increasingly suppressed by HIV then there is a higher incidence of allergic-type reactions. SD is an allergic contact dermatitis to the yeast *Malassezia furfur* which is a normal skin commensal. SD classically affects the scalp, eyebrows, nasal creases, moustache and anterior chest. Adherent greasy scales cover underlying inflammatory eczema which may be very itchy (Figure 15.2). Management is aimed at reducing the numbers of yeast on the skin and suppressing the eczema. Ketoconazole shampoo can be used to wash the body and scalp once/twice weekly to reduce yeast carriage. Twice-daily topical steroids (± miconazole) can be used to control the dermatitis. In refractory cases systemic imidazoles can be effective. However, if the patient's immune system reconstitutes with HAART SD usually abates.

Psoriasis

It is estimated that 5% of HIV patients develop psoriasis and of those 50% suffer from psoriatic arthropathy. The pathophysiology of psoriasis is complex; however there is a general consensus that it is a T-cell mediated autoimmune disease. The paradox in HIV is that immune dysregulation of T-cells goes hand in hand with severe, extensive and refractory psoriasis, indicating that there are likely to be other cells involved in the development of psoriasis such as Th17. Care is needed in managing patients with HIV and psoriasis as conventional immunosuppressive treatments should be avoided. Intensive topical treatment with steroid/calcipotriol formulations can be effective.

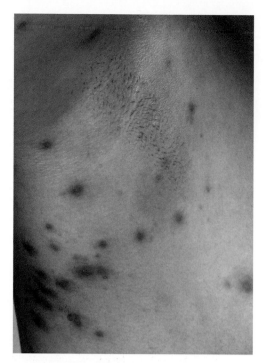

Figure 15.3 Eosinophilic folliculitis.

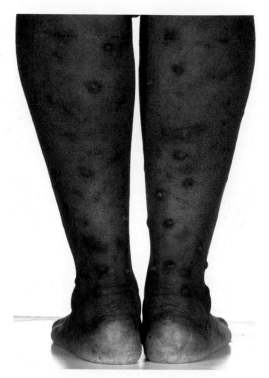

Figure 15.4 Nodular prurigo.

Eosinophilic folliculitis

Eosinophilic folliculitis (EF) is an intensely pruritic condition of unknown aetiology that tends to occur when the CD4 count falls below 250 cells/μL. Speculation that the causative agent is *Demodex*, a commensal skin mite that lives in the perifollicular region, is based on responses to antiparasitic treatments including permethrin and ivermectin. Clinically patients present with multiple discrete, erythematous, perifollicular papules and pustules affecting the face and trunk (Figure 15.3). Differential diagnoses include *Staphylococcus* or *Pityrosporum* folliculitis and acne. Microbiological swabs are negative in EF. Peripheral eosinophilia and raised IgE may be noted. HAART therapy can help if the CD4 count rises above 250 cells/μL. UVB phototherapy can be very effective. Topical corticosteroids may reduce pruritus. Systemic indomethacin, minocycline and itraconazole have also been used.

Nodular prurigo

Non-specific pruritus is common in HIV patients, 30% developing itchy nodular lesions on the skin called nodular prurigo. The cause is unknown. Classically, small red papules develop on the trunk and limbs which itch intensely and through scratching chronic nodules form (Figure 15.4). Nodular prurigo can be very aggravating and persistent. Relief from pruritus may be gained by regular applications of emollients. Potent topical steroids applied daily under occlusion of wraps or body suits may flatten lesions and relieve itching. UVB phototherapy and amitriptyline can also be used.

Infections

Fungal infections

Superficial dermatophyte and yeast infections are frequently more extensive in HIV patients with a higher incidence of dissemination

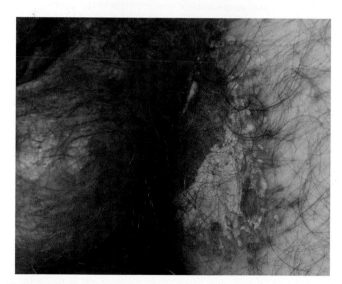

Figure 15.5 Flexural *Candida* infection.

systemically. Deep fungal infections that are not normally seen in healthy individuals occur in AIDS patients as opportunistic infections. *Cryptococcus neoformans* and *Histoplasma capsulatum* may cause inflammatory papular and necrotic lesions, particularly in the later stages of the disease.

Candidiasis is common and often associated with secondary bacterial infections. The oral mucosa can be extensively infected with *Candida albicans* that spreads to the pharynx and oesophagus. Clinically there are extensive white plaques on a background of erythema. Candidiasis of the skin has a predilection for the flexures where classically there is confluent erythema with peripheral satellite lesions (Figure 15.5). Patients may complain of

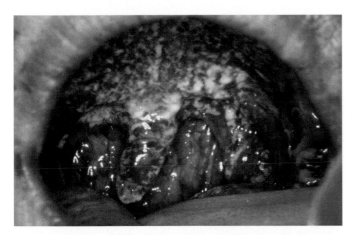

Figure 15.6 Pseudomembranous *Candida*.

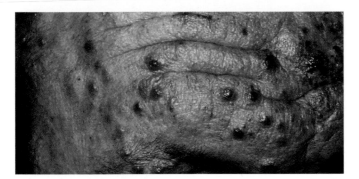

Figure 15.7 Bacillary angiomatosis.

cutaneous discomfort and itching and oral ulceration and dysphagia (Figure 15.6). Women with HIV can develop severe vulvovaginitis caused by chronic candidiasis.

Bacterial infections

Impetigo caused by *Staphylococcus aureus* may be severe with large bullous lesions associated with strains producing exfoliative toxins A/B. Erythrasma (*Corynebacterium*) may be persistent and recurrent in the flexural areas and often mistaken for a superficial fungal infection.

Bartonella henselae and B. quintana infections can cause bacillary angiomatosis (BA) in AIDS patients, who present with multiple small haemangioma-like papules on the skin and mucous membranes. Skin lesions develop slowly over several weeks (Figure 15.7), and visceral organs may also be affected – most commonly the liver. The differential diagnosis usually includes Kaposi's sarcoma. Blood cultures are usually diagnostic but the laboratory must be alerted to the possibility of *Bartonella* as blood cultures must be incubated for 3 weeks under specific conditions. Skin biopsy for histology is usually diagnostic. *Bartonella* are highly sensitive to macrolide antibiotics which are bacteriostatic and therefore an anti-angiogenic effect through down-regulation of endothelial cells has been postulated as the mechanism of action in BA. The treatment of choice is erythromycin 500 mg qds for up to 12 weeks. Azithromycin 500 mg on the first day and then 250 mg daily for 5 days is also highly effective.

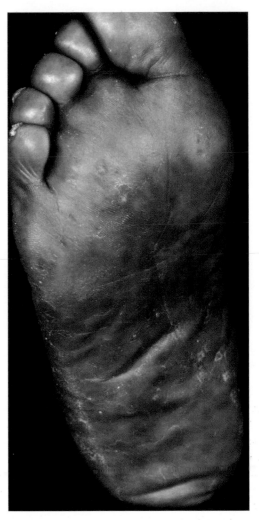

Figure 15.8 Secondary syphilis.

Syphilis

Approximately 12 million new cases of syphilis infection are reported each year according to the WHO, with a notable resurgence in many parts of the world where the incidence was previously low. Between 20 and 70% of patients in the USA and Europe are co-infected with HIV and syphilis simultaneously. Syphilis is caused by the spiral bacterium (spirochaete) *Treponema pallidum*. Syphilis is the great mimicker of other diseases and in the context of HIV infection presentations may be atypical.

Classically a painless genital ulcer develops 3–4 weeks after transmission via sexual intercourse. Secondary syphilis presents with a rash, fever, arthralgia and lymphadenopathy 4–8 weeks after the initial infection. The rash is usually asymptomatic and characteristically affects the trunk, palms and soles. Early lesions are usually annular erythematous macules that fade to a greyish-brown (Figure 15.8). Serological testing for syphilis should be performed to confirm the diagnosis. Primary/secondary syphilis should be treated with a single dose of intramuscular benzathine penicillin 2.4 megaunits, or intramuscular procaine penicillin 600 000 units daily for 10 days. Latent syphilis requires prolonged treatment.

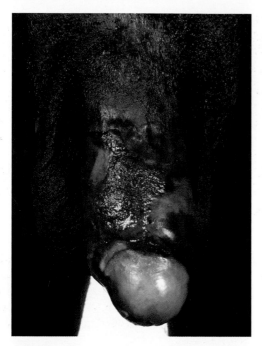

Figure 15.9 HSV (immune reconstitution inflammatory syndrome, IRIS).

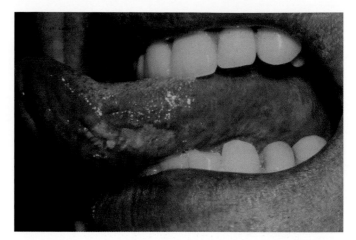

Figure 15.10 Oral hairy leukoplakia.

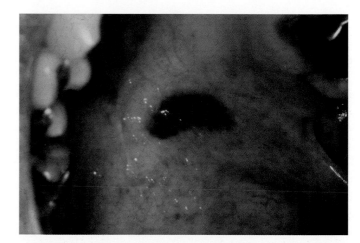

Figure 15.11 Kaposi's sarcoma on the hard palate.

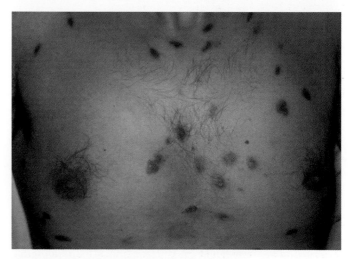

Figure 15.12 Kaposi's sarcoma on the trunk.

Mycobacteria may produce widespread cutaneous and systemic lesions. Varieties of mycobacteria that do not normally infect the skin may cause persistent necrotic papules or ulcers.

Viral infections

Herpesviruses

Herpesvirus types 1, 2 and 3 including herpes simplex (oral/genital) and herpes zoster infections may be unusually extensive, with large individual lesions in patients with HIV. Herpes zoster (shingles) classically spreads to involve adjacent dermatomes. Occasionally persistent ulcerated lesions are seen with resultant squamous cell carcinoma which can arise in any chronic ulcer. Herpes simplex virus (HSV) infections may be particularly severe and recurrent such that patients require secondary long-term prophylaxis. In the context of HAART, an immune reconstitution inflammatory syndrome (IRIS) can occur in association with genital HSV with florid debilitating inflammatory reactions leading to extensive and persistent painful ulceration (Figure 15.9).

Epstein-Barr virus (EBV) is human herpesvirus type 4. Ninety per cent of adults have evidence of past infection with EBV which remains latent in the body in B-cells. In 30–50% of AIDS patients EBV enters a replicative phase leading to oral hairy leukoplakia (OHL). OHL is characterized by overgrowth of epithelial plaques on the sides of the tongue (Figure 15.10) with a verrucous grey/white surface. Biopsies from OHL show a lack of host Langerhans cells which may account for the lack of immune response to the virus. Looking for OHL in the mouth can be a very quick and simple way of assessing potential immunosuppression in a previously undiagnosed individual in the clinic or field setting. OHL has also been reported in the context of haematological malignancy and after organ transplantation.

Kaposi's sarcoma (KS). Human herpesvirus type 8 is thought to be the causative agent in KS. In AIDS patients lesions usually affect the face, oral cavity and perineum (Figures 15.11 & 15.12). Early lesions may be erythematous-violaceous patches or papules which progress to firm nodules or plaques with a purplish-brown

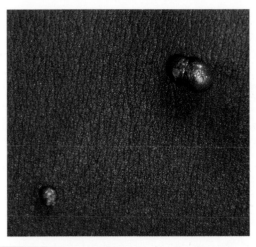

Figure 15.13 Molluscum contagiosum.

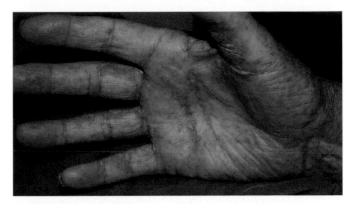

Figure 15.15 Crusted scabies.

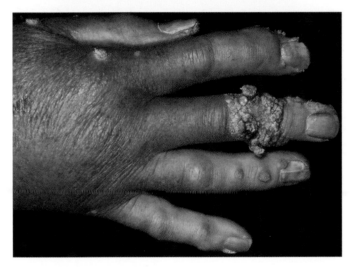

Figure 15.14 Human papillomavirus warts: extensive.

discolouration. Lesions may eventually ulcerate. KS koebnerizes (occurs at sites of skin trauma) and secondary lymphoedema may occur, particularly in affected limbs. Histology from skin/mucosal lesions can be diagnostic. Cutaneous therapy is directed at haemostasis, restoring function, improving the cosmetic appearance and debulking advanced disease. A variety of measures can be considered such as excision, radiotherapy, pulsed-dye laser and intralesional chemotherapy (vinblastine, vincristine and bleomycin).

Other viruses

Molluscum contagiosum infections are frequent in HIV patients. Individual lesions may be larger than usual (giant molluscum) and they may be extensive. Mollusca are readily identified as firm papules with an umbilicated centre (Figure 15.13). The differential diagnosis of large mollusca-like lesions in the context of HIV includes fungal infections due to cryptococcus and histoplasmosis. If the diagnosis is in question then a skin biopsy for histology analysis can be very helpful.

Human papillomavirus (HPV) warts may be numerous and large in HIV patients (Figure 15.14). Perianal and genital warts can be particularly troublesome and may be associated with intraepithelial neoplasia of the cervix and sometimes invasive perianal squamous cell carcinoma. With immune reconstitution HPV warts tend to resolve, but in the meantime they may respond to wart therapies including salicylic acid, cryotherapy, imiquimod and diphencyprone therapy.

Infestations

Scabies in HIV patients may present with classic burrows on the fingers and genitals or as widespread crusted (Norwegian) scabies which is highly contagious (Figure 15.15). Patients present with hyperkeratotic papules and plaques with relatively little inflammation (helping to distinguish it from psoriasis). Itching may be mild or intractable. Microscopic examination of the crusts is a simple rapid diagnostic test. Topical treatment with 5% permethrin (two applications 7 days apart) may be effective, but ivermectin 200 micrograms/kg as a single dose (or repeated after 7 days) may be needed in refractory/crusted and recurrent infestations.

Drug rashes

HIV patients frequently take multiple medications, many of which have a reputation for causing drug rashes (sulphonamides and antibiotics). Nonetheless the frequency of drug rashes in HIV patients is extremely high (10 times higher than in the general population) especially at CD4 counts below 200 cells/μL. This is partially explained by the fact that HIV itself affects the metabolism of many drugs. The majority of drug rashes occur within 7–20 days after starting the offending drug, and take the form of toxic erythema (maculopapular eruption) which is usually mild and resolves when the medication is stopped.

However, severe life-threatening drug reactions such as toxic epidermal necrolysis (TEN) are 1000 times more common in HIV-positive individuals. In HIV patients TEN has been reported in association with nevirapine, abacavir and co-trimoxazole. Clinically patients present with rapid, widespread (>30% of skin surface area), painful, full-thickness skin necrosis which is associated with a 25–30% risk of mortality (Figure 15.16).

Other drug rashes in HIV patients include pigmentation of nails/tongue/skin (zidovudine, clofazimine), mucosal ulceration

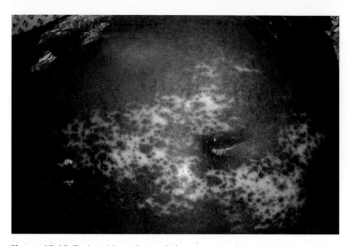

Figure 15.16 Toxic epidermal necrolysis.

(zalcitabine, foscarnet), diffuse erythema (abacavir), phototoxic rashes (St John's wort), Stevens–Johnson syndrome (co-trimoxazole, dapsone) and TEN.

Further reading

Adler MW. *ABC of AIDS*, 5th edn. BMJ Publishing Group, London, 2001.
Colven R. Update on HIV/AIDS. *An issue of Dermatologic Clinics*, 1st edn. Saunders, Philadelphia, 2006.

CHAPTER 16

Fungal Infections

OVERVIEW

- Fungi can cause infections of the epidermis and mucosae, and therefore the skin, hair, nails and orogenital tract may be affected.

- There are two types of fungal infection in humans – the dermatophyte moulds and yeasts.

- Fungal infections are more common in hot climates and in immunosuppressed individuals.

- A diagnosis of fungal infection is confirmed by culture of skin scrapings, but rapid PCR and ELISA tests are increasingly used.

- Clinical features vary according to the site and causative fungus. For example, endothrix fungi that infect the hair shaft give a different picture from those that remain on the hair surface.

- Tinea corporis should be distinguished from other cutaneous disorders including erythrasma, seborrhoeic dermatitis and pityriasis versicolor.

- Onychomycosis (fungal infection of the nails) affects mainly adults and may be chronic in those working in damp environments. Chronic infection of the toenails occurs mainly in men and is difficult to clear.

- *Candida*, a yeast, causes lesions in the mucous membranes and flexures where it must be differentiated from psoriasis, seborrhoeic dermatitis and contact dermatitis.

- Deep fungal infection occurs in diabetics, patients who are debilitated and the immunosuppressed.

Introduction

One million species of fungi are currently recognized of which 300 are pathogenic to humans and of these over three-quarters primarily infect the skin and subcutaneous tissues. Superficial fungal pathogens cause some of the most common and the rarest infections known to man. Historically superficial fungal infections have caused minimal disease in temperate climates, with the most severe outbreaks occurring in the tropics and subtropics. However, global boundaries are becoming increasingly indistinct and therefore diseases more widespread, due to a combination of human migration

and population dynamics. The use of potent immunosuppressant and antimicrobial drugs has increased the incidence of fungal infective episodes. Currently there is emerging resistance to antifungal medications and to date no human fungal vaccine exists.

Some fungi live on the skin as part of the normal skin flora whilst others come into contact with the skin through the environment and animals. Superficial fungal infections attack the epidermis, mucosa, nails and hair, and are divided into two groups: moulds (e.g. dermatophytes) and yeasts (e.g. *Candida*).

Yeasts that comprise part of the normal skin flora can become pathogenic due to a change in the host's immune system. This allows the yeast to disseminate throughout the body causing serious life-threatening disease. Conversely mycoses that originate as systemic infections can become deposited in the skin via haematogenous spread.

Investigations

Diagnosis of fungal infections can be made by taking skin scrapings, nail clippings, scalp brushings and skin biopsies for mycological analyses (Box 16.1). A moistened bacterial swab taken from the affected skin and inoculated into standard fungal media can be a useful additional test. Expert mycologists who perform fungal microscopy may be able to make an immediate diagnosis through recognition of characteristic fungal features. Macroscopic patterns

---

Box 16.1 **Principles of diagnosis**

- Consider a fungal infection in any patient with itchy, dry, scaly lesions
- Skin samples are taken by scraping the edge of the lesion with a scalpel held at right angles to the skin and collected onto a piece of dark paper
- Nail clippings should be taken from the nail including subungal debris
- Laboratories will report initially on direct microscopy but culture results take 2–4 weeks
- Lesions to which steroids have been applied are often quite atypical because the normal inflammatory response is suppressed – *tinea incognito*
- Wood's light (ultraviolet light) can reveal *Microsporum* infections of hair, as they produce a green-blue fluorescence

---

ABC of Dermatology, 5th edition. Edited by P. K. Buxton and R. Morris-Jones.
© 2009 Blackwell Publishing, ISBN: 978-1-4051-7065-9.

of fungal growth from cultures may also lead to species diagnoses; however fungi are usually slow to grow. Modern fungal diagnostics are moving towards the use of rapid PCR tests and ELISA which can rapidly process numerous specimens simultaneously. Some mycology reference laboratories may also be able to provide a sensitivity profile to antifungal drugs from any fungal strain isolated.

General features of fungi in the skin

Superficial dermatophyte infections are named according to the body site affected: tinea capitis (scalp), tinea corporis (body), tinea cruris (groin) and tinea pedis (feet). Fungal infections invariably cause itching; the skin may be dry and scaly or in flexural areas wet maceration can result.

Zoophilic (animal) fungi generally produce a more intense inflammatory response with deeper indurated lesions (Figure 16.1) than fungal infections due to anthropophilic (human) species. Some lesions have a prominent scaling margin with apparent clearing in the centre leading to annular or ring-shaped lesions – hence the term 'ringworm'.

Children below the age of puberty are susceptible to scalp ringworm, termed tinea capitis. In many inner city areas the most common fungus isolated is caused by a human species *Trichophyton tonsurans*, but fungi from animals (cattle, dogs, and cats) can also occur. Infection from dogs and cats with a zoophilic fungus (*Microsporum canis*) to which humans have little immunity can occur at any age. *Adults* typically are more commonly affected by tinea pedis. Tinea cruris in the groin is seen mainly in men, and

fungal nail infections (onychomycosis) are particularly common in the elderly and debilitated.

Scalp and face

Tinea capitis (scalp ringworm) mainly affects pre-adolescent children. The main fungal pathogens isolated include *Trichophyton*, *Microsporum* and *Epidermophyton*. Fungi may penetrate the hair shaft itself (endothrix infections which are characterized by multiple patchy areas of alopecia, minimal scaling and inflammation) or remain on the outside (ectothrix in which there are numerous broken-off hairs and partial alopecia). In favus infections due to *T. schoenleinii* there is a mixed picture with multiple adherent yellow crusts leading to extensive alopecia. *T. tonsurans* (endothrix) is currently the most common infection in the UK.

Clinically features are highly variable: diffuse scaling, grey patches, black dots (broken-off hairs), multiple pustules, kerion formation and occipital lymphadenopathy. A *kerion* is an inflamed, boggy, pustular lesion on the scalp that occurs when there is a brisk inflammatory response. This settles with antifungal treatment and does not require surgical drainage (Figures 16.2–16.4).

Scalp brushings should be taken to isolate the fungal pathogens from index cases and close family contacts. Parents may have tinea corporis on the shoulder/neck area where their child's infected head has come to rest.

Topical antifungals are unable to penetrate the hair shaft sufficiently to eradicate endothrix infections and therefore systemic antifungal agents are required for rapid clinical and mycological cure. Oral griseofulvin (10 mg/kg if over 1 month of age) is the current FDA approved treatment. It is effective for the treatment of *Microsporum* infections when given for 8–10 weeks and has minimal side-effects. However, there is increasing evidence that oral terbinafine has a comparable safety profile and greater efficacy against *T. tonsurans* and is half the cost. Terbinafine is given daily for 1 month (dosage according to weight: <20 kg 62.5 mg; 20–40 kg 125 mg; > 40 kg 250 mg daily). Ideally repeat scalp brushings should be taken after treatment to ensure mycological cure.

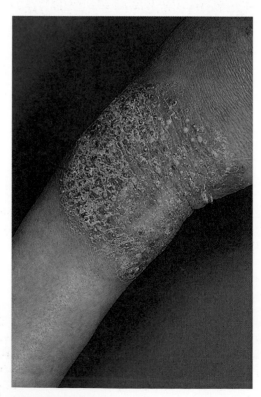

Figure 16.1 Animal ringworm.

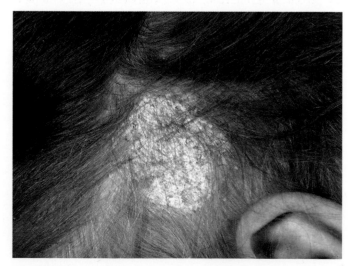

Figure 16.2 Tinea capitis: *Microsporum*.

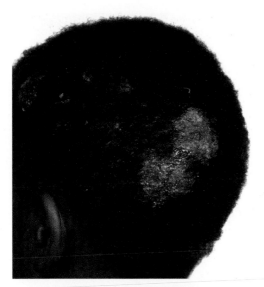

Figure 16.3 Tinea capitis – *Trichophyton tonsurans*.

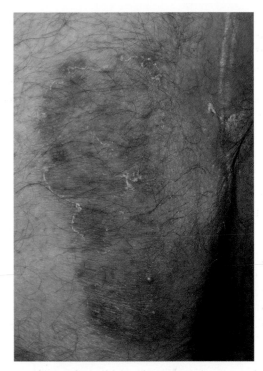

Figure 16.5 Tinea incognito.

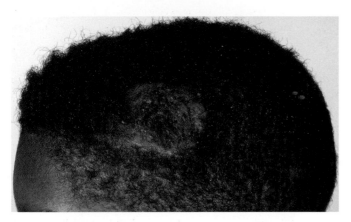

Figure 16.4 Kerion on scalp.

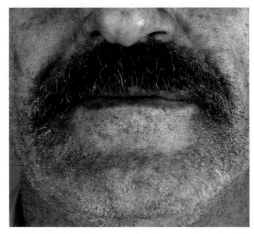

Figure 16.6 Seborrhoeic dermatitis.

Tinea incognito is the term used for the indistinct appearance of a superficial fungal infection on the skin caused by use of topical/ systemic steroids. Therefore because the typical clinical features of the fungal infection (raised scaly margin with inflammation) are lost, the diagnosis becomes more difficult (Figure 16.5). The groin, hands, and face are sites where this is most likely to occur. Management is to stop the steroids and treat with topical antifungal agents.

Seborrhoeic dermatitis (SD) is an allergic contact dermatitis to the yeast *Malassezia furfur* which is part of the normal skin flora; therefore the condition is usually chronic. SD most frequently affects the hair-bearing skin (scalp, eyebrows, moustache and anterior chest) and nasal creases (Figure 16.6). There is marked scaling with associated eczema and adherent greasy scales. SD may be very itchy. It should be explained to patients that the problem will always tend to recur following treatment, which is aimed at reducing the numbers of yeast on the skin and controlling the eczema. Ketoconazole shampoo can be used to wash the body and scalp once weekly to reduce yeast numbers. Twice-daily topical steroids (± miconazole) can be used to treat the eczema. In refractory cases systemic imidazoles can be effective.

Feet (and hands)

Tinea pedis or athlete's foot is a common disease mainly affecting adults. It is easily acquired in public swimming pools or showers and industrial workers appear to be particularly predisposed to this infection. Tinea pedis is very itchy and can affect any part of the foot (Figure 16.7) but frequently occurs between the toes where the skin becomes macerated. Across the plantar and dorsal aspects of the feet there is usually a dry, scaling rash occasionally with vesicles

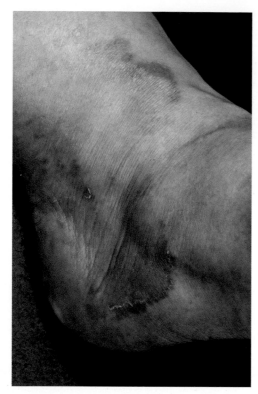

Figure 16.7 Tinea pedis.

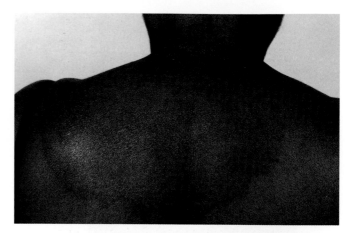

Figure 16.8 Tinea corporis.

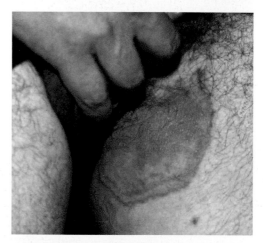

Figure 16.9 Tinea cruris.

at the active margins. The hands may be similarly affected. The condition needs to be differentiated from psoriasis and eczema and therefore scrapings for mycology can be helpful. Terbinafine 1% cream twice daily for 2–4 weeks is usually effective but recurrent infections may occur.

Trunk

Tinea corporis also causes pruritus. Lesions tend to be erythematous with a well-defined scaly edge (Figure 16.8). In the groin (tinea cruris) (Figure 16.9) there may be extension onto the adjacent thighs and abdomen. Intense erythema and satellite lesions suggest a *Candida* infection. The differential diagnosis includes erythrasma (Figure 16.10) due to *Corynebacterium minutissimum* which may require a systemic erythromycin/tetracycline. Terbinafine 1% cream is the most effective topical treatment for tinea corporis/ cruris; other agents include miconazole, clotrimazole, ketoconazole and econazole for 2–4 weeks. If systemic therapy is required itraconazole 100 mg daily for 2 weeks (or 200 mg for 1 week) may be effective.

In countries without access to antifungal drugs simple measures such as antiseptic paints – Neutral Red or Castellan's paint – can be used. Whitfield's ointment (benzoic acid ointment) is easily prepared and is reasonably effective for superficial fungal infections.

Pityriasis versicolor affects the upper back, chest and arms. It usually becomes apparent when the skin is exposed to the sun as these areas fail to tan. Well-defined macular lesions of variable colour (hence the name 'versicolor') from pale tan to darker brown are covered with fine

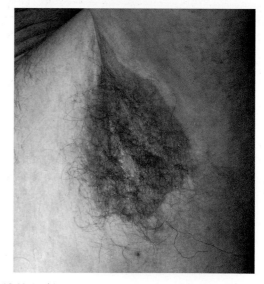

Figure 16.10 Erythrasma.

scale (Figure 16.11). The differential diagnosis includes seborrhoeic dermatitis, pityriasis rosea and vitiligo. In skin scrapings the causative organism *Malassezia furfur* can be readily identified.

Topical selenium sulphide (Selsun®) and topical ketoconazole 2% cream applied once daily for 2 weeks reportedly cures between

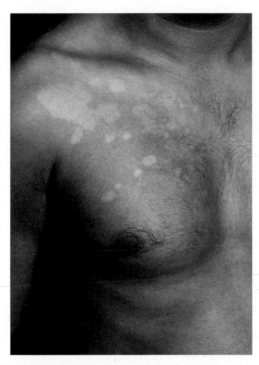

Figure 16.11 Pityriasis versicolor.

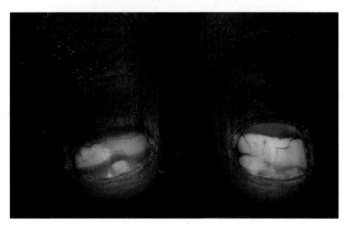

Figure 16.12 Onychomycosis.

70 and 80% of patients, but one-third relapse. Systemic treatment with ketoconazole (200 mg once daily for 2 weeks), fluconazole (300 mg once weekly for 2 weeks) or itraconazole (200 mg once daily for 7 days) give comparable results.

Nails

Onychomycosis affects mainly adult toenails. Nail plates become thickened, brittle and white to yellow (Figure 16.12). The distal nail plate is usually affected initially with spread proximally to involve the nail fold. In psoriasis of the nail the changes occur proximally and tend to be symmetrical and are associated with pitting and other evidence of psoriasis elsewhere.

Topical treatment should be considered for a single nail or very mild distal nail-plate onychomycosis. Agents available include amorolfine and ciclopirox olamine 8% nail lacquer solutions, sodium

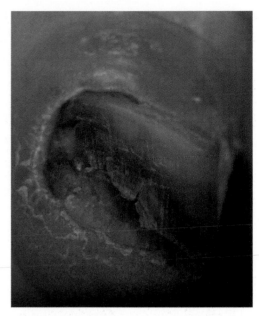

Figure 16.13 Chronic paronychia.

pyrithione, bifonazole/urea, imidazoles and allylamines. Systemic therapy is with terbinafine 250 mg daily for 16 weeks (toenails) or 8 weeks (fingernails), or itraconazole 'pulsed' therapy (200 mg twice daily for 1 week per month, total of 4 months).

Chronic paronychia occurs around the nails of individuals involved in 'wet-work' who repeatedly put their hands in water (such as child carers, chefs, dentists, nurses and hairdressers). Other predisposing factors include diabetes, poor peripheral circulation and removal of the cuticle. There is erythema and swelling of the nail fold, often on one side with brownish discolouration of the nail (Figure 16.13). Pus may be exuded. There is usually a mixed infection including *Candida albicans* and bacteria.

Pushing back the cuticles should be avoided. This is commonly a long-term condition, lasting for years. The hands should be kept as dry as possible, an azole lotion applied regularly around the nail fold, and in acute flares a course of erythromycin prescribed.

Yeast infections

Candida infection may occur in the flexures of infants, elderly or immobilized patients, especially under the breasts and abdominal skin folds. This should be differentiated from: (a) psoriasis, which does not itch; (b) seborrhoeic dermatitis, a common cause of a flexural rash in infants; and (c) contact dermatitis/discoid eczema. *Candida* intertrigo is symmetrical and 'satellite' pustules or papules outside the outer rim of the rash are typical (Figure 16.14). Yeast, including *Candida albicans*, may be found in the mouth and vagina of healthy individuals. Clinical lesions in the mouth – white buccal plaques or erythema – may develop. Predisposing factors include general debility, impaired immunity (including HIV), diabetes mellitus, endocrine disorders and corticosteroid treatment. Vaginal candidosis or thrush is a common (occasionally recurrent) infection of healthy young women, leading to itching, soreness and a mild discharge.

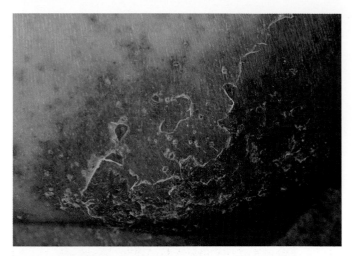

Figure 16.14 Candida infection in the groin.

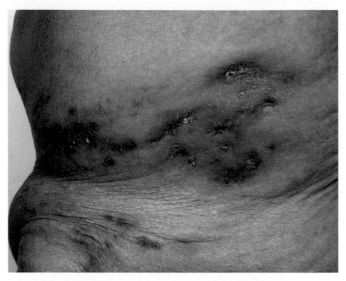

Figure 16.15 Deep fungal infection.

The majority of superficial *Candida* infections can be treated using topical antifungals including clotrimazole, miconazole and nystatin in various formulations including pastilles, lozenges, oral gel, mouthwashes, pessaries, creams and lotions. Many patients find systemic treatments more convenient such as fluconazole 150 mg as a single dose or itraconazole 200 mg twice for 1 day. Some drugs interact with azole drugs, the main ones being terfenadine, astemizole, digoxin, midazolam, cyclosporin, tacrolimus and anticoagulants.

Deep fungal infections

Fungal infections of the deeper tissues are rare in healthy individuals and usually only affect those who have underlying medical problems or are immunocompromised by illness or medication. Some infections that involve deeper skin tissues include histoplasmosis, cryptococcosis, sporotrichosis, *Fusarium* spp. and *Penicillium marneffei*. In HIV patients papules resembling molluscum contagiosum may be the earliest feature of deep fungal infections.

In tropical countries deep fungal infections are more common. These are described in Chapter 18. They should be considered in any patient from a tropical country with chronic indurated and ulcerating lesions (Figure 16.15).

Further reading

Midgley G, Clayton Y, Hay RJ. *Diagnosis in Color. Medical Mycology.* Mosby-Wolfe, London and St Louis, 1997.

Richardson M, Johnson E. *Pocket Guide to Fungal Infection*, 2nd edn. Blackwell Publishing, Oxford, 2006.

Seal DV, Hay RJ, Middleton KR. *Skin and Wound Infection. Investigation and Treatment in Practice.* Blackwell Publishing, Oxford, 2000.

CHAPTER 17

Insect Bites and Infestations

OVERVIEW

- Bites can cause a local skin reaction and/or systemic disease in humans through the transmission of parasites, bacteria or viruses.

- Patients with delusions of parasitosis believe that their skin is infested by insects when none are present. Treatment is difficult and requires sympathy and tact.

- A generalized anaphylactic reaction to an insect sting can be life-threatening. Patients known to be at risk should carry a preloaded syringe of adrenaline to use when reactions occur.

- Biting insects such as mosquitoes, midges, bedbugs, fleas, sandflies, mites, ticks and lice can transmit parasites to humans.

- Worldwide scabies is the most common infestation. Female mites burrow though the epidermis, laying eggs which hatch into larvae. Intense itching results.

- Other infestations include head lice and body lice (which transmit trench fever and typhus). Pubic lice may be associated with other sexually transmitted diseases.

- Cutaneous larva migrans occurs when larvae from the dog/cat hookworm penetrate human skin causing a superficial creeping eruption.

Box 17.1 **Clinical features of bites**

- Exposed skin sites, especially lower limbs
- Clustering or linear lesions
- Papules, nodules, urticated lesions
- Blisters or ulceration
- Excoriations with secondary bacterial infection

Box 17.2 **Risk factors for bites**

- Outdoor activities
- Travel
- Poor-quality accommodation
- Contact with animals
- Recent death of a family pet

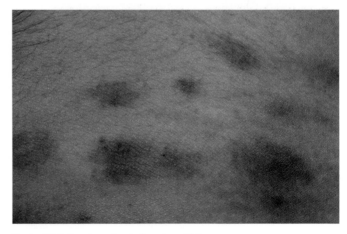

Figure 17.1 Papular urticaria from insect bites.

Insect bites and stings

When insects bite, they inject their saliva into the skin and ingest blood, which usually causes a localized area of discomfort and itching (Figure 17.1). Stinging insects inject venom through the sting that causes a more severe local reaction. More serious effects are due to (a) reactions from the bite or sting itself or (b) the introduction of parasites.

Most cases of bites from fleas, midges and mosquitoes are readily recognized (Box 17.1) and cause few symptoms apart from discomfort. Occasionally an allergic reaction confuses the picture, such as large bullae (Figures 17.2 & 17.3). Persuading patients that their recurrent itching spots are due to flea bites can be difficult and they may reject the suggestion (Box 17.2). Some patients develop a persistent insect bite reaction (Figure 17.4).

Delusions of parasitosis

Patients are convinced that they have an infestation when they do not. Often they will bring small packets or jars containing 'insects' (Figure 17.5). Examination shows these to be pickings of keratin, cotton or thread etc. Sympathy and tact will win patients' confidence; derision and disbelief will merely send them elsewhere for a further medical opinion. Antipsychotic drugs may help to dispel

ABC of Dermatology, 5th edition. Edited by P. K. Buxton and R. Morris-Jones.
© 2009 Blackwell Publishing, ISBN: 978-1-4051-7065-9.

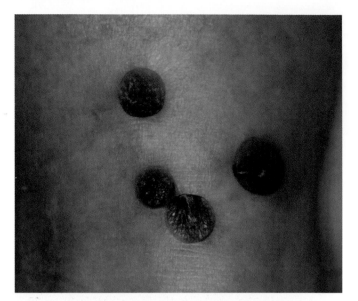

Figure 17.2 Blisters resulting from insect bites.

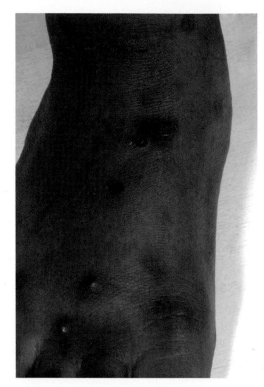

Figure 17.4 Persistent insect bite reaction.

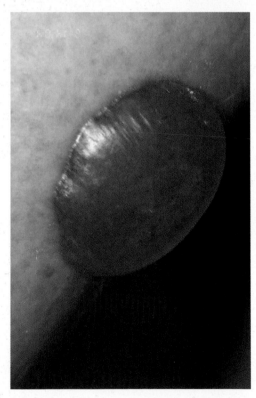

Figure 17.3 Bulla bite reaction.

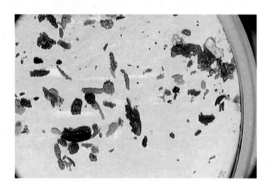

Figure 17.5 Parasitophobia specimens.

reaction may occur. In severe reactions medical attention is usually sought.

Management of bite reactions

- Over-the-counter preparations can be used in the majority of cases, such as bite-soothing spray, lidocaine and hydrocortisone ointment.
- Antihistamine creams (crotamiton, doxepin) or tablets (cetirizine, desloratadine) can help to reduce itching.
- If blisters are present they can be deflated with a sterile needle.
- Topical steroids such as Betnovate ointment twice daily can be applied to reduce inflammation, swelling and itching.
- If bite reactions are secondarily infected topical or oral antibiotics may be needed. Topical fucidin ointment or Fucibet cream (a combination steroid and antibiotic) can be used twice daily. Flucloxacillin usually covers secondary staphylococcal infections (erythromycin in penicillin-sensitive patients).

the delusion of parasitic infestation and should be used in conjunction with advice from a psychiatrist if possible. Drugs such as risperidone can be of benefit but care must be taken due to potential side-effects particularly if the patient has epilepsy or cardiovascular disease.

Allergic reaction to bites

Commonly, insect bite reactions cause local irritation and rarely (often to stings rather than bites) a generalized anaphylactic

Table 17.1 Skin lesions associated with insect bites.

Rash morphology	Differential diagnosis	Vectors (organisms)
Maculopapular	Human typhus Rocky mountain spotted fever Scrub typhus Relapsing fever	Human louse (*Rickettsia*) Ticks (*Rickettsia*) Mites (*Rickettsia*) Lice/ticks (*Borrelia recurrentis*)
Vesicular	Rickettsial pox	Mouse/louse (*Rickettsia*)
Annular	Lyme disease	Tick/blackfly (*B. burgdorferi*)
Nodules (pruritic)	Onchocerciasis	Blackfly (*Filaria, Onchocerca volvulus*)
Nodules (ulcerating)	Leishmaniasis	Sand fly (*Leishmania*)
Necrotic lesions	Tick typhus	Ticks (*Rickettsia*)
Facial flushing	Yellow fever/ dengue	*Aedes* mosquito (*Arbovirus*)

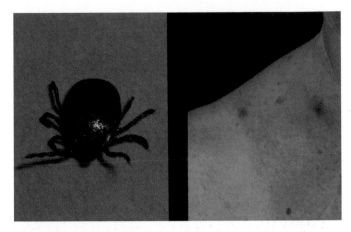

Figure 17.6 Tick bite reaction.

- In very severe cases a short course of oral prednisolone may be needed (30 mg daily for 5 days).

Prevention of bites

Keep the skin covered with clothing (especially dark colours), wear insect repellent (WHO recommends Icaridin* (Autan®, chemical KBR 3023) and DEET), sleep under bed nets off the ground.

Insect bites transmitting parasites

The identity of the biting insect can be important information if a parasitic infection is suspected. Insects that bite humans include mosquitoes, midges, bed bugs, fleas, sand flies, mites, ticks and lice. Each insect has its own specific distribution, preferred location, seasonal activity and preferred skin sites. All these factors can help to pinpoint the offending insect (see Table 17.1).

It may therefore be significant to know where the patient has been and their activities. Travel to tropical areas raises the possibility of parasite infection, while Lyme disease may occur from walking in endemic areas. Handling grain at harvest time may lead to harvest mite (*Pyemotes* spp.) bites.

Lyme disease

Tick and mosquito bites can lead to infection with *Borrelia burgdorferi*, causing arthropathy, fever and a distinctive rash (erythema chronicum migrans) (Figures 17.6 & 17.7).

If the patient is unwell and has visited an area where Lyme disease is endemic (parts of the USA and Europe) or gives a history of a tick bite then check serology for *Borrelia burgdorferi*. Do not wait for the results, however, but treat with doxycycline 100 mg twice daily for 10–30 days. Children under 8 years and pregnant or breastfeeding women should be given amoxicillin instead.

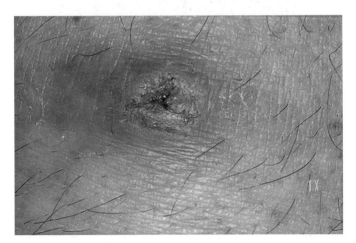

Figure 17.7 Erythema chronicum migrans in Lyme disease.

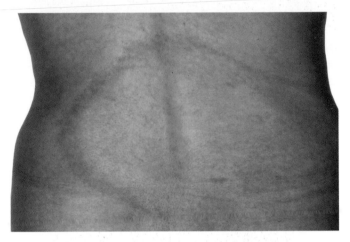

Figure 17.8 Spider bite (Nigeria).

Spider bites

Bites from spiders found in the tropics and subtropics can be quite severe (Figure 17.8). The bite of the brown recluse spider (found in parts of the USA) can become necrotic resembling pyoderma gangrenosum (i.e. a necrotic ulcerated lesion). Some spiders inject venomous neurotoxins that may be fatal, for example bites from

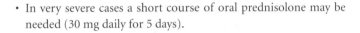

the 'black widow' (*Latrodectus mactans*), 'fiddleback'(*Loxosceles veclusa*), and *Atrax* species found in Australia.

European spiders may cause a painful bite reaction, but they are not venomous. However, with increasing transportation of fresh produce from topical and subtropical countries to Europe there are incidents of venomous spiders arriving by ship in consignments of fruit.

Wasp and bee stings

The Hymenoptera are a large order of insects, which inject venom through the sting apparatus. Both bee and wasp venom contains histamine, mast cell-degranulating peptide, phospholipase A2 and hyaluronidase. Wasp venom also contains antigen-5, and bee venom melittin and acid phosphatase. Local reactions are usually insignificant but generalized systemic reactions with massive respiratory tract oedema can be fatal.

Treatment

Mild local reactions can be treated with oral antihistamines. If an anaphylactic reaction is developing subcutaneous adrenaline 1:1000 0.5 mL should be given (repeated every 30 minutes if necessary).

Desensitization with venom extract carried out in a specialized unit is effective in those sensitive to bee venom.

Infestations

Scabies (*Sarcoptes scabiei*)

The most common infestation worldwide is scabies which causes intense itching that characteristically keeps those affected awake at night. The female mite burrows into the epidermis and lays eggs which hatch into larvae within a few days. See Box 17.3.

Transmission occurs due to close personal contact (at least 15 minutes of skin-to-skin contact) with an infected individual. The first symptoms of itching occur 2 weeks later when the immune system reacts to the proteins in the mites, eggs and faeces in the skin. Most infestations in immunocompetent individuals carry 10 adult mites, but in crusted scabies mite numbers will be in the hundreds due to failure of the host's immune system.

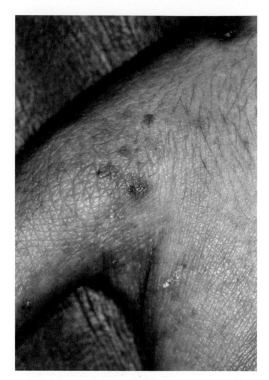

Figure 17.9 Scabies burrows.

Diagnosis

Scabies infestations may be difficult to diagnose due to the wide variation in clinical presentations. However, key points in the history include several individuals in the same household/institution/classroom/ward being affected simultaneously by a rash that is intensely itchy at night. Clinically burrows can be seen, especially in the finger-web spaces and on the genitals. Burrows are linear palpable ridges on the skin with a black speck indicating the position of the mite (Figure 17.9), which can be teased out of its burrow using a sterile needle and mounted onto a microscope slide. Patients often have a widespread papular rash, which is due to a reaction to the infestation, with multiple excoriation marks which can become secondarily infected with staphylococcus.

Scabies in children

Babies and young children infested with scabies characteristically present with erythematous cutaneous papules and nodules in the axillae and on the soles of the feet (Figures 17.10 & 17.11). It is not unusual for the lesions to blister. Classic burrows are rarely seen in this age-group.

Crusted scabies

Crusted scabies can look similar to dry scaly skin rashes such as psoriasis and eczema, and consequently can be misdiagnosed. Patients are usually immunosuppressed or elderly and do not complain of itching, as their immune cells are not reacting against the mite proteins. Consequently mite numbers are usually in the hundreds. Clinically patients have a crusted fine scaling on the skin which is superficial with very little erythema (unlike psoriasis and eczema) (Figure 17.12). If the diagnosis is missed then numerous

> ### Box 17.3 Scabies – points to note
>
> - There may be very few burrows, though the patient has widespread itching
> - The distribution of the infestation is characteristically the fingers, wrists, nipples, abdomen, genitalia, buttocks and ankles
> - Close personal contact is required for infestation to occur; for example, within a family, through infants in playgroups, and through regular nursing of elderly patients
> - Itching may persist even after all mites have been eliminated; itching papules on the scrotum and penis are particularly persistent

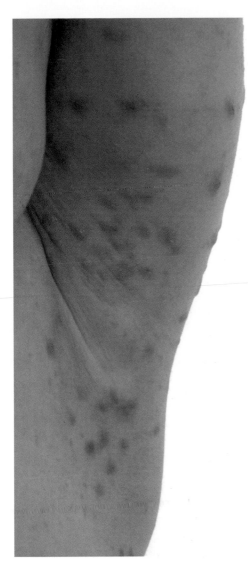

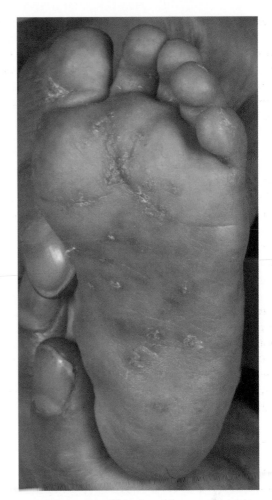

Figure 17.11 Scabies on sole of foot in an infant.

Figure 17.10 Scabies nodules in a child.

close contacts such as nurses and carers develop classic scabies and small outbreaks can occur.

Management (Box 17.4)

A full explanation of how to use topical therapy is essential if infestations are to be successfully managed. The most common cause of treatment failure is incorrect use of insecticides. Patients should be told that they and all their close personal contacts need to be treated at the same time, the lotions should be applied from the neck downwards (although the head and neck of babies should also be treated), the treatment left on overnight, and then repeated after 7 days. They should pay particular attention to the web spaces and genital areas. They should reapply the lotion after washing their hands.

Towels, bedding and underwear should be washed. Patients should be warned that the skin itching will take 6–8 weeks to subside. Persistent itching often leads patients to conclude that the mites are still active and they subsequently treat themselves repeatedly, leading to an irritant dermatitis. The itching resolves when

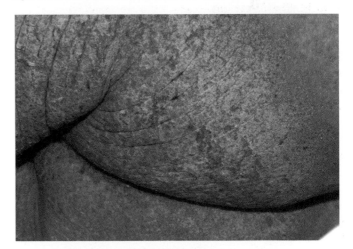

Figure 17.12 Crusted scabies on buttocks.

the mites, eggs and faeces have been removed from the skin by the host's immune cells.

Lice

Head lice

Head lice have infested humans for thousands of years. They have a worldwide distribution and can affect anyone. Children are the most common hosts. The exact prevalence is difficult to estimate with 0.1% to 66% of schoolchildren shown to be infected in different areas of rural Africa and 11% in Australia.

Lice are transmitted by head-to-head contact, and on combs, brushes and hats. Girls are more commonly affected than boys; this is thought to be due to their close contact with others during play. Mild itching may be the only symptom of head lice. Careful inspection of the hair close to the scalp may reveal adult lice and nits (white empty egg cases) in infested individuals (Figure 17.13). Fine-toothed combs can aid detection.

Management
- Only treat individuals with live lice visible on the scalp. Fine-toothed nit-combs can be used to comb out lice and eggs

> **Box 17.4 Management of scabies**
>
> - First-line treatment for scabies is 5% permethrin cream left on overnight, two applications 7 days apart. Adults apply from neck downwards; babies/infants apply to all the skin
> - Second-line is 0.5% malathion lotion left on overnight, (applied as above)
> - Ivermectin 200 micrograms/kg, two doses 7 days apart (named-patient basis), can be given to immunocompromised patients and those with crusted scabies (avoid in patients less than 15 kg and in pregnancy).
> - If you suspect genuine resistance (i.e. the treatment has been carried out according to your instructions), then switch to a different class of insecticide.
> - Pruritus can be alleviated with menthol in aqueous cream, crotamiton or doxepin. In severe cases a topical steroid can be applied twice daily to settle persistent nodular skin reactions.
> - If permethrin and malathion are not available then 10% sulphur in yellow soft paraffin is effective and safe; 25% benzyl benzoate emulsion may also be used.

over a basin ('bug-busting'). An application of hair conditioner usually allows the comb to pass more easily through the hair. Wet combing alone (30 minutes every 3 days for 2 weeks) has been shown to be inferior to insecticides, but in highly motivated families it can be very successful.

- First-line treatment is permethrin 1–5% crème rinse applied to dry hair and left on overnight. This should be repeated after 7 days.
- Alternative agents include phenothrin 0.5% or malathion 0.5% (applied as above).
- Combinations of insecticides and bug-busting can be used.

Body lice
Body lice are the vectors of several human pathogens including *Bartonella quintana* (agent of trench fever, bacillary angiomatosis and endocarditis) and *Rickettsia prowazekii* (agent of typhus). Body lice tend to affect individuals from poorer economic backgrounds and those sleeping rough. The lice live in the host's clothes and bite the skin. Close inspection, especially of the clothing seams, reveals the adults and eggs. Infested individuals have a widespread papular eruption with excoriations. If the patient has a fever or constitutional symptoms then the possibility of louse-borne systemic infection should be raised.

Management
- Wash clothing in hot water or 'tumble-dry' to kill adults and eggs.
- Treat the skin reactions with a moderately potent topical steroid, plus topical antibiotic if secondarily infected with bacteria.
- Take bloods for culture and serology if louse-borne systemic disease is suspected. Refer to cardiologists if endocarditis is suspected.

Pubic lice
These lice prefer the sparser hair-bearing sites on the skin such as the pubic, axillary and eyelash areas (Figure 17.14). The so-called crab lice are slow moving and are spread by close personal contact. Check the patient for other sexually transmitted diseases.

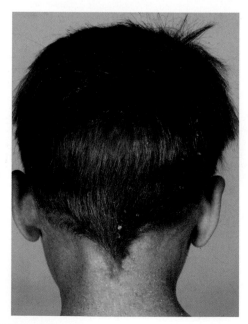

Figure 17.13 Head lice.

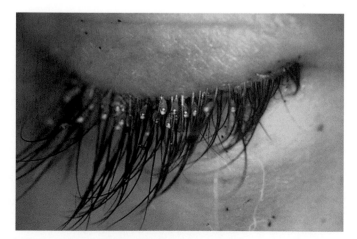

Figure 17.14 Pubic lice on eyelashes.

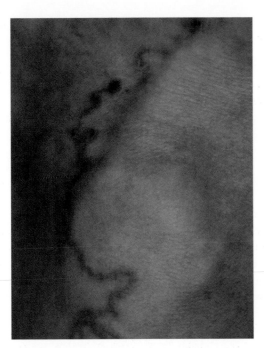

Figure 17.15 Cutaneous larva migrans.

Management
- Use topical permethrin 5% cream or 0.5% malathion to the skin from the neck downwards, left on overnight, repeated after 7 days.
- If the eyelashes are involved use petrolatum only, as insecticides can damage the eyes.

Cutaneous larva migrans

Larvae from nematodes such as the dog/cat hookworm (*Ancylostoma caninum*) and *Strongyloides* parasites accidentally penetrate human skin and then wander aimlessly, unable to invade the deeper tissue causing a superficial creeping eruption (Figure 17.15). In their animal host the larvae eventually make their way to the gut to complete their lifecycle. Treat the patient with albendazole 400 mg daily for 3 days, or ivermectin as a single dose of 200 mg/100 kg body weight.

Further reading

www.dermnet.com
www.phmeg.org.uk

CHAPTER 18

Tropical Dermatology

OVERVIEW

- The majority of tropical diseases are due to infections and infestations, a large proportion involving the skin.

- Hot humid conditions in the tropics and frequent lack of effective healthcare means skin diseases are common and recurrent.

- Pyogenic bacteria commonly involve the skin, causing impetigo and erysipelas.

- The intensity and type of immune response to tropical diseases such as leprosy and leishmaniasis determine the clinical manifestations.

- Cutaneous fungal infections can be very florid, persistent and recurrent. Tinea imbricata, nigra, piedra and favus are specifically found in the tropics.

- In deep fungal infections there is chronic inflammation in the subcutaneous tissues. These include chromoblastomycosis, mycetoma, blastomycosis and histoplasmosis.

- The most common infestations affecting the skin are scabies and lice. Others include tungiasis, myiasis, onchocerciasis, loiasis (*Loa loa*) and dracunculiasis.

Introduction

Tropical dermatology is a diverse topic covering a multitude of different skin diseases many of which are infections and infestations. This chapter will concentrate on tropical diseases involving the skin (bacterial, viral, protozoan, helminth and arthropod related). Health workers in the tropics and subtropics may be familiar with many of the cutaneous presentations in the local population. However, due to the relative ease of world travel more visitors who are immunologically naïve may present locally with atypical features or florid disease. In addition when these individuals return home they can present to their family medical practitioner who may be unfamiliar with tropical skin diseases.

Hot humid conditions in the tropics and subtropics provide an ideal environment for the proliferation of many organisms. Up to

ABC of Dermatology, 5th edition. Edited by P. K. Buxton and R. Morris-Jones.
© 2009 Blackwell Publishing, ISBN: 978-1-4051-7065-9.

50% of the local population is estimated to be affected by a skin disease in the tropics, the majority being infections or infestations such as impetigo, tinea and scabies. Many of these conditions are amenable to treatment. However the hot humid conditions, overcrowding, poverty and the lack of resources mean that skin diseases are common and frequently recurrent. Local simple therapies can be very effective and may be administered by those with only minimal training. Healthcare infrastructure in the tropics is improving although many areas still suffer from lack of basic medicines and trained healthcare personnel.

Many tropical dermatoses have distinctive clinical features. Skin changes may result from the presence of the organisms, ova or larvae, or a reaction in the skin to disease at a distant site.

Bacterial infections

Individuals living and travelling in the tropics are prone to *Staphylococcus aureus* infections on the skin in the form of impetigo (see Chapter 13). Bacterial infections may arise secondary to minor trauma or may be superimposed on any other skin disease. Clinical features include erythema, exudates, vesicles/bullae and crusting. Impetigo is highly contagious and many family members may be infected.

Deeper infections mainly caused by *Streptococcus* result in erysipelas or cellulitis which may be accompanied by systemic symptoms. The face and limbs are most frequently affected. Deep infections may occur following minor trauma or impaired barrier function due to pre-existing skin diseases such as tinea, scabies, atopic eczema or dermatitis.

The skin changes are characterized by marked erythema and tissue swelling. The patient may have systemic symptoms such as fever, rigors and malaise. Individuals who do not have immediate access to antiseptics or antibiotics may develop severe skin changes and ultimately bacteraemia.

Leprosy

Leprosy is caused by *Mycobacterium leprae* which results in a chronic granulomatous infection of the skin and peripheral nerves. Leprosy is endemic in Africa, south-east Asia, the Indian subcontinent and South America. Aerosols from the nasal mucosa are thought to be the mode of transmission between humans, but animal reservoirs do exist (nine-banded armadillo, chimpanzees and some monkeys).

The incubation period is highly variable (6 months to 40 years) with a mean of 4–6 years.

There is a spectrum of clinical disease (Figure 18.1) depending on the patient's cell-mediated immunity to *M. leprae*. Patients whose immune systems respond poorly have clinical disease characterized by numerous skin lesions with numerous mycobacteria (multibacillary). Patients whose immune systems are responding well to the infection have very few mycobacteria present (paucibacillary) in isolated skin lesions. These two ends of the spectrum are referred to as tuberculoid leprosy (good immune response) and lepromatous leprosy (poor immune response). Clinical intermediates exist and these are termed 'borderline' cases (Figures 18.2–18.5).

Diagnosis

Typical clinical findings are as follows.

- In tuberculoid leprosy (TT) there is a single anaesthetic patch or plaque with a raised border.
- In lepromatous leprosy (LL) there are widespread symmetrical shiny papules, nodules and plaques which are not anaesthetic.

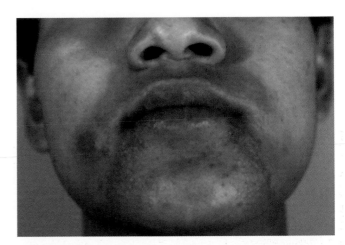

Figure 18.3 Tuberculoid leprosy.

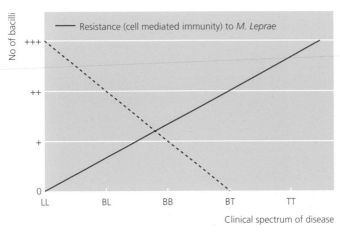

Figure 18.1 Spectrum of clinical disease in leprosy. BB, mid-borderline leprosy; BL, borderline lepromatous leprosy; BT, borderline tuberculoid leprosy; LL, lepromatous leprosy; TT, tuberculoid leprosy.

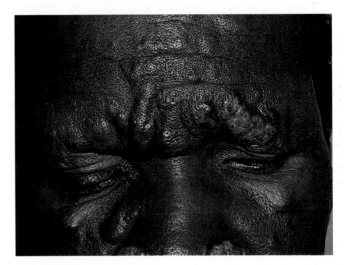

Figure 18.4 Lepromatous leprosy.

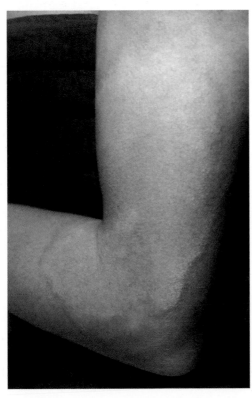

Figure 18.2 Tuberculoid leprosy: hypopigmented patches.

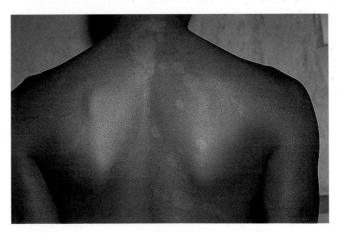

Figure 18.5 Borderline leprosy.

- In borderline leprosy (BT, BB, BL) there are varying numbers of lesions, few in BT and numerous in BL. They may be widespread but are asymmetrical. BB is mid-borderline leprosy.
- Palpably enlarged cutaneous nerves (great auricular nerve in the neck, the superficial branch of the radial nerve at the wrist, the ulnar nerve at the elbow, the lateral popliteal nerve at the knee, and the sural nerve on the lower leg).
- Glove and stocking sensory loss leads to secondary changes through trauma such as blisters, erosions and ulcers on anaesthetic fingers/toes.
- Deformity due to invasion of the peripheral nerves with leprosy bacilli, a leprosy reaction or recurrent trauma to anaesthetic limbs.

Slit skin smears measure the numbers of bacilli in the skin (bacterial index, BI – see Box 18.1) and the percentage of these that are living (morphological index, MI).

Treatment
Paucibacillary leprosy (BI of 0 or 1+):
- rifampicin 600 mg once a month (supervised)
- dapsone 100 mg daily
- for 6 months.

Multibacillary leprosy (BI of 2+ or more):
- rifampicin 600 mg once a month (supervised)
- clofazamine 300 mg once a month (supervised)
- clofazamine 50 mg/day
- dapsone 100 mg/day
- for 12 months.

Cutaneous leishmaniasis
Leishmaniasis affects approximately 12 million people worldwide and is found in over 80 countries (in the 'Old World' in Africa, Asia and Europe and in the 'New World' in Central and South America). Leishmaniasis is caused by *Leishmania* protozoan parasites transmitted by the bite of the female sandfly (usually at night). Rarely in humans transmission via blood transfusion, congenital passage and sexual intercourse have been reported. Animal reservoirs include dogs, rodents, foxes and jackals. Clinically leishmaniasis is classified into cutaneous, mucocutaneous and visceral, depending on the parasite's ability to proliferate at a particular temperature. Therefore the amastigote parasites may remain in the skin or be carried by macrophages to internal organs. There are many different

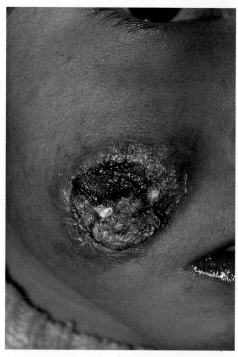

Figure 18.6 Acute leishmaniasis.

species of *Leishmania* parasites, each restricted to a particular geographical region (Box 18.2).

Cutaneous lesions usually on exposed skin sites develop within weeks of the sandfly bite. Children are more frequently affected than adults. Several family members may be affected simultaneously, often bitten by the same sandfly. Painless erythematous papules leading to nodules and eventually ulceration can classically be seen. The clinical presentation varies according to the host's nutritional state, their immunity and the *Leishmania* species involved. Spontaneous resolution may occur after 2–10 months, but latent reactivation after several years in an area of minor skin trauma means leishmaniasis can be an unpredictable disease.

Mucosal involvement may occur in isolation or concurrently with cutaneous lesions, and in some cases there may be a delay of up to 20 years between the appearance of cutaneous and mucosal lesions. Mucosal lesions may be painful and can lead to nasal obstruction, congestion, tissue destruction and bleeding.

Acute leishmaniasis
A red nodule like a boil ('Delhi boil', 'Balkan sore') occurs at the site of the bite. The nodules enlarge and may ulcerate (moist and exudative or dry and crusted) (Figure 18.6). Lesions usually

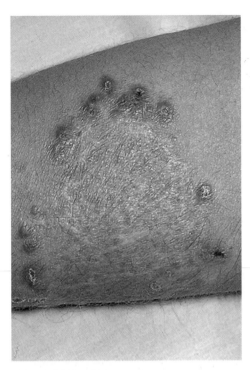

Figure 18.7 Chronic leishmaniasis.

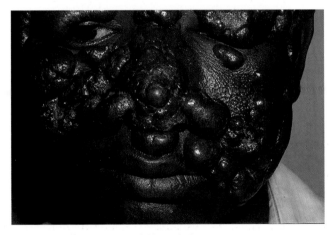

Figure 18.8 Diffuse cutaneous leishmaniasis.

heal spontaneously after approximately 1 year leaving a pale cribriform scar.

Chronic leishmaniasis

In a patient with good cell-mediated immunity, after the acute leishmaniasis has healed, new granulomas appear at the edge of the scar; these do not heal spontaneously (Figure 18.7).

Diffuse cutaneous leishmaniasis

This is leishmaniasis in a patient with no immunity to the organism (equivalent to lepromatous leprosy). Extensive skin nodules occur with numerous organisms (Figure 18.8).

Diagnosis

Diagnosis is usually made from a history of travel to an endemic area and clinical appearances of the lesions. Skin biopsy stained with Giemsa will demonstrate the parasites in over 50% of cases and modern polymerase chain reaction (PCR) techniques can be useful in determining the species responsible which can help to guide management.

Leishmaniasis skin testing is used in some countries where killed parasites are injected into the dermis and the reaction measured at 48 hours. This is, however, not positive in acute infections and in endemic areas is often positive in over 70% of the population. If visceral leishmaniasis is suspected then serology testing with an indirect fluorescent antibody test (IFAT)/Western blot or ELISA can be highly specific and sensitive.

Treatment

A proportion of cutaneous lesions will heal spontaneously or resolve following simple treatments such as cryotherapy, heat treatment or surgery.

Pentavalent antimonials sodium stibogluconate (Pentostam) or meglumine antimoniate are the main therapeutic agents used to treat leishmaniasis in most countries. Intralesional stibogluconate (1–3 mL injected into the base of the lesion leading to blanching – two injections a few days apart are often sufficient) or local applications of paromomycin can be effective for isolated cutaneous lesions. Systemic stibogluconate i.v./i.m. (200 mg test dose followed by 20 mg/kg daily) should be used until healing occurs (usually 2–3 weeks, although some experts consider four treatments sufficient).

Amphotericin B deoxycholate and liposomal amphotericin B (AmBisome) 0.5–3 mg/kg given on alternate days have been shown to be highly affective but must be administered intravenously and can be expensive. An alternative agent is pentamidine 2–4 mg/kg on alternate days (maximum 15 doses). Miltefosine is the first highly effective oral preparation for the treatment of leishmaniasis. A 28-day treatment course leads to 90% cure rates. It is currently used in India, Colombia and Germany, and although it is generally well tolerated it is teratogenic. There is some evidence that itraconazole and ketoconazole can be effective for treating leishmaniasis.

Superficial fungal infections

The warm moist conditions in the tropics and subtropics are ideal for the survival and proliferation of fungal species in the environment and on the skin. Cutaneous fungal infections can be very florid, persistent and recurrent (Figure 18.9). There are also many fungal infections that are specifically found in the tropics. These include tinea imbricata, tinea nigra, piedra and favus (Table 18.1).

Superficial dermatophyte fungal infections (see Chapter 16) generally present with itching. Lesions often expand slowly from a small focus on the skin to form rings or annular lesions, where the edge is active and there is central clearing. The margins are usually palpable and the lesions scaly.

Tinea imbricata due to *Trichophyton concentricum* is characterized by superficial concentric scaling rings spreading across the trunk (Figure 18.10). The condition is frequently chronic and relapsing. It occurs mainly in Central/South America and Asia. Topical Whitfield's ointment may be effective or oral griseofulvin or terbinafine.

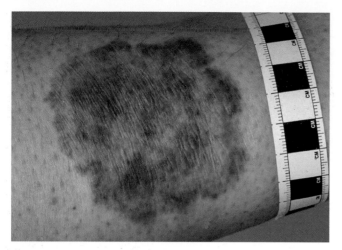

Figure 18.9 Superficial fungal infection.

Table 18.1 Tropical fungal infections of the skin.

Superficial cutaneous infection	Black/white piedra, tinea nigra, *Malassezia* yeast
Cutaneous infection	Tinea, *Trichophyton*, *Scytalidium*, *Candida*
Subcutaneous infection	Sporotrichosis, chromoblastomycosis, mycetoma
Systemic infection with cutaneous signs	*Fusarium*, *Penicillium marneffeii*, *Histoplasma*, lobomycosis, blastomycosis

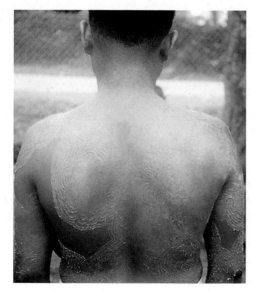

Figure 18.10 Tinea imbricata.

Tinea nigra caused by *Cladosporium werneckii* occurs in the tropical areas of America, Asia, and Australia. The pigmented fungus invades the stratum corneum usually through contact with contaminated soil, vegetation or sewage. Hyperpigmented brown or black macules are seen most commonly on the palms and soles.

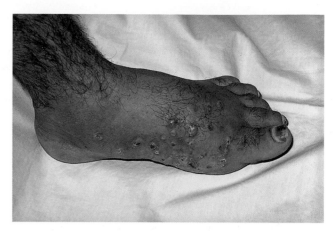

Figure 18.11 Madura foot.

Treatment with keratolytic agents (salicylic acid preparations and topical retinoids) can be effective due to the very superficial nature of the infection. Topical antifungals such as terbinafine, miconazole, ketoconazole and clotrimazole are also effective.

Piedra is a fungal infection of the hair producing hard nodular lesions on the hair shaft. The lesions may be black (due to *Piedraia hortae*) or white (due to *Trichosporum beigelli*). The nodules consist of clumps of fungal hyphae that can be difficult to remove from the hair shaft when the fungus is pigmented. Hair removal has traditionally been used to clear infections. Salicylic acid, formaldehyde preparations and antifungal creams are also effective. Re-infection rates are high.

Favus is widespread throughout the Mediterranean, the Middle East and tropics, but is rare in Africa. It is due to an endothrix fungus – *Trichophyton schoenleinii* – which causes a thick yellow crust usually on the scalp, but nails and glabrous skin may also be affected. The confluent areas of yellow adherent crusts are frequently secondarily infected with bacteria and have an unpleasant odour. Erythematous areas of scarring occur that must be differentiated from lichen planus and other causes of scarring alopecia. Prolonged systemic treatment with griseofulvin, terbinafine and itraconazole is usually effective.

Deep fungal infections

In these conditions there is chronic inflammation in the subcutaneous tissues leading to granulomatous and necrotic nodules.

Mycetoma (Madura foot)

This is a chronic granulomatous infection of the dermis and subcutaneous fat caused by various species of fungus (eumycetoma) or bacteria (actinomycetoma). Endemic areas include Asia, Africa and South America. Mycetoma most commonly occurs on the foot of an agricultural worker but any skin site can be affected. Traumatic implantation is thought to be the mode of transmission of the organism into the subcutis. Patients most commonly present with a swollen foot and multiple discharging sinuses (Figure 18.11). The infective 'grains' can be seen as tiny dark or pale bodies within the discharging purulent exudate. These can be teased out with a sterile needle and identified by microscopy and culture. Many fungal species (*Acremonium*, *Fusarium*, *Aspergillus*, *Madurella*, *Exophilia*) and actinomycetes bacteria (*Nocardia*, *Actinomadura*, *Streptomyces*) have been implicated in the aetiology of mycetoma. Identification of the organism is important as this guides treatment.

Diagnosis

- Examination of the discharging grains (colour will give a clue as to the cause).
- Culture of the grains to identify the causative fungus or bacterium.
- If no grains can be found a skin biopsy may be needed.
- Radiological imaging may demonstrate bone involvement.

Treatment

Fungal mycetoma
A combination of medical and surgical treatment is frequently recommended for these difficult infections.

- Surgical excision of affected tissue if disease is limited. Amputation if extensive.
- Ketoconazole (200–400 mg daily) or itraconazole (200 mg twice daily) for at least 12 months. In addition the newer agent posaconazole 800 mg daily for up to 34 months has been shown to be highly effective.

Bacterial mycetoma
Two drugs may be used for a synergistic effect.

- Sulphamethoxazole/trimethoprim mixture 960 mg twice daily (for up to 2 years).
- Other agents include dapsone, streptomycin, rifampicin, amikacin and imipenem.

Chromoblastomycosis

This is a chronic granulomatous condition that mainly affects the legs. Chromoblastomycosis results from traumatic implantation of a variety of parasitic fungi including *Fonsecaea*, *Cladosporium* and *Philalophora* into the skin. The disease is characterized by large spreading verrucous nodules or plaques from the site of implantation (Figure 18.12). In some cases the whole of the lower leg can be affected, with blockage of lymphatic ducts leading to an elephantiasis-type appearance.

Diagnosis is usually straightforward with typical fungal Medlar bodies being visualized on microscopy from a scraping or skin biopsy. Treatment has been extremely difficult in the past; cryosurgery has been used with some success as has itraconazole 200 mg twice daily. However recent reports of cure rates around 80% with posaconazole 800 mg daily are highly encouraging. Healing usually occurs with depressed pale scarring. In refractory cases surgery may be required.

Blastomycosis

This condition is caused by invasion of the lymphatic system, lungs and skin by the fungus *Paracoccidioides brasiliensis*. The widespread

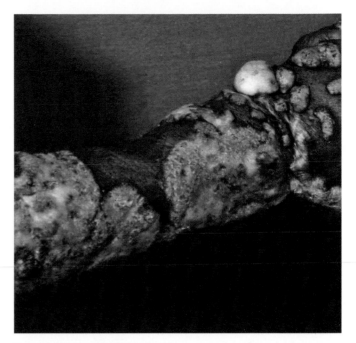

Figure 18.12 Chromoblastomycosis.

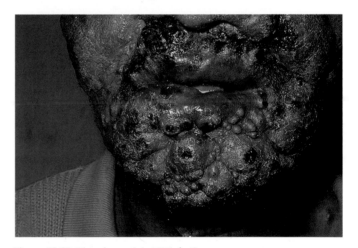

Figure 18.13 Histoplasmosis in HIV infection.

cutaneous lesions, which vary in appearance and distribution, must be differentiated from tuberculosis and other mycoses such as sporotrichosis, chromoblastomycosis and coccidiomycosis. It occurs in Central and South America.

Histoplasmosis

Histoplasma capsulatum is the fungal organism responsible for histoplasmosis. Two forms of the fungi exist: *H. capsulatum var. capsulatum* and *H. capsulatum var. duboisii*. The former mainly North American form causes respiratory disease, and the latter skin and bone disease in West Africa. The cutaneous form leads to nodules and ulcers at the site of traumatic implantation that can progress to deeper tissues leading to bony involvement. The disease is usually treated with itraconazole or amphotericin B (Figure 18.13).

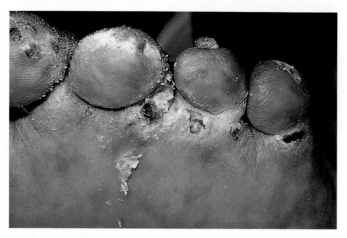

Figure 18.14 Tungiasis.

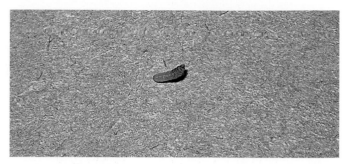

Figure 18.15 Myiasis: papule.

Infestations

Tungiasis

Invasion of the skin by sand fleas (*Tunga penetrans*) causes tungiasis in tropical areas of Africa, America and India. Pregnant female fleas burrow into the plantar skin especially under the toes and toenails (Figure 18.14). A marked inflammatory reaction occurs at the skin site leading to encapsulation of the parasite. Clinically lesions can appear white with a black central dot – not dissimilar to a plantar wart. Dermoscopy can help to visualize the central plugged opening of the fleas burrow. The release of flea eggs through the central opening may be seen if you are lucky.

The disease can usually be prevented by wearing shoes and keeping skin exposure to a minimum. (Vaseline with 10% kerosene applied daily can prevent the tunga flea from penetrating.)

Removal of the flea is both diagnostic and therapeutic. The flea can be winkled out with a pin or sterile needle (most individuals in endemic areas perform this themselves). If the fleas are very extensive, soak the feet in kerosene or treat with a single dose of ivermectin 200 micrograms/kg body weight.

Subcutaneous myiasis

Invasion of the skin by the larvae of the tumbu (mango) fly (*Cordylobia anthropophaga*) in central and southern Africa causes myiasis. The fly lays her eggs on clothes laid out to dry; these hatch out 2 days later on contact with the skin when the clothes are worn. The larvae burrow into the skin causing a red painful or itchy papule/nodule, predominantly on the trunk, buttocks and thighs (Figure 18.15).

Other flies that cause myiasis:
- *Dermatobia hominis* – tropical Bot fly, in Mexico, central, and south America with tender nodules developing on the scalp, legs, forearms and face
- *Aucheronia* sp. – Congo floor maggot, in central and southern Africa; bites of the larvae cause intense irritation
- *Callitroga* sp. in central America causing inflamed lesions with necrosis.

Preventative measures include ironing clothes before wearing them to kill the eggs. Treatment of skin lesions with an application of petroleum jelly or grease causes the larvae either to suffocate or crawl out of the skin.

Filariasis

Thread-like helminths ('filum' from the Latin: thread) cause an infestation in humans when transmitted by insect vectors such as mosquitoes. There are many different species of filarial worms that live in the lymphatics and connective tissue. The basic life cycle starts in humans when the fertilized eggs develop into microfilariae. These are taken up by insect vectors (intermediate hosts) in which further development occurs; the mature stages are then inoculated back into humans when the insects bite.

Three diseases are caused by filarial worms.
- Lymphatic filariasis due to *Wuchereria bancrofti*, which liberate microfilariae into the bloodstream.
- Onchocerciasis due to *Onchocera volvulus*. The microfilariae are liberated into the skin and subcutaneous tissues.
- Loiasis due to *Loa loa*, in which microfilariae are found in the blood.

Lymphatic filariasis affects 120 million people in 73 countries (34% in sub-Saharan Africa). The adult worms can live for up to 4–6 years in the lymphatic vessels leading to dilatation, tortuosity and malfunction. Lymphoedema results in the draining tissues, usually the legs, genitalia and breasts (Figure 18.16). Individuals may be asymptomatic for long periods with adult worms producing thousands of microfilariae each day. These are picked up by mosquitoes when they take a blood meal and are passed on to the next host when they feed again.

The diagnosis can be confirmed by examining a thick blood smear taken at midnight. More conveniently detection of filarial antigens can be done at any time and takes just 5 minutes to complete. Fingerprick blood is placed on an immunochromatographic filariasis card to detect circulating *W. bancrofti* antigens. PCR techniques are highly sensitive and can detect one microfilaria in 1 mL of blood.

Treatment

In endemic areas the whole community should be treated with a single dose of two of the following three drugs once a year for 4–6 years:
- ivermectin 400 micrograms/kg body weight
- diethylcarbamazine (DEC) 6 mg/kg body weight
- albendazole 600 mg.

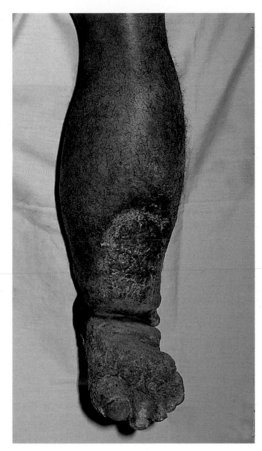

Figure 18.16 Lymphoedema of the legs in filariasis.

The chronic lymphoedema can be improved by keeping the legs moving and raising the legs when sitting, and secondary bacterial infection can be prevented by regular washing and moisturizing of the skin.

Onchocerciasis

Onchocerciasis (river blindness) occurs in Africa south of the Sahara and in Central America. It is due to *Onchocerca volvulus* transmitted by the bite of blackflies *Simulium damnosum* which breed by fast-flowing rivers. The inoculation of microfilariae by the bite of a blackfly causes intense local inflammation and is followed by an incubation period of 1–2 years. The adult worms live in nodules around the hips and in themselves cause no harm. However they produce thousands of microfilariae each day which travel to the skin and eyes. In the skin they produce a very itchy rash which looks like lichenified eczema. On the lower legs there is often spotty depigmentation (Figure 18.17). Involvement of the eyes causes blindness.

Risk factors for being infected
- Living, working or playing near fast-flowing rivers.
- Not wearing enough clothes so that the skin is exposed to insect bites.
- The construction of dams leading to less breeding of black-flies within the dam itself but increased breeding in the dam spillways.

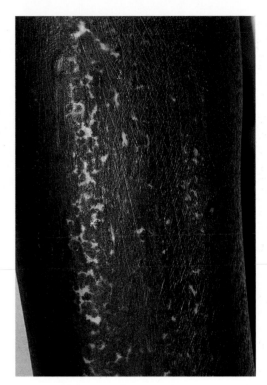

Figure 18.17 'Leopard skin' in onchocerciasis.

Diagnosis
The microfilariae can be demonstrated by skin snips or slit-lamp examination of the eyes. Skin snips are usually taken from six sites (iliac crests, scapulae and calf bilaterally). Very superficial samples of skin (without drawing blood) are taken and placed in saline; within an hour the microfilariae can be seen on microscopy. Removal of a skin nodule can reveal the adult worms. PCR to show parasite DNA and ELISA tests are now available in some countries.

Treatment
Spray the breeding areas with insecticides. An annual dose of iver-mectin (400 micrograms/kg for 4–6 years) should be taken by all those living in endemic areas to prevent the release of microfilariae from the adult worms.

Loiasis (*Loa loa*)
Loiasis occurs in the rain forests of central and West Africa. It is transmitted by mango flies, deer and horseflies. The adult worms live in the subcutaneous tissues where they can be seen in the skin and under the conjunctivae. The microfilariae are only found in the blood. A hypersensitivity to the worms shows itself as swelling of the skin, particularly of the wrists and ankles (Calabar swellings), which is itchy and erythematous.

Diagnosis
- Thick blood film to look for microfilariae (sample taken between 10 am and 2 pm).
- Adult worms can be identified by soft-tissue ultrasound examination.
- Immunoassay for antigen detection may be the most reliable test.

Treatment

- A single dose of ivermectin 400 micrograms/kg body weight or a 3- week course of albendazole 400 mg/kg body weight/twice daily.
- Diethylcarbamazine citrate (DEC) should be avoided as this can cause death as a result of a reaction to toxins from the rapid destruction of the microfilariae.

Dracunculiasis

Dracunculus medinensis or 'Guinea worm' is a nematode that infests the connective tissue of humans. It is acquired from drinking fresh water containing the intermediate host, a copepod (*Cyclops*) that contains the parasitic larvae. From the gastrointestinal tract the female mature nematode migrates to the subcutaneous tissue, usually of the lower leg. Papules develop at the skin site containing the female worm and numerous microfilariae which are released on contact with water. Treatment consists of very carefully extracting the worm by winding it onto a stick (a few cm/day) over several weeks (adults can be 1 m long). Symptomatic treatment of secondary infection and allergic reactions is also required. If the adult worm dies in the extremity it may become encased in calcium, causing chronic pain and leg swelling.

To prevent exposure to the larvae water should be filtered or boiled before drinking. Swimming in fresh water in endemic areas should be avoided, in order to break the life cycle.

Further reading

Lucchina LC, Wilson M *et al. Colour Atlas of Travel Dermatology.* Blackwell Publishing, Oxford, 2006.

Tyring SK, Lupi O, Hengge UR. *Tropical Dermatology.* Churchill Livingstone, Oxford, 2005.

CHAPTER 19

Hair and Scalp

Samantha Bunting, David Fenton

OVERVIEW

- Hair is an important part of the image that an individual presents to the world and inappropriate growth or distribution can have disturbing effects.

- Hair grows in a cyclic manner. A long growth phase involving most of the hair is followed by a period of arrested growth and shedding of the hair.

- Excess or diminished growth of hair may indicate underlying disease. Hypertrichosis, an excessive growth of hair, may be due to endocrine or metabolic changes or drugs. Hirsutism is defined as increased growth in the beard area in females.

- Hair loss or alopecia may be associated with scarring and loss of hair follicles. It may be generalized or localized; with or without inflammation.

- In telogen effluvium all the scalp hair enters a resting phase at the same time and is subsequently shed, causing disconcerting, but temporary, baldness.

- There may be inflammatory changes in the scalp and hair follicles that may be due to primary skin conditions or bacterial or fungal infection.

Introduction

Human hair plays a significant role in the self-image of an individual and the image they present to the world. Healthy hair conveys a sense of well-being, vitality and youthfulness and as such it cannot be overestimated how devastating diseases affecting this vital organ can be. Excess hair growth in females, particularly in prominent sites such as the face, is not only an embarrassment but may indicate underlying systemic disease.

Hair cycle

Hair is a modified type of keratin and is produced by the hair matrix, which is equivalent to the epidermis. Three types of hair occur in humans.

1 Lanugo hair covers the fetus in utero and is normally shed before birth. This is long and silken.

2 Vellus hair covers the whole body (sparing the palms and soles only) and is short, fine and non-pigmented.

3 Terminal hair is limited to the eyebrows, lashes and scalp until puberty; following puberty secondary terminal hair develops in the axillae, pubic region and on the central chest in men in response to androgens. It is coarser than vellus hair and tends to be darker and longer.

The hair follicle is unique among epidermal structures in that it grows in cycles (Figure 19.1). There are three phases.

1 Anagen – the active growth phase, which typically lasts 1000 days depending on predetermined genetic factors (as opposed to body hair which lasts from 1 to 6 months).

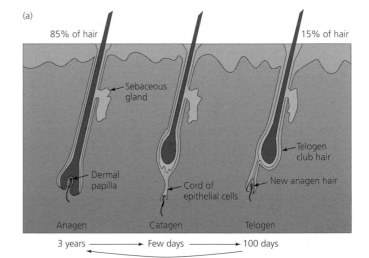

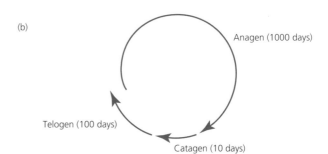

Figure 19.1 (a) Diagrammatic cross-section of hair at various growth phases. (b) Hair growth cycle.

ABC of Dermatology, 5th edition. Edited by P. K. Buxton and R. Morris-Jones.
© 2009 Blackwell Publishing, ISBN: 978-1-4051-7065-9.

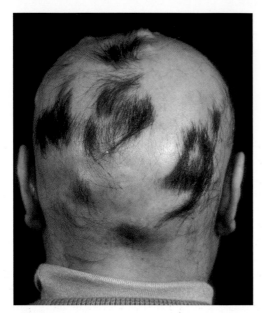

Figure 19.2 Alopecia areata.

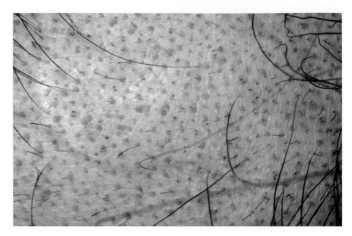

Figure 19.3 Exclamation mark hairs.

2 Catagen – the short growth arrest phase, approximately 10 days.
3 Telogen – the resting phase, lasting approximately 100 days irrespective of location.

The ratio of anagen to telogen hairs is 9:1 reflecting the fact that only a few hairs at a time are in catagen phase. On average, 100 hairs are shed per day although seasonal variation does occur.

Hair loss

Hair loss or alopecia can be divided into non-scarring and scarring types depending on the underlying pathological process and these can then be further categorized according to distribution, either diffuse or localized.

Alopecia areata and other non-scarring alopecias

Alopecia areata (AA) is an organ-specific autoimmune disease which leads to non-scarring alopecia. It affects 0.15% of the population and can affect any hair-bearing part of the body. Extensive involvement may lead to total scalp hair loss (alopecia totalis), total body hair loss (alopecia universalis) or localized hair loss along the scalp margin (ophiasis).

AA typically presents with smooth round or oval patches of non-scarring hair loss on the scalp (Figure 19.2). Exclamation mark hairs, when present, are diagnostic of AA. These characteristic hairs break at their distal point as they taper and lose pigment proximally giving them the appearance of an exclamation mark and occur at the periphery of patches of alopecia (Figure 19.3). Nail abnormalities, predominantly pitting or roughening, may occur in association with this condition (Figure 19.4). Other organ-specific autoimmune disorders such as vitiligo and thyroiditis are occasionally associated with AA.

The age of onset is usually in the first two decades. The course of AA is difficult to predict. Poor prognostic markers include:
- childhood onset of disease
- atopy

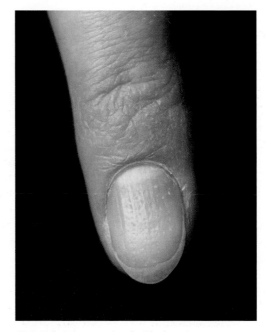

Figure 19.4 Nail pitting associated with alopecia areata.

- ophiasis (band of alopecia in occipital region)
- nail dystrophy
- family history of other autoimmune disorders
- presence of autoantibodies.

Trichotillomania, traction alopecia, telogen effluvium, androgenetic alopecia and tinea capitis should all be excluded by clinical examination, appropriate mycology and skin biopsy where there is diagnostic difficulty. In AA the hair follicle is not injured and maintains the potential to regrow hair should the disease go into remission. There is, however, no cure for AA and no universally proven treatment to stimulate hair regrowth and sustain remission. It is unclear if any of the treatment options available alter the course of the disease. Treatment is therefore guided by the extent of the disease and the age of the person being treated.

Current treatments include the following.

Topical/intralesional corticosteroids. Potent topical corticosteroids can be used on the scalp for 2–3 months to localized patches of alopecia. Intradermal injection of triamcinolone diluted with local anaesthetic can be used. This may stimulate localized regrowth of hair. Unfortunately it often falls out again and there is a risk of causing atrophy. Topical steroid lotion can be used but results are variable.

Systemic immunosuppression for example psoralens taken by mouth plus exposure to ultraviolet light A (PUVA); systemic corticosteroids.

Contact sensitization using either irritants (dithranol or retinoids) or allergens (diphencyprone).

Topical minoxidil (also used in combination with corticosteroids).

Other non-scarring alopecias

Androgenetic alopecia

Androgenetic alopecia is synonymous with male-pattern baldness and is the most prevalent form of hair loss, affecting some 50% of Caucasian males to some extent by the age of 50. It also affects a significant number of women. It causes hair loss over the temples (frontal recession) or vertex in men; women experience thinning over the vertex usually without frontal recession (Figure 19.5). The hair loss in androgenetic alopecia is the result of changes in the hair cycle from long anagen and short telogen to long rest and short growth phase. Over time, the follicles become smaller, producing shorter and finer hairs. These changes in hair cycle are androgen dependent and genetically determined. The clinical features are easily recognizable. In premenopausal women there may be other signs of androgenization to suggest underlying polycystic ovarian syndrome.

There is currently no cure for androgenetic alopecia and few treatments have been shown to be effective. Two drugs which are currently licensed to promote hair growth in men with androgenetic alopecia are oral finasteride and topical minoxidil. Hair transplants represent a last resort in those in whom medical therapy

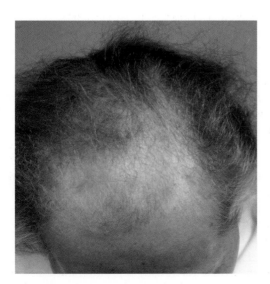

Figure 19.5 Female androgenetic alopecia.

Table 19.1 Causes of telogen effluvium.

Hormonal (e.g. pregnancy)
Nutritional
Drugs
Systemic disease (e.g. inflammatory bowel disease)
Stress (e.g. after febrile illness, post-operative)

fails; hair follicles are harvested from the occiput or sides of the scalp by excising a strip of skin and follicular units are dissected out and implanted into the bald areas. Topical minoxidil and oral anti-androgens may also be effective in female androgenetic alopecia.

Telogen effluvium

In the normal scalp each hair follicle passes through the growth cycle independently, or asynchronously. However, following a number of stimuli the majority of hair follicles may enter the resting phase (telogen) at the same time (synchronously) resulting in diffuse shedding approximately 2 months after the triggering event, often described as the hair 'falling out by the roots'. This is usually an acute self-limiting phenomenon; however a chronic telogen effluvium may occur (Table 19.1).

Postfebrile alopecia refers to hair loss as a result of a high swinging fever above 39°C. It has been reported in a wide range of infectious diseases (including glandular fever, influenza, malaria and brucellosis) and inflammatory bowel disease.

Dietary factors such as iron deficiency and hypoproteinaemia may play a role in diffuse alopecia and may be accompanied by nail dystrophy.

The assessment of a patient with suspected telogen effluvium should include investigations based on the history and physical examination. The patient's iron status should be checked and iron replacement should be implemented to achieve serum ferritin of 70 micrograms/L. Ultimately the condition will resolve once the precipitating factor has been removed and reassurance is all that is required.

Tinea capitis

Tinea capitis (see Chapter 16) is a fungal infection, which causes patchy usually non-scarring hair loss associated with short broken-off hairs, scaling and erythema of the underlying skin (Figure 19.6). It occurs almost exclusively in children. The most common fungi causing disease in urban areas are *Trichophyton tonsurans* (spread from human to human by direct contact) and *Microsporum canis* (caught from kittens or puppies). The diagnosis can be confirmed by taking hair pluckings and performing microscopy to look for spores inside the hair shaft; culture identifies the underlying organism. Scalp brushings can be taken and the bristles directly inoculated into the culture medium. Tinea capitis due to *Microsporum canis* fluoresces green under Wood's light.

Kerion formation (Figure 19.7) is an inflamed, boggy, pustular lesion on the scalp that may result from tinea infections (cattle ringworm in rural areas and human *T. tonsurans* in urban areas). This swelling will resolve with systemic antifungal treatment and should not be surgically drained.

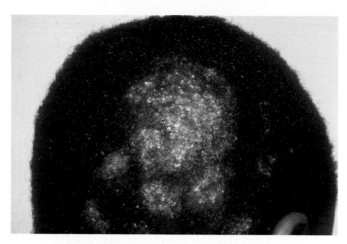

Figure 19.6 Tinea capitis.

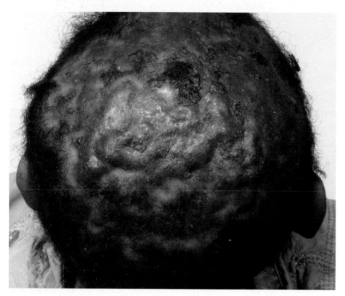

Figure 19.7 Kerion.

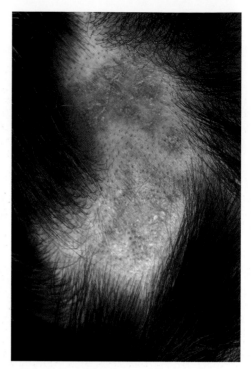

Figure 19.8 Discoid lupus erythematosus.

Oral griseofulvin or terbinafine are given daily for 4–6 weeks. Secondary bacterial infection should be treated with appropriate antibiotics (usually flucloxacillin to cover for *S. aureus*). If infection is due to *Microsporum canis* it is important to treat the affected pet.

Scarring alopecia

The scarring alopecias are characterized by permanent hair loss due to replacement of hair follicles by scar tissue. Scarring alopecia may be primary or secondary, depending on whether the hair follicle acts as the primary target or is damaged incidentally by non-follicular events. Permanent alopecia may also occur in conditions not traditionally considered as scarring processes such as in traction alopecia or trichotillomania in which follicular drop-out may occur.

Primary causes

These are best considered according to the underlying pathological process and skin biopsy can be very helpful in establishing a diagnosis.

Lymphocytic disorders

Discoid lupus erythematosus and lichen planopilaris are both causes of scarring alopecia associated with a lymphocytic inflammatory infiltrate histologically. Both conditions may be associated with cutaneous findings elsewhere which may be diagnostic of the underlying disease. In lupus affecting the scalp, scarring alopecia is associated with scaling, erythema and the presence of follicular plugging (Figure 19.8). Lichen planopilaris is characterized clinically by perifollicular erythema, follicular spines and scarring (Figure 19.9). Skin biopsy with direct immunofluorescence is helpful in confirming the underlying diagnosis in those patients where there is diagnostic doubt. Treatment options include oral antimalarials, corticosteroids and systemic retinoids.

Pseudopelade of Brocq is the label given to patients with a non-inflammatory scarring alopecia in the absence of any other underlying pathology on biopsy. It may represent end-stage lichen planopilaris.

Neutrophilic disorders

Dissecting folliculitis presents with multiple painless boggy nodules, typically on the vertex or occiput, which frequently discharge purulent exudate. Superficial pustules are often seen. This condition is mostly seen in young black males who may also suffer from acne and hidradenitis suppurativa. Treatment options include oral antibiotics (usually tetracyclines), oral corticosteroids, dapsone and isotretinoin.

Folliculitis decalvans is a rare form of recurrent folliculitis which leads to patches of scarring; crusting and tufting of the hairs may be seen, where multiple hairs emerge from a single follicle (Figure 19.10). Topical and oral antibiotics with antistaphylococcal activity are the mainstay of therapy, supporting the

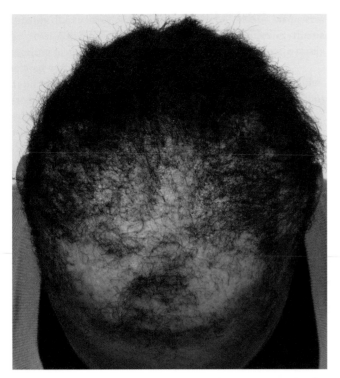

Figure 19.9 Lichen planopilaris.

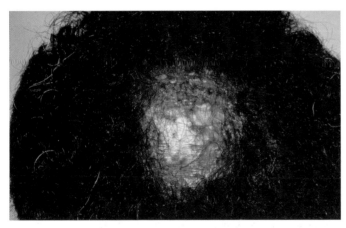

Figure 19.10 Folliculitis decalvans.

Table 19.2 Secondary causes of scarring alopecia.

Post-traumatic
 Burns
 Radiotherapy
Neoplasia (e.g. squamous cell carcinoma, lymphoma, sarcoma)
Infection (e.g. TB, syphilis, kerion)

hypothesis that this condition is due to an abnormal host response to *S. aureus*. Rifampicin 300 mg twice daily and clindamycin 300 mg twice daily for 12 weeks is often effective.

Secondary causes of scarring alopecia

Many well-recognized secondary causes of scarring alopecia exist (Table 19.2). Treatment is directed at the cause.

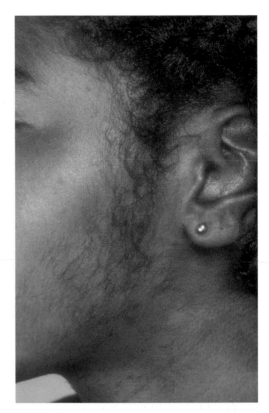

Figure 19.11 Hirsutism.

Excessive hair

Two patterns of hair overgrowth are recognized: hirsutism and hypertrichosis.

Hirsutism

This is defined as increased growth of the terminal hairs in androgen-sensitive areas such as the beard and moustache regions in females (Figure 19.11). The presence of terminal hair in a male distribution is not necessarily a sign of disease, and the determination of whether a patient has hirsutism must take into account the normal pattern of hair growth for the patient's racial origin. The patient's cultural and social background plays a major factor in determining how much facial and body hair is cosmetically acceptable. Whilst hirsutism is most noticeable on the face, it may also affect other androgen-responsive areas such as the thighs, the back and the abdomen.

The assessment of the patient with hirsutism must include a general examination to identify an underlying endocrine abnormality, particularly if there is a relatively short history associated with amenorrhoea and signs of virilization. Features suggestive of virilization in addition to hirsutism include deepening of the voice, increased muscle bulk and cliteromegaly, an extremely sensitive sign. These features suggest a more sinister underlying cause. A list of the causes of hirsutism is given in Table 19.3.

Management

As a general rule if the periods are normal, so are the hormone levels. Over-investigation should be avoided once it is clear that

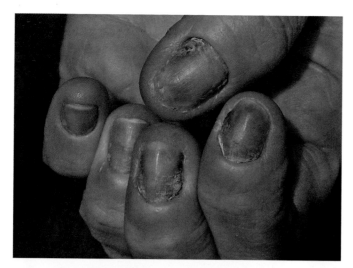

Figure 20.9 Yellow nail syndrome.

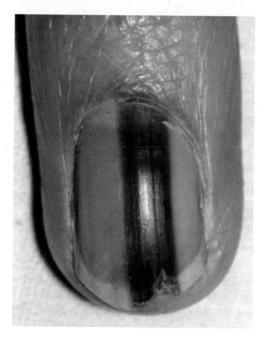

Figure 20.10 Melanonychia in a person with white skin. Could be a naevus or a subungual melanoma.

Thickened nail from trauma or fungal infection.

Brown colour or melanonychia refers to a brown streak in the nail due to pigment production in the nail matrix (Figure 20.10). The melanin source may be benign or malignant. Dark-skinned races have prominent benign multiple brown streaks. Pale-skinned people have a higher chance of a melanonychia representing a malignant process (melanoma). Slight discolouration of the nails may be seen in Addison's disease caused by adrenal insufficiency.

Minocycline and zidovudine can result in melanonychia.

Longitudinal pigmented streaks result from increased melanin deposition in the nail plate (Box 20.1).

Box 20.1 **Pigmented streaks in nails**

Single
Melanocytic naevi or lentigo
Subungual melanoma
Trauma

Multiple
Racial
Drugs
Addison's

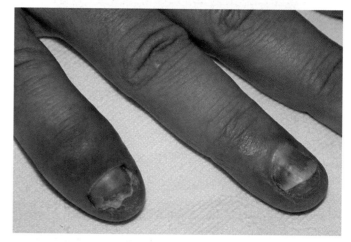

Figure 20.11 Nail psoriasis with onycholysis, pitting and arthritis of the distal interphalangeal joint of the little finger.

Longitudinal brown streaks are frequently seen in individuals with racially pigmented skin. This is rare in Caucasians and whilst it may still represent a benign process it is important that isolated brown streaks in the nail of pale-skinned people are seen by a specialist for an expert diagnosis to exclude the possibility of subungual melanoma. This is associated with Hutchinson's sign in which pigmentation extends into the surrounding tissues, particularly the cuticle. Adrenal disease may rarely be associated with longitudinal streaks.

Common dermatoses and the nail unit

Psoriasis is one of the most common dermatoses with nail involvement. About 80% of people with psoriasis will have some nail features at some point in the course of their disease. The features include pitting, transverse ridges, onycholysis, oily spots, subungual hyperkeratosis (Figure 20.11) and chronic paronychia. At times, disease may be sufficiently severe as to result in loss of function through pain and the inability to sustain pressure or undertake fine manipulation.

Eczema may be associated with brittle nails that tend to split. Thickening and deformity of the nail occurs in eczema or contact dermatitis, sometimes with transverse ridging. Pitting can also be seen. Nail bed changes are less common than in psoriasis, although

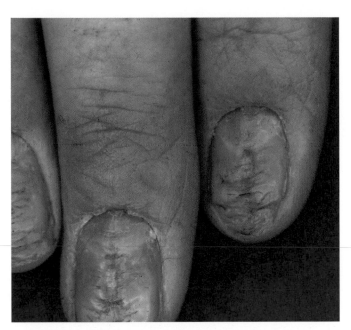

Figure 20.12 Eczema causing inflammatory matrix changes and nail dystrophy disproportionate to the nail fold inflammation.

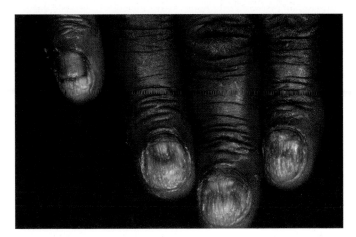

Figure 20.13 Lichen planus.

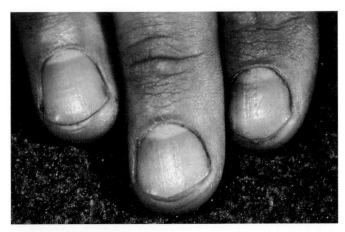

Figure 20.14 Nail dystrophy with alopecia areata comprising multiple small, regular, pits.

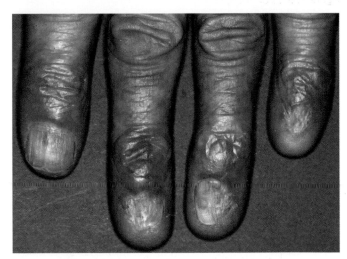

Figure 20.15 Dystrophy due to lupus.

allergic contact sensitivity where allergen is sequestered beneath the nail can produce dramatic acute and chronic nail bed disease (Figure 20.12).

Lichen planus can result in many features mimicking psoriasis, but in its most characteristic form produces atrophy of the nail plate which may completely disappear. The cuticle may be thickened and grow over the nail plate, known as pterygium formation (Figure 20.13).

Alopecia areata is associated with changes in the nails in about 30% of cases. Features include ridging, pitting, leuconychia and friable nails. Where the nails are friable, it is referred to as 'trachyonychia' and may involve any or all of the nails – known as '20-nail dystrophy' (Figure 20.14).

Darier's disease is associated with dystrophy of the nail and longitudinal streaks which end in triangular-shaped nicks at the free edge (see Figure 20.6). On the skin there may be the characteristic brownish scaling papules on the central part of the back, chest and neck. These are made worse by sun exposure.

Autoimmune conditions such as pemphigus and pemphigoid may be associated with a variety of changes including ridging, splitting of the nail plate, and atrophy and shedding in some or all of the nails.

Discolouration of the nail and friability are associated with *lupus erythematosus* (Figures 20.15 & 20.16).

Infection

Bacterial infection of periungual tissues

Infection of the nail unit may affect the soft tissues or the nail plate. The proximal and lateral nail folds are typically affected by *Staphylococcus aureus* or less commonly *Streptococcus* or Gram-negative organisms. Treatment is with drainage of any pus collection and systemic antibiotics, modified after initiation by culture results.

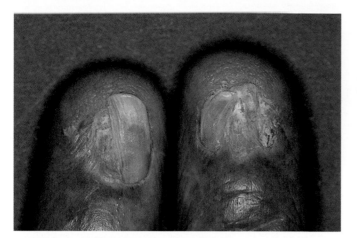

Figure 20.16 Pterygium formation with lupus.

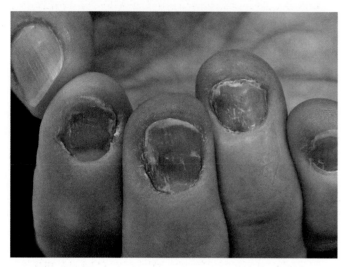

Figure 20.17 Chronic paronychia with alteration of nail plate shape and discolouration secondary to nail fold inflammation and microbial colonization.

The nail bed may become infected as a result of onycholysis (Figure 20.17). *Candida* and *Pseudomonas* are the most common agents, where their growth is promoted by the damp warm character of the onycholytic space. Treatment may entail clipping back the nail to expose the nail bed, avoidance of wet work, drying beneath the nail with a hair dryer daily and the use of antimicrobials. Topical antimicrobial treatment can be as gentamicin eye drops used beneath the nail, or as part of a long-term regimen to prevent relapse undertaking daily 5-minute soaks with vinegar or sodium hypochlorite solution. Ultimately, cure relies on management of the onycholysis.

Fungal nail infection

Nail plate infection with dermatophyte fungi is mainly associated with nail bed involvement and typically in a previously traumatized nail. Dermatophyte nail fungal infection is usually of the toenails rather than the fingernails and involvement of nearby skin should be sought and treated, especially between the 4th and 5th toes. It is important to confirm the presence of fungus before

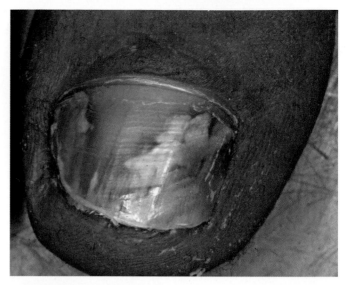

Figure 20.18 Fungal infection.

considering treatment as nail psoriasis, eczema and trauma can all look similar. The diagnosis is confirmed by taking generous clippings of nail plate and subungual debris for microscopy and culture (Figure 20.18). Positive culture is a prerequisite for systemic treatment.

Culture will determine if the fungus is a dermatophyte such as *Trichophyton rubrum*, or a non-dermatophyte. The latter are more difficult to treat effectively and therapy should be guided by a dermatologist or someone with specialist knowledge of onychomycosis.

Treatment of dermatophyte onychomycosis is optional based on patient preference and clinical factors. Systemic treatment with terbinafine is likely to ultimately achieve a normal nail in about 50% of patients. This figure will be slightly increased by concomitant use of topical amorolfine lacquer weekly.

Trauma

Acute trauma is usually either a crush or leverage injury. Crush injury is typically associated with subungual bleeding. Where this involves more than 50% of the nail area, drainage is indicated to relieve pain and reduce the risk of compression, using an opened red hot paper clip or a nail drill, usually available in emergency departments. Leverage injuries lead to complete or partial lifting of the nail plate, with nail avulsion in the latter instance. It is best to clean the nail and return it *in situ* to act as a dressing to the wounded nail bed. It will need to be held in place by a dressing or cyanoacrylate glue. It will eventually drop off when the new nail generates beneath.

Chronic trauma of the toenails is typically due to poorly fitting footwear, where the free edge of the nail is brought into repeated contact with the shoe. This is most marked when footwear is pointed or there is a high heel, creating a force on the foot downwards into the toe of the shoe. Trauma between toes and footwear can also arise with well-fitting shoes in activities such as step aerobics, hill walking (downwards) and long-distance running. The

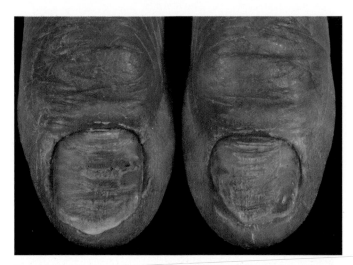

Figure 20.19 Chronic rubbing trauma to the proximal nail fold leads to a 'habit-tic' pattern of longitudinal dystrophy.

initial effect of chronic trauma is asymptomatic bleeding. Later there is thickening and yellow discolouration of the nail. Over many years, the shape of the nail matrix is altered and the nail may grow upwards and lose nail bed attachment. With marathon running it is not uncommon for people to shed nails after the event.

Chronic trauma of the fingernails arises through 'habit tic' picking (Figure 20.19), manicure or occupational repetitive trauma, such as cardboard box assembly.

In all instances of chronic trauma, management relies on identification of the cause and its avoidance. For some patterns of self-inflicted trauma, it is not easy to persuade the patient of their role in the process. Physical protection of the nail and nail fold with occlusive dressing, sometimes supplemented with steroid ointment, can be helpful in instances of fingernail problems.

General diseases affecting the nails

Nail changes in systemic illness

Acute illness
Acute illness results in a transverse line of atrophy known as a Beau's line. Shedding of the nail, onychomedesis, may occur in severe illness.

Chronic illness
Clubbing affects the soft tissues of the terminal phalanx with swelling and an increase in the angle between the nail plate and the nail fold. There is chronic swelling of periungual tissues with increased vasculature associated with an increase in the transverse and longitudinal curvature of the nail (see Figure 20.7). At the base of the nail the angle with the nail fold is lost due to the swelling and the nail fold has a 'boggy' consistency. It is due to systemic or inherited factors which mean that it affects all nails, although the changes in the toes are less obvious than in the digits of the hands. It is associated with chronic respiratory disease, cyanotic heart disease and

occasionally inflammatory bowel disease. It can be hereditary and may be unilateral in association with vascular abnormalities.

Cyanosis Where cyanotic heart disease or fibrotic or cavitating pulmonary disease is the underlying cause, the nail bed may be cyanosed. In idiopathic variants, or where there is underlying inflammatory bowel and liver disease it can be a normal pink colour.

Splinter haemorrhages occur beneath the nail and are usually the result of minor trauma. They are also associated with a wide range of general medical conditions including subacute bacterial endocarditis and severe rheumatoid arthritis.

Lesions adjacent to the nail

Viral warts are the most common tumour arising in the nail folds and nail bed with secondary effects on the nail plate. In childhood these usually resolve without treatment. In adults, resolution is less predictable. Topical, surgical, laser and chemotherapeutic options are available but all have a significant failure rate with possible complications of pain, infection and scarring in the more aggressive treatments.

Myxoid pseudocysts arise through damage to the synovial capsule which allows escape of synovial fluid in the subcutaneous tissue. This is usually secondary to osteoarthritis although it can be caused by specific trauma. The fluid collects on the dorsal aspect of the digit, beneath the proximal nail fold but above the matrix, or beneath the matrix. Where the location impinges on the nail matrix, nail plate growth will be altered to reflect the pattern of pressure (Figure 20.20). Careful ligature of the defect in the synovial capsule can be curative, but has a relatively high failure rate in the toes.

Naevi may occur adjacent to the nail and a benign melanocytic naevus can produce a pigmented streak. Subungual melanoma may produce considerable pigmentation of the nail and often causes pigmentation of the cuticle, Hutchinson's sign. Sometimes subungual melanoma is amelanotic so there are no pigmentary changes and any rapidly growing soft tumour should raise suspicions of this condition.

Subungual exostosis can cause a painful lesion under the nail (Figure 20.21). It is confirmed by X-ray examination. Lateral and plane views are needed to ensure that a subtle bony protuberance is not missed. A large part of the pathology is the cartilaginous cap which is radiolucent.

Glomus tumours arise as dermal tumours beneath the nail. They are characterized by pain which is worse in the cold and at night. Pain can be diminished by elevating the limb. When the tumour is in the nail bed there may be minimal or nil clinical changes. When it is located beneath the matrix, pressure upon the matrix will alter matrix function. This causes a red streak in the nail, which ultimately may wear through the nail and produce a split. Treatment is by surgical excision.

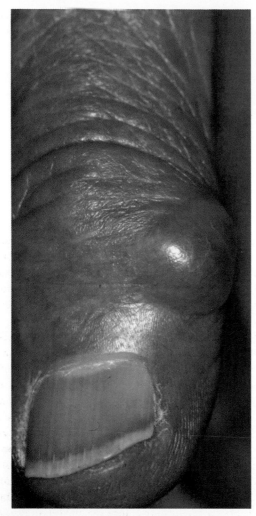

Figure 20.20 Mucoid cyst, also called myxoid pseudocyst.

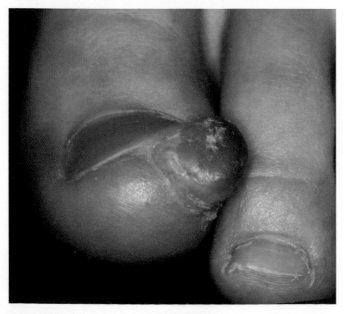

Figure 20.21 Subungual exostosis of the big toe.

Periungual fibrokeratomas appear as firm fibrous lumps that may be spherical or elongated. Nail growth is altered by pressure on the nail matrix. They are associated with tuberous sclerosis but this is unlikely with single lesions in an adult. However, a full examination and family history should be carried out to ensure that the diagnosis has not been missed. Patients presenting with multiple tumours are more likely to have tuberous sclerosis. Surgery can be effective in fibromas causing functional impairment or pain.

Treatment of nail conditions

Inflammatory and infective nail conditions often occur when there has been inadequate hand or foot care. The principles of care of the nails are as follows.

- Keep nails short. Do not cut toenails too short for fear of precipitating ingrowing nail.
- Dry hands and feet carefully after washing, especially between digits.
- Wear gloves when undertaking wet work, gardening or work entailing contact with solvents or abrasive materials.
- Ensure well-fitting footwear with a high 'box' (the space at the end to accommodate the toes).
- Use emollients to prevent drying of the skin and treat early tinea pedis with topical antifungal creams.

Tumours require surgical management which is best provided by a dermatological surgeon or a plastic or orthopaedic surgeon with expertise in hand or foot surgery.

Severe systemic inflammatory diseases can be associated with nail changes that may be severe enough to affect function and quality of life. In these instances systemic therapies such as ciclosporin, methotrexate, retinoids, prednisolone or biologics may be warranted. The nature of nail growth means that benefit of therapy may not be seen for 2–3 months, but once the inflammatory disease is suppressed it is possible to discontinue therapy and await further improvement. Systemic therapy may be given as pulses which make it possible to reduce the risk of side-effects and to maximize cost benefit.

Further reading

Baran R, Dawber RPR, de Berker DAR, Haneke E, Tosti A, eds. *Baran and Dawber's Diseases of the Nails and Their Management*, 3rd edn. Blackwell Science, Oxford, 2001.

de Berker DA, Baran R, Dawber RP. *Handbook of Diseases of the Nails and their Management*. Blackwell Scientific Publications, Oxford, 1995.

CHAPTER 21

Benign Skin Tumours

OVERVIEW

- Skin cells can proliferate in a benign controlled manner, known as hyperplasia, or as an uncontrolled, dysplastic growth to produce cancer.

- Benign skin lesions are common and generally have a well-defined appearance. Any sudden increase in size, irregularity or bleeding may suggest malignant change.

- Benign skin lesions are generally asymptomatic but may bleed persistently (pyogenic granuloma) or cause pain (poroma and glomus tumour). Some benign tumours are disfiguring and cause psychological problems.

- Benign pigmented tumours include seborrhoeic warts, which are well defined with a warty rough dull surface, freckles (lentigines) and skin tags.

- Pigmented naevi may be congenital (present at birth) or acquired. The vast majority remain benign. However, change in colour, texture, size or new satellite lesions developing may indicate malignant change. Numerous benign lesions consist of papules, nodules and plaques.

- Benign vascular lesions include naevi such as port wine stain, cavernous haemangioma and naevus flammeus neonatorum.

- The most common acquired vascular lesions are spider naevi, Campbell de Morgan spots (cherry haemangiomas) and pyogenic granulomas.

Introduction

Any cell within the skin can proliferate to form a benign lump or skin tumour. In general a proliferation of cells can lead to hyperplasia (benign overgrowth) or dysplasia (malignancy/cancer). This chapter considers benign lesions which by definition are harmless, but may cause symptoms such as pain, itching and bleeding or may be a cosmetic nuisance. Many benign skin lesions are pigmented which can lead to a high level of anxiety for patients and occasionally medical staff as they may be confused with malignant melanoma.

Pattern recognition plays a valuable role in the correct diagnosis of benign skin lesions. The clinical features of any lesion can be

a useful guide to distinguishing the benign from the malignant. However if there is uncertainty as to the nature of any skin lesion after clinical examination then a diagnostic biopsy for histology is essential. The old adage 'if in doubt cut it out' may be appropriate if there is diagnostic uncertainty and skin experts are not available locally to see the patient.

Benign cutaneous lesions are almost universally present on the skin of adults and are therefore so common that most are ignored and are never brought to medical attention. Nonetheless, the sudden appearance of new lesions, symptoms such as itching, pain or bleeding or the unsightly nature of lesions may bring them to the attention of the affected individual and thus the local practitioner. Reassurance is usually all that is needed. However, in some instances benign skin lesions need removal, for example if they bleed persistently (pyogenic granulomas), they repeatedly catch on clothing (protuberant benign moles) or they cause pain (poroma on the foot), etc. Some individuals are deeply affected by the cosmetic appearance of their benign skin lesions and these may therefore need removal on psychological grounds.

From a medical practitioner's point of view we need to decide whether a lesion can be safely left or should be treated. This chapter concentrates on the correlation between clinical and pathological features of common benign tumours which should ease their diagnosis (Table 21.1). Chapter 22 examines premalignant and malignant skin tumours.

Pigmented benign tumours

Seborrhoeic warts

Seborrhoeic warts are increasingly common with increasing age. Lesions are most frequently seen on the trunk, face and neck in sizes varying from 0.5 to 3.0 cm in diameter. Seborrhoeic warts may be barely palpable, protuberant or pedunculated (Figures 21.1 & 21.2). They always have a warty dull surface. Colours are highly variable from pale tan through to dark brown. When deeply pigmented, inflamed or growing they can appear to have some malignant characteristics which may cause anxiety. Seborrhoeic keratoses, however, have some characteristic features which include:

- well-defined edge
- warty, papillary surface, often with keratin plugs
- raised above surrounding skin to give a 'stuck on' appearance.

ABC of Dermatology, 5th edition. Edited by P. K. Buxton and R. Morris-Jones.
© 2009 Blackwell Publishing, ISBN: 978-1-4051-7065-9.

Table 21.1 Differential diagnosis of common benign skin tumours.

Clinical features	Differential diagnoses
Pigmented	Seborrhoeic keratoses, dermatosis papulosa nigra, freckles (lentigines), solar lentigo, melanocytic naevus, blue naevus, Mongolian blue spot, dermatofibroma, apocrine hidrocystomas (r)
Vascular	Naevus flammeus, strawberry naevus, port-wine stain, spider naevi, Campbell de Morgan spots, pyogenic granuloma
Papules	Skin tags (fibroepithelial polyps), milia, sebaceous gland hyperplasia, dermatosis papulosa nigra, syringomas, trichoepitheliomas (r), apocrine hidrocystomas (r)
Nodules	Dermatofibroma, lipoma, angiolipoma, epidermoid cyst, pilar cyst, pilomatrixoma (r), poroma (r), intradermal naevus, apocrine hidrocystomas (r)
Plaques	Naevus sebaceus, epidermal naevus, inflammatory linear verrucous epidermal naevus (ILVEN), seborrhoeic keratoses

r, rare.

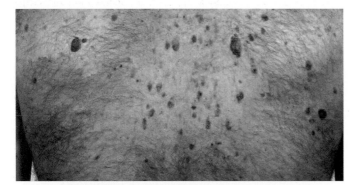

Figure 21.1 Seborrhoeic warts.

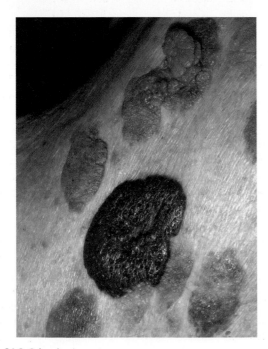

Figure 21.2 Seborrhoeic warts.

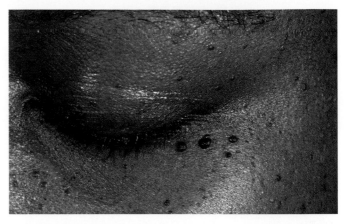

Figure 21.3 Dermatosis papulosa nigra.

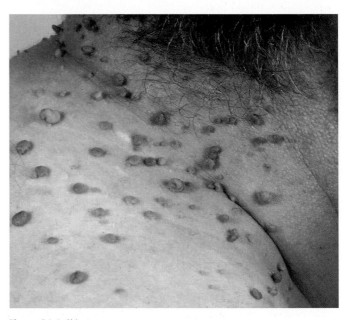

Figure 21.4 Skin tags.

Dermatosis papulosa nigra (DPN)

These lesions are usually multiple small pigmented papules seen on the face of adults with black skin (Figure 21.3). DPN is very common with up to one-third of individuals with skin type VI affected. Frequently there is a strong familial tendency towards the condition. Typically the lesions occur on the cheeks, forehead, neck and chest. Histologically they resemble seborrhoeic keratoses; however some experts think they arise from a developmental defect in the follicular unit. No treatment is needed, but if patients find the lesions cosmetically unacceptable then light electrodesiccation and gentle curettage can effectively remove lesions. New ones will inevitably form, however (see Chapter 23).

Skin tags

Skin tags may be pigmented but are usually straightforward to diagnose. They are frequently multiple and more commonly occur at sites of occlusion where the skin may be rubbed by skin or clothing/jewellery in the axillae, neck, groin and under the breasts (Figure 21.4). Histologically some are in fact pedunculated

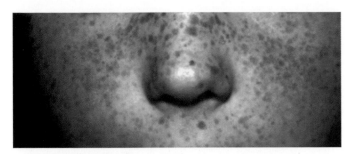

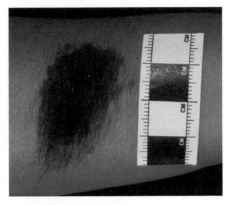

Figure 21.5 Lentigines.

Figure 21.6 Congenital melanocytic naevus.

seborrhoeic warts whilst others simple papillomas (fibroepithelial polyps).

Lentigines (freckles)

Patients often refer to solar-induced freckles as 'sun spots' or 'liver spots'. Lentigines are small macular well-demarcated pigmented lesions that usually occur on sun-exposed skin (Figure 21.5). They first appear in childhood and generally increase in number with increasing age. Lentigines are more common in individuals with fair rather than dark skin types. The colour of the lentigines varies from pale tan to almost black which usually corresponds to the amount of melanin pigment produced by the increased number of melanocytes. In contrast to moles where the melanocytes form nests (naevi), the melanocytes in lentigines line up along the basement membrane.

Benign lentigines may also occur on the lip and genital mucosa. Labial lentigines may be associated with Peutz–Jeghers syndrome (an inherited condition with gastrointestinal polyps), Laugier–Hunziker syndrome (which has associated nail pigmentation) and LAMB (lentigines, atrial myxoma, mucocutaneous myxomas and blue naevi). In LEOPARD syndrome (lentigines, electrocardioconduction defects, ocular hypertelorism, pulmonary stenosis, abnormal genitalia, retardation of growth and deafness) lentigines are characteristically seen on the neck and trunk.

Melanocytic naevi

The majority of moles are benign and can be safely ignored. However, knowing which are potentially harmful or malignant can be difficult for inexperienced practitioners. Clinical features of benign moles will be considered in this chapter to aid their diagnosis. Malignant moles are considered in Chapter 22.

The term naevi is derived from the Greek word meaning 'nest'. A proliferation of melanocytes forms these nests at different levels in the skin resulting in moles. If the nests of melanocytes are confined to the dermoepidermal junction then the mole is referred to as 'junctional naevus', if they are in the dermis only – 'intradermal naevus' and if present in the epidermis and dermis – 'compound naevus'. Naevi may be congenital ('birth mark') or acquired, usually in early childhood. The number of moles usually remains static in adulthood with a decline after the sixth decade.

Congenital melanocytic naevi

Between 1 and 2% of neonates have a congenital naevus present at birth. Similar lesions can appear during the first 2 years of life that look histologically identical to congenital moles. Melanocytes are derived from neural crest cells; during embryogenesis they migrate into the skin and central nervous system. Congenital naevi are thought to result from an anomaly of melanocyte development or migration. Congenital naevi are classified according to their size: small are <1.5 cm, medium 1.5–19.9 cm and giant >20 cm in diameter. Congenital naevi usually grow in proportion to the growth of the child, and their colour varies from pale brown to black. With increasing age congenital naevi often develop hair and become more protuberant (Figure 21.6).

Giant lesions can cover a considerable area of the trunk and buttocks, such as the bathing trunk naevi, and these are the most likely to undergo malignant change (approximately 5%). The majority of congenital naevi are, however, benign. If malignancy is suspected due to a sudden change in size, colour, border and development of new satellite lesions then surgical excision would be indicated. Surgical removal of very large lesions may be difficult, and tissue expanders, staged operations and skin grafting are often needed. Attempts at curettage or laser removal have both been advocated as alternatives to excision, but recurrence is more likely.

Mongolian blue spots are congenital skin lesions that result from collections of melanocytes deep in the skin, usually present on the back. The lesions are macular and large and may be multiple. The condition is most common in black and Asian skin (Figure 21.7).

Acquired melanocytic naevi

These are moles acquired during childhood. The main stimulus to their formation is thought to be solar radiation and a genetic susceptibility. These moles have a variable appearance determined by the depth of the melanocytes and the cellular type.

Junctional naevi are flat macules with melanocytes proliferating into nests that sit along the dermoepidermal junction (Figure 21.8).

Compound naevi have clusters of melanocytes at the dermoepidermal junction and within the dermis. These naevi are raised and pigmented (Figure 21.9). The surface of the naevus may be thrown into folds due to the melanocyte proliferations, giving a papillary appearance.

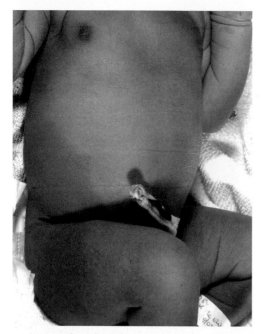

Figure 21.7 Mongolian blue spot.

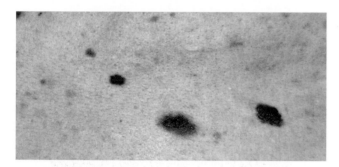

Figure 21.8 Junctional naevus.

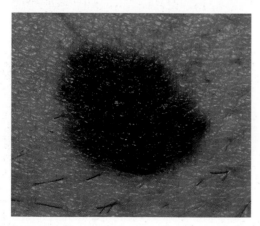

Figure 21.9 Compound naevus.

In a purely *intradermal naevus* the junctional element is lost, and nests of melanocytes are found within the dermis alone. These naevi are frequently non-pigmented and most commonly occur on the face (Figure 21.10).

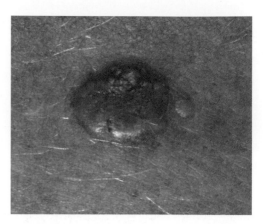

Figure 21.10 Intradermal naevus.

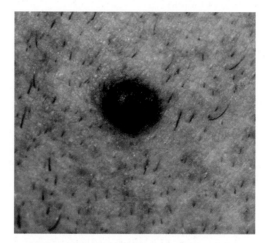

Figure 21.11 Blue naevus.

Blue naevus is a collection of deeply pigmented melanocytes situated deep in the dermis, which accounts for the deep slate-blue colour (Figure 21.11).

Spitz naevus presents as a fleshy pink papule in children. It is composed of large spindle cells and epitheloid cells with occasional giant cells, arranged in nests (Figure 21.12).

Halo naevus consists of a melanocytic naevus with a surrounding halo of depigmentation (Figure 21.13). Patients may have several halo naevi simultaneously. They are thought to be associated with the presence of antibodies against melanocytes, which can cause the entire naevus to disappear eventually.

Becker's naevus is an area of increased pigmentation, often associated with increased hair growth, which is usually seen on the upper trunk or shoulders (Figure 21.14).

Dermatofibroma

These are firm discrete nodules arising in the dermis, usually on the legs of women. Initially lesions may appear red or light brown but usually mature into a firm brown papule with a ring of darker peripheral pigment (Figure 21.15). Lesions may be itchy or even

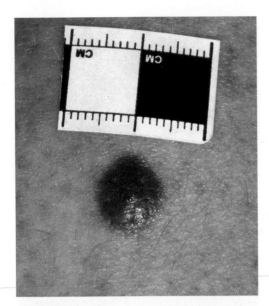

Figure 21.12 Spitz naevus.

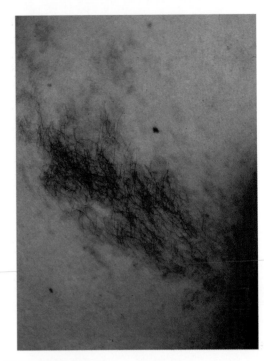

Figure 21.14 Becker's naevus.

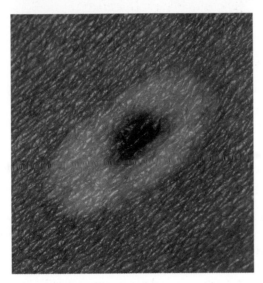

Figure 21.13 Halo naevus.

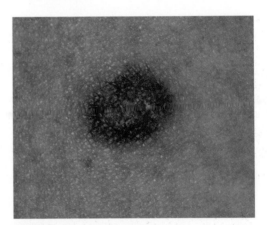

Figure 21.15 Dermatofibroma.

painful. The underlying pathophysiology is poorly understood; some authors believe they arise at the site of insect bites or minor trauma whilst others believe them to be a true benign tumour of fibroblasts.

Benign vascular tumours

The most common benign vascular malformations and tumours are described and their management options discussed.

Naevus flammeus neonatorum refers to 'stork marks' or 'salmon patches' present at birth most commonly at the glabella, eyelids and nape of the neck (Figure 21.16). Up to one-third of neonates are affected. Lesions on the neck persist for life; however facial lesions usually fade or completely disappear by the age of 2 years.

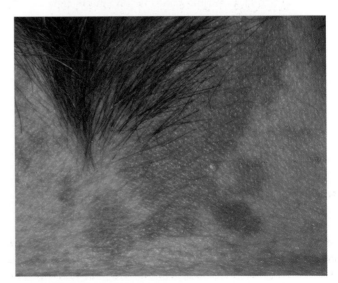

Figure 21.16 Naevus flammeus neonatorum.

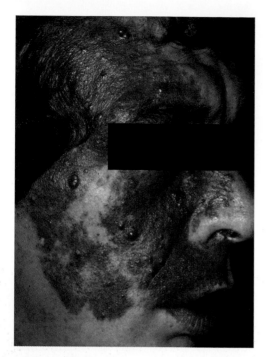

Figure 21.17 Sturge–Weber syndrome.

Port-wine stains are capillary malformations of the superficial dermal blood vessels that are present at birth. Therefore they are not strictly neoplasms but are discussed here for convenience. They most commonly occur on the head and neck. Lesions may initially be a pale pink colour but darken with increasing age through red to purple. Capillary malformations increase in size proportionally with the growth of the child and tend to persist. Port wine stains on the face are usually unilateral with a sharp midline border (Figure 21.17). In time the affected area becomes raised and thickened due to a proliferation of vascular and connective tissue. If the area supplied by the ophthalmic or maxillary divisions of the trigeminal nerve is affected there may be associated angiomas of the underlying meningies with epilepsy – Sturge–Weber syndrome. Patients should have an MRI scan with gadolinium enhancement to visualize neural involvement. Klippel–Trenaunay syndrome usually presents with a capillary malformation associated with limb overgrowth and varicosities. In addition lesions of the limb may be associated with arteriovenous fistulae: the so-called Parkes–Weber syndrome.

Capillary malformations may be treated with a pulsed-dye laser which targets oxyhaemoglobin (see Chapter 24). The ideal age for treatment is difficult to determine. Some experts feel laser treatment should be undertaken before the first birthday, but a general anaesthetic may be necessary. The outcome of laser treatment depends on the size, location and depth of vessels in the skin, but most lesions require multiple treatments. Patients can be offered cosmetic camouflage.

Cavernous haemangiomas/strawberry naevi are true benign vascular neoplasms which grow out of proportion to the growing neonate. These lesions usually appear at birth or during the first few weeks of life and rapidly enlarge at around 6 months of age (Figure 21.18).

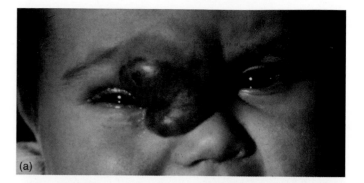

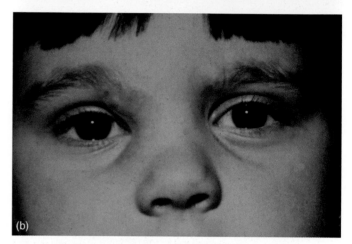

Figure 21.18 Cavernous haemangioma. (a) At 5 months of age. (b) At 5 years of age.

The exact cause is unknown; however, several theories exist including speculation that they may arise from endothelial cells breaking away from the placenta. Lesions may be single (80%) or multiple and are more common in infants whose mothers underwent chorionic villous sampling. Clinically a soft vascular swelling is found, most commonly on the head and neck. The lesions resolve spontaneously in time and do not require intervention unless recurrently bleeding or interference with visual development occurs. Interventions include surgery, laser treatment, prednisolone and sclerotherapy (see Chapter 24).

Spider naevi consist of a central vascular papule with fine lines radiating from it (Figure 21.19). They are more common in children and women. Large numbers may raise the possibility of liver disease or an underlying connective tissue disorder such as systemic sclerosis.

Campbell de Morgan spots (cherry haemangiomas) are discrete red papules 1–5 mm in diameter. They occur in up to 50% of adults, are usually multiple and occur most frequently on the trunk (Figure 21.20).

Pyogenic granuloma is poorly named as it is not infectious but a lobular capillary haemangioma. The usually single vascular lesion grows rapidly and easily bleeds with minor trauma (Figure 21.21). The bleeding can be profuse and recurrent. Lesions may arise at the site of trauma, often on the digits. Distinction from amelanotic

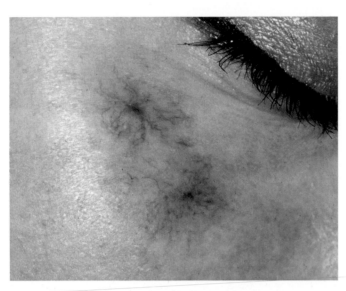

Figure 21.19 Spider naevi.

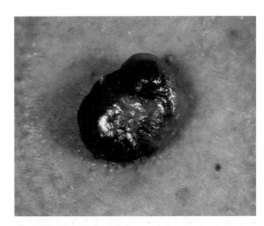

Figure 21.21 Pyogenic granuloma.

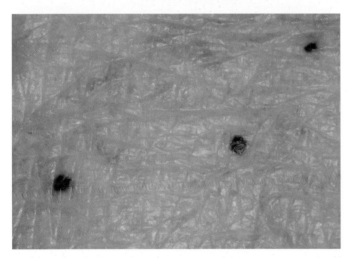

Figure 21.20 Campbell de Morgan spots.

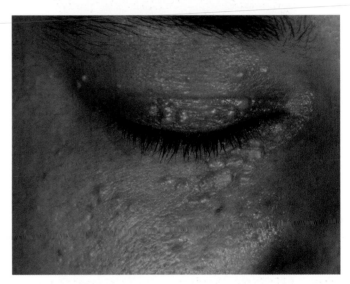

Figure 21.22 Syringomas.

melanoma is important. Although benign, pyogenic granulomas need to be removed surgically by curettage and cautery as they rarely resolve spontaneously (see Chapter 23).

Benign tumour papules

These commonly include skin tags (fibroepithelial polyps – see above), dermatosis papulosa nigra (see above), syringomas, trichoepitheliomas, apocrine hidrocystomas, milia and sebaceous gland hyperplasia.

Syringomas are benign adnexal tumours of the eccrine glands. Lesions are usually multiple, slow-growing, small and flesh coloured, and usually appear on the face around puberty (Figure 21.22). The trunk and groin areas may also be affected. Treatment on cosmetic grounds is surgical with shave removal or cautery of the lesions.

Trichoepitheliomas are benign adnexal tumours of hair follicle origin. These may resemble syringomas as they are also small, often

multiple and occur on the face and scalp (Figure 21.23). Surgical removal or laser treatment can help to alleviate the cosmetic appearance but lesions tend to be multiple and may recur.

Apocrine hidrocystoma are benign adnexal tumours of apocrine glands that form papules or nodules around the eyes. Lesions are usually solitary and may be translucent or pale through to black (lipofuscin pigment).

Milia are small keratin cysts consisting of small white papules found on the cheek and eyelids. Milia are common on the cheeks of newborns, and secondary milia may occur following skin trauma or inflammation (Figure 21.24). These minute cysts are harmless and require no treatment. They can be removed under topical anaesthetic with a sterile needle.

Sebaceous gland hyperplasia is a benign hamartomatous enlargement of the sebaceous glands and therefore not a tumour. However these small papules are not infrequently confused with benign skin tumours and basal cell carcinomas, and therefore are discussed here (Figure 21.25). Turnover of sebocyte cells within the glands decreases

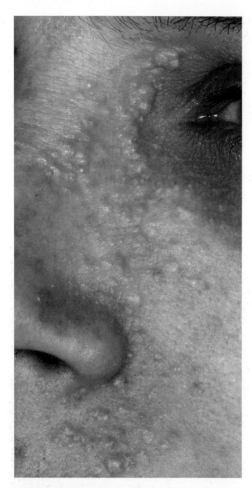

Figure 21.23 Trichoepitheliomas.

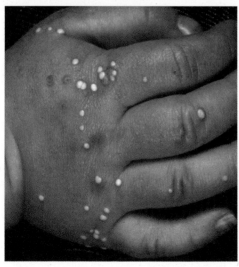

Figure 21.24 Milia.

with increasing age leading to hyperplasia. This is particularly prominent in patients who are immunosuppressed with ciclosporin. There is an increased frequency of sebaceous gland hyperplasia reported with Muir–Torré syndrome. Patients develop sebaceous adenomas/carcinomas in association with systemic malignancies.

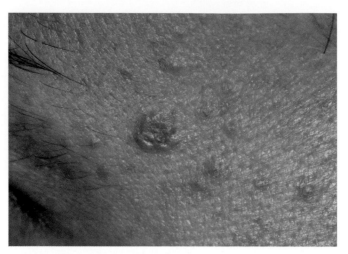

Figure 21.25 Sebaceous gland hyperplasia.

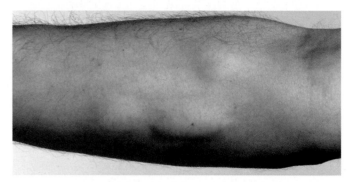

Figure 21.26 Lipoma.

Benign tumour nodules

Lipomas are common slow-growing benign subcutaneous tumours of fat. They may be congenital or acquired, single or multiple (Figure 21.26). Lipomas are usually asymptomatic but they may classically cause pain when they are associated with Dercum's disease (postmenopausal women who may be obese, depressed or alcoholic with multiple painful lipomas on the lower legs). *Angiolipomas* may also be painful.

Benign painful tumours in the skin: 'BENGAL'
- *B*lue rubber bleb naevus
- *E*ccrine spiradenoma
- *N*eurilemmoma/neuroma
- *G*lomus tumour
- *A*ngiolipoma
- *L*eiomyoma.

Epidermoid cysts (previously called sebaceous cyst) are common. They are soft, well-defined, mobile swellings usually on the face, neck, shoulders or chest. There may be an obvious central punctum (Figure 21.27). These are not derived from sebaceous glands and therefore the term sebaceous cyst should not be used. Epidermoid cysts arise due to a proliferation of epidermal cells in the dermis

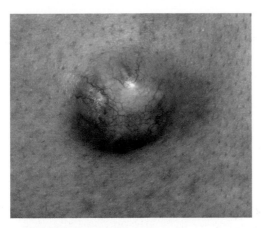

Figure 21.27 Epidermoid cyst.

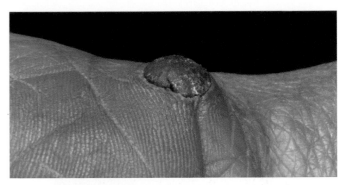

Figure 21.29 Eccrine poroma.

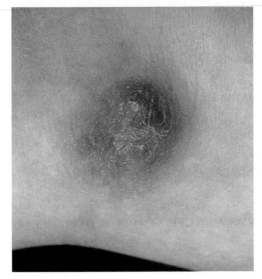

Figure 21.28 Pilomatrixoma.

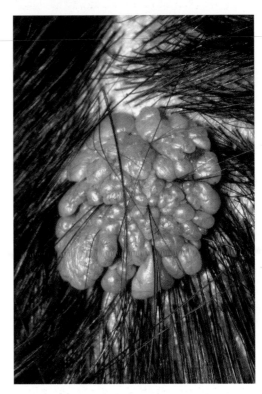

Figure 21.30 Naevus sebaceous.

derived from the hair follicle. They may become inflamed or infected causing discomfort and discharge (thick yellow material that has a bad odour) but are generally asymptomatic. If cysts are troublesome they can be completely excised or removed by punch extrusion (see Chapter 23).

Pilar cysts on the scalp are very common and frequently multiple. Clinically they can resemble epidermoid cysts but they do not have a punctum. They are derived from hair follicles. Surgical removal may be necessary in some cases, when the tumour usually 'shells out' very easily.

Pilomatrixoma is a benign tumour of the hair matrix. A very hard slow-growing lump usually presents on the head/neck of a child (Figure 21.28). Lesions may be a few centimetres in diameter. Spontaneous regression is not usually observed, and although they are benign most tumours are excised for histology.

Poromas may be apocrine- or eccrine-derived benign tumours of the skin. These nodular lesions are slow growing but may be painful

(Figure 21.29). Rarely lesions may undergo malignant transformation. Surgical excision of poromas is the treatment of choice.

Benign tumour plaques

Naevus sebaceous is a warty, well-defined plaque of 0.5–2 cm in diameter that mainly occurs on the scalp. Lesions may be present at birth or appear during childhood and slowly increase in size. In neonates a hairless yellow plaque may be seen on the scalp (Figure 21.30). As the lesion matures it may become verrucous and occasionally a trichoblastoma may develop within it. This is a benign tumour that may be misdiagnosed histologically as a basal cell carcinoma. Very large lesions may be associated with internal disorders.

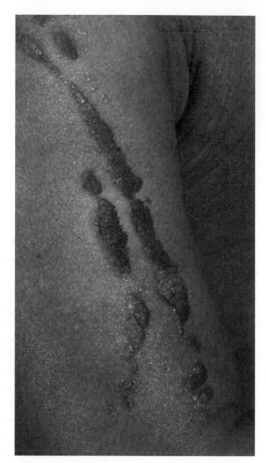

Figure 21.31 Epidermal naevus.

Epidermal naevi are congenital lesions that may be linear or clustered and appear as warty brown papular lesions on the skin (Figure 21.31).

Inflammatory linear verrucous epidermal naevus (ILVEN) may be present at birth or appear during the first 5 years of life, most commonly on the lower limb or trunk. Lesions are warty and brown and are usually linear or clustered. Lesions may become red and inflamed and may be mistaken for eczema (Figure 21.32). Topical steroids and emollients may help to relieve itching and dryness.

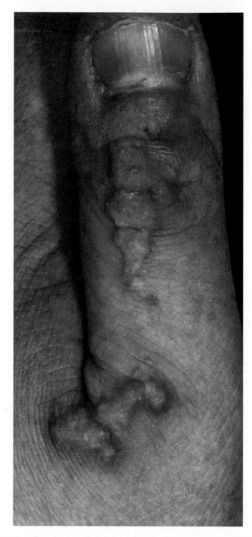

Figure 21.32 Inflammatory linear verrucous epidermal naevus (ILVEN).

Further reading

Leboit PE, Burg G, Weedon D, Sarasin A. *Pathology and Genetics of Tumours of the Skin* (IARC WHO Classification of Tumours). WHO, Lyon, 2005.
Mackie RM. *Skin Cancer: An Illustrated Guide to the Etiology, Clinical Features, Pathology and Management of Benign and Malignant Cutaneous Tumours*, 2nd edn. Martin Dunitz, London, 1996.

CHAPTER 22

Premalignant and Malignant Skin Tumours

OVERVIEW

- Skin cancers are amongst the most common malignancies and arise when there is there is an uncontrolled proliferation of undifferentiated dysplastic cells.

- In premalignant lesions there is abnormal growth of cells but not complete dysplastic change. This occurs in actinic keratoses and Bowen's disease.

- Squamous cell carcinoma develops in previously normal skin or pre-existing lesions such as actinic keratoses or Bowen's disease.

- Basal cell carcinoma (BCC) is the most common cancer in humans, occurring most commonly on the face. Clumps of dysplastic basal cells form nodules that expand and break down to form an ulcer with a rolled edge.

- The carcinogenic effect of the sun is an important cause of skin cancer and is a major factor in the high incidence of malignant melanoma.

- Pigmented naevi or moles are usually benign but the signs of malignant change must be recognized.

- Malignant melanoma is a malignant tumour of melanocytes. A major risk factor is high-intensity UV exposure, particularly in childhood.

- Melanoma occurs in various forms; superficial spreading melanoma is the most common. Other types include lentigo maligna melanoma, nodular melanoma, acral melanoma and amelanotic melanoma.

- The prognosis of melanoma depends on the depth of invasion.

Introduction

Malignancies of the skin are amongst the most common cancers known to man. In benign tumours there is a proliferation of well-differentiated cells with limited growth, whereas in a malignant tumour the dysplastic cells are undifferentiated and expand in an uncontrolled manner. The carcinogenic effect of the sun is thought to play an important role in many types of skin cancer. One hundred years ago a tanned skin pointed to working outdoors. Nowadays many individuals deliberately seek the sun for the

purposes of tanning. Longer holidays, cheap flights and a fashion to be tanned may all have contributed to the doubling incidence of malignant melanoma over the past decade.

However, recently there has been an increasing global awareness concerning the dangers of strong sunlight. Public health campaigns such as 'slip slop slap' ('*slip* on a shirt, *slop* on sunscreen, and *slap* on a hat') in Australia have been very successful at modifying people's behaviour in the sun. High-intensity ultraviolet (UV) light can lead to sunburning episodes in fair-skinned individuals, and this is thought to be a risk factor for malignant melanoma, the most serious form of skin cancer.

The visible nature of skin cancer means detection should be straightforward by the trained eye, although histological confirmation is essential. Early recognition of malignant skin tumours by medical practitioners is essential in order that patients suffer minimal morbidity and avoid skin cancer-induced mortality.

Premalignant skin tumours

Actinic keratoses

Actinic keratoses (AKs) occur on exposed skin, particularly in those who have worked outdoors or have been exposed to short intervals of high-intensity UV. AKs occur on the face (including the lip), dorsal hands, distal limbs and bald scalp, particularly in those with fair skin and increasing age (Figure 22.1). Clinically their appearance varies from a rough area of skin to a raised keratotic lesion. The edge is irregular and they are usually less than 1 cm in diameter. Histologically AKs have altered keratinization which may lead to dysplasia and eventually invasive squamous cell carcinoma. Malignant change may be suspected in an AK that suddenly grows rapidly, becomes painful or inflamed.

Management

Treatment with liquid nitrogen (cryotherapy) by a medical practitioner is usually effective for individual lesions with cure rates of around 70% (see Chapter 23). Various topical preparations that can be applied by patients themselves are currently available. 5-Fluorouracil (5-FU) 5% cream is useful for larger or multiple AKs, and is applied once daily for 4–6 weeks. The 5-FU kills any dysplastic keratinocytes and therefore produces brisk inflammation at the application site. Patients may therefore need to stop using the cream for a few days during the treatment course if discomfort is severe.

ABC of Dermatology, 5th edition. Edited by P. K. Buxton and R. Morris-Jones.
© 2009 Blackwell Publishing, ISBN: 978-1-4051-7065-9.

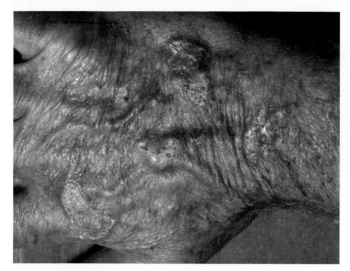

Figure 22.1 Actinic keratoses.

Imiquimod 5% is an immunomodulatory preparation that recruits immune cells to the area of skin where it is applied, thus attacking the dysplastic cells. Imiquimod is applied three times a week for 4 months. There is some evidence that memory T-cells are induced by this therapy, resulting subsequently in lower numbers of clinical AKs.

Topical non-steroidal anti-inflammatory diclofenac has been shown to be effective against AKs if it is used regularly twice daily for 3 months. This treatment seems to produce less skin irritation than 5-FU or imiquimod.

Photodynamic therapy (PDT) (see Chapter 24) has been shown to be as effective as 5-FU.

Any lesions not responding to the above measures should be biopsied to check for invasive malignancy.

Bowen's disease

Bowen's disease is squamous cell carcinoma (SCC) *in situ*; in other words SCC in the epidermis with no evidence of dermal invasion. Bowen's disease is more common in the elderly and is seen most frequently on the trunk and limbs. Risk factors for Bowen's disease include solar radiation, human papillomasvirus warts (HPV 16), radiotherapy, ingestion of arsenic in 'tonics' and exposure to chemicals. Clinically Bowen's disease is characterized by well-defined, erythematous macules with slight crusting (Figure 22.2). Lesions enlarge slowly and may reach up to 3 cm in diameter. After many years invasive carcinoma may develop. Bowen's disease may be confused with a patch of eczema or superficial basal cell carcinoma. Erythroplasia of Queyrat is a similar process occurring on the glans penis or prepuce.

Skin biopsy can confirm the diagnosis histologically. Management includes excision, curettage and cautery, cryotherapy, 5-FU, imiquimod 5% and photodynamic therapy (see Chapters 23 & 24).

Malignant skin tumours

Basal cell carcinoma (BCC)

This is the most common cancer in humans with a lifetime risk of around 30%. Known risk factors for BCC include increasing

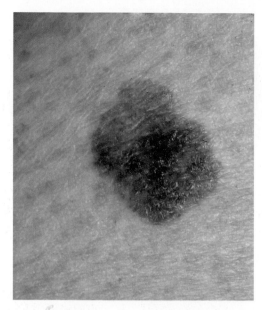

Figure 22.2 Bowen's disease.

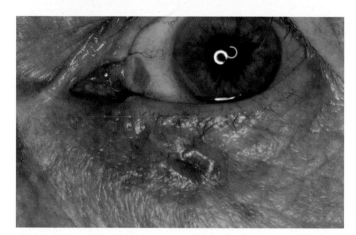

Figure 22.3 Nodular-type basal cell carcinoma below the eye.

age, fair skin, high-intensity UV exposure, radiation, immunosuppression, previous history of BCCs and congenital disorders such as Gorlin's syndrome. Sun-exposed skin in the 'mask area' of the face is most frequently affected. Typically lesions start as small papules that slowly grow. Lesions often have a 'pearly' shiny translucent quality. Colour varies from clear to deeply pigmented. The tumour is composed of masses of dividing basal cells that have lost the capacity to differentiate any further. As a result no epidermis is formed over the tumour and the surface breaks down to form an ulcer, the residual edges of the nodule forming the characteristic 'rolled edge'. Once the basal cells have invaded the deeper tissues the rolled edge disappears.

BCC types

Nodular appear as small papules or nodules with a rolled edge and frequently a central depression that may become ulcerated. The nodules are pearly and may have dilated telangiectatic vessels on their surface. Some BCCs appear more cystic in nature (Figures 22.3–22.5).

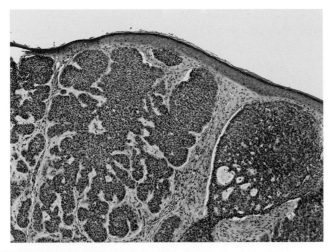

Figure 22.4 Nodular basal cell carcinoma histology.

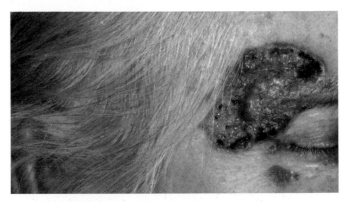

Figure 22.7 Pigmented basal cell carcinoma.

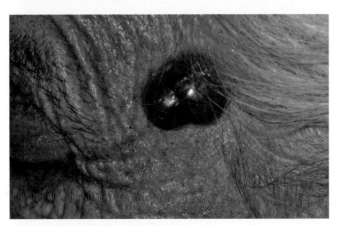

Figure 22.5 Cystic basal cell carcinoma.

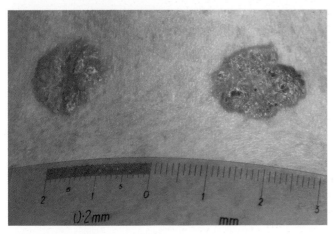

Figure 22.6 Superficial basal cell carcinoma.

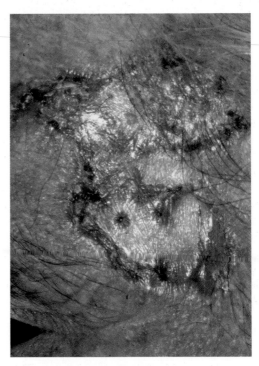

Figure 22.8 Morphoeic basal cell carcinoma.

Morphoeic or sclerosing type appears as a superficial atrophic scar in the skin. There is loss of the normal skin markings and the edge is usually indistinct (Figure 22.8). This can lead to incomplete excision of these infiltrative BCCs and therefore Moh's micrographic surgery may be indicated (see Chapter 23) to ensure surgical cure.

Management of BCC

The diagnosis is confirmed histologically which also provides information on the behaviour of the tumour cells – superficial, micro- or macronodular and invasive. The site, size and histological appearances guide therapy. Treatment options include excision (including Moh's micrographic surgery), excision and grafting, curettage and cautery, radiotherapy, cryotherapy, imiquimod 5% and photodynamic therapy for large superficial BCCs (see Chapters 23 & 24). Therapy options are frequently discussed with the patient at a multidisciplinary skin cancer meeting including dermatologists, plastic

Superficial appear as a patch on the skin, often on the trunk. They may be mistaken for a patch of eczema or tinea, but are not usually pruritic and slowly enlarge (Figure 22.6). A firm 'whipcord' edge may be present.

Pigmented can lead to confusion with naevi, seborrhoeic keratoses and melanoma (Figure 22.7).

surgeons, oculoplastic surgeons, oncologists and specialist cancer nurses.

As a general rule surgical scars will improve with time compared to radiotherapy sites which tend to deteriorate cosmetically. Surgery is frequently preferable around the eyes and other vital structures where identifying clear tumour margins is desirable. Large nasal tip lesions may be more optimally treated with radiotherapy as this can be a difficult site for grafting.

Squamous cell carcinoma (SCC)

Squamous cell carcinoma is the second most common form of skin cancer after basal cell carcinoma (BCC). Risk factors for SCC are similar to those for BCCs but in addition SCC may develop in any chronic wound or scar (Marjolin's ulcer), and human papillomaviruses (HPV) are thought to play a significant role in the pathogenesis. Transplant patients who are medically immunosuppressed seem to be particularly susceptible to the development of SCCs which may be HPV mediated.

Dysplastic proliferations of abnormal keratinocytes may arise *de novo* or in pre-existing skin lesions such as actinic keratoses or Bowen's disease. By definition SCCs have invasive tumour cells within the dermis. Seventy per cent of lesions occur on the head and neck. Clinical suspicion of an SCC arises when lesions are rapidly growing, painful and markedly hyperkeratotic (Figures 22.9–22.11). SCCs are usually nodular with surface changes including crusting, ulceration or the formation of a cutaneous horn. Some lesions can be verrucous and therefore mistaken for viral warts, or indeed arise from a chronic viral wart.

Keratoacanthoma is thought to be a variant of SCC, and current thinking dictates these should be treated as if they are indeed SCCs. These lesions typically appear rapidly over a few weeks and have a characteristic central crater within the nodule (Figure 22.12). They may spontaneously regress leaving a significant scar which has led to debate about their exact nature and how they should be managed. Histologically they look malignant and most specialists feel comfortable treating them as for an SCC.

Regional lymph nodes should be palpated to look for local metastases for any lesions suspicious of a SCC, in addition involvement of other organs such as the liver, lung or brain may occur. A CT scan may be indicated for very large or aggressive lesions before decisions concerning management.

Management of SCC

Management of these patients should ideally be discussed at a multidisciplinary team meeting with the patient (see above under management of BCC).

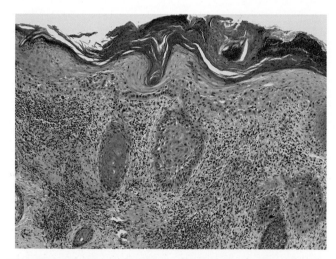

Figure 22.11 Squamous cell carcinoma histology.

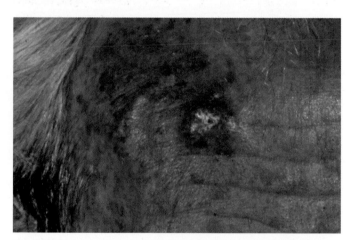

Figure 22.9 Squamous cell carcinoma: early stages.

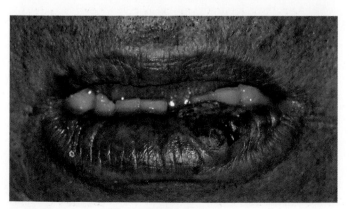

Figure 22.10 Squamous cell carcinoma on the lip.

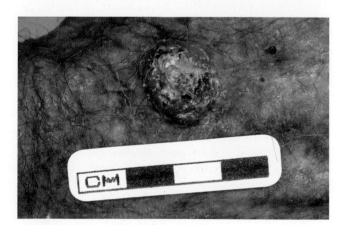

Figure 22.12 Keratoacanthoma.

Surgical options. Ideally lesions should be excised with a 4–6 mm margin. Skin grafting may be required depending on the size of the lesion and the site. Tumour curettage and cautery (three passes over the affected area) can be highly successful in experienced hands.

Medical options. Radiotherapy can provide excellent results for tumours not amenable to surgery. Radiotherapy does, however, involve multiple trips to the hospital and symptoms of pain at the site during healing. In patients who develop multiple SCCs such as renal transplant patients secondary prophylaxis may be considered with oral retinoids. These have been shown to reduce the number of new lesions appearing if taken indefinitely.

Moles/naevi: benign or malignant?

The term naevus (mole) is derived from the Greek word meaning 'nest' which is formed by a proliferation of melanocytes. Benign moles show little change and remain static for years. Any change may indicate that a mole is becoming more active or even transforming into a melanoma. Size, shape and colour are the main features, and it is change in these that is most important. The ABCDE acronym is a useful guide for assessing the malignant potential of a mole: *a*symmetry, *b*order (irregular), *c*olour (irregular), *d*iameter (>0.5cm), *e*volving (Box 22.1). Any symptoms such as itching, crusting, ulceration or bleeding may also indicate malignant transformation. Patients can be educated about what changes to look for in their own moles so they can alert their local practitioner about any changes. Examine all the patient's skin and look for any mole that 'stands out from the crowd'.

Dysplastic naevi

These are moles that look atypical ('funny-looking moles'). They are often deeply pigmented and have an irregular margin (Figure 22.13). Clinically and histologically they have features of very early malignant change and therefore could progress to malignant melanoma. Fifty per cent of superficial spreading malignant

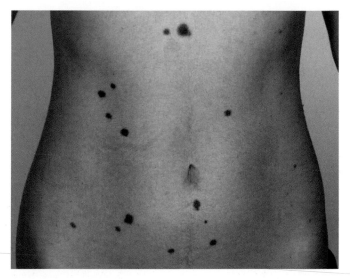

Figure 22.13 Dysplasic naevi.

melanomas are thought to arise from pre-existing moles, many of which are atypical.

Some patients have multiple atypical moles and may have the so-called *dysplastic naevus syndrome*. Usually there is a family history of dysplastic moles. During adolescence these patients acquire multiple pigmented moles most frequently on the trunk. Compared to normal moles these naevi are larger and their pigment more heterogeneous. These patients often need regular monitoring by a skin specialist.

Malignant melanoma (MM)

Melanoma is an invasive malignant tumour of melanocytes. Melanoma accounts for 4% of skin tumours but is responsible for 75% of skin cancer deaths. Most cases occur in white adults over the age of 30. Females are more commonly affected than males in the USA but this trend is reversed in Australia. Solar radiation is a known carcinogen and is considered to be the main risk factor for MM, particularly intermittent unaccustomed and high-intensity UV exposure particularly in childhood. Other risk factors include light skin tones, poorly tanning skin, red or fair-coloured hair, light-coloured eyes, female sex, increasing age, a personal or family history of MM and congenital defect of DNA repair (xeroderma pigmentosum). The presence of giant congenital melanocytic naevi, one to four dysplastic naevi, multiple common moles, actinic lentigines and change in a mole are additional risk factors for MM.

Incidence

The incidence of melanoma has tripled over the past 20 years. In Australia, 1 in 35 women and 1 in 25 men will develop melanoma during their lifetime. In Europe there are 63 000 new cases of malignant melanoma diagnosed each year, accounting for 2% of all cases. In the USA the lifetime risk of developing MM is estimated to be 1 in 60.

Sun exposure

The highest incidence of melanoma occurs in countries near the equator with high-intensity UV throughout the year. However,

---

Box 22.1 **The ABCDE of malignant pigmented lesions**

- *Asymmetry* – if you draw an imaginary line through the centre of a mole in any axis and both halves match then the mole is symmetrical and likely to be benign. *Growth* – benign pigmented naevi continue to appear in adolescents and young adults. Any mole increasing in size in an adult over the age of 30 may be a melanoma
- *Border* – benign moles usually have an even, regular outline. Any indentations such as scalloped edges may indicate malignant change, such that one part of the mole is growing
- *Colour* – variation in colour may be a sign of dysplasia or malignant change in a mole. Melanomas may be intensely black and show very variable colour within a single lesion from white to slate blue, with all shades of black and brown. Amelanotic melanomas shows little or no pigmentation
- *Diameter* – apart from congenital naevi most benign moles are less than 1 cm in diameter. Any lesion growing to over 0.5 cm should be carefully checked. However, some malignant melanomas are small – 0.1–0.2 cm
- *Evolving* – a mole changing over time

skin type and the regularity of exposure to sun are also important. The incidence is higher in fair-skinned people who have concentrated high-intensity exposure on holiday than those with darker skin types who have regular exposure throughout the year. Sunburning episodes are thought to be a risk factor for MM. The most frequent site of MM in women is the legs whilst in men it is the trunk. This is thought to be a direct consequence of behaviour in the sun, i.e. women expose their legs and men remove their shirts.

Pre-existing moles

It is rare for ordinary moles to become malignant but congenital naevi and multiple dysplastic naevi are more likely to develop into malignant melanoma. Fifty per cent of MM is thought to arise in pre-existing moles.

Types of melanoma

Clinically there are five main types of melanoma.

Superficial spreading melanoma is the most common type. It is common on the back in men and on the legs in women. As the name implies the melanoma cells spread superficially in the epidermis, becoming invasive after months or years. The margin and the surface are irregular, with pigmentation varying from brown to black (Figure 22.14). There may be surrounding inflammation and signs of regression – pale areas within it. Nodules may appear within the tumour when it becomes invasive which worsens the prognosis (Figure 22.15).

Lentigo maligna melanoma occurs characteristically on the face of elderly people. Initially there is a slowly growing, irregular pigmented macule (lentigo maligna) that is present for many years (Figure 22.16) before a melanoma develops (Figure 22.17). Malignant change may be suspected if a darker colour develops within the macule.

Nodular melanoma presents as a dark nodule from the start without a preceding *in situ* epidermal phase (Figure 22.18). It is more common in men than women and is usually seen in people in their

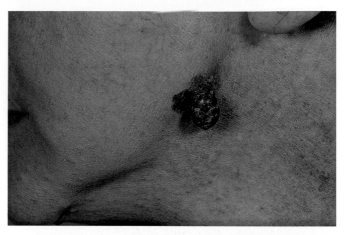

Figure 22.15 Malignant melanoma nodule developing within an SSMM.

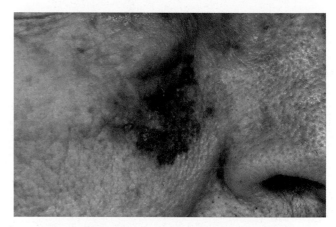

Figure 22.16 Lentigo maligna.

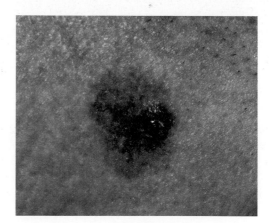

Figure 22.17 Lentigo maligna melanoma.

fifties and sixties. This tumour is in a vertical growth phase from the start and therefore has a correspondingly poor prognosis.

Acral melanoma occurs on the palm and soles and near/under the nails. Benign pigmented naevi may also occur in these sites and it is important to recognize early dysplastic change (ABCDE – as above). A very important indication that discolouration of the nail is due to melanoma is 'Hutchinson's sign': pigmentation of the nail

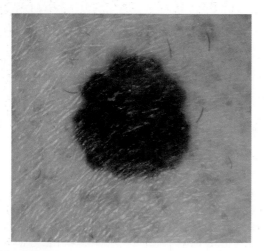

Figure 22.14 Superficial spreading malignant melanoma.

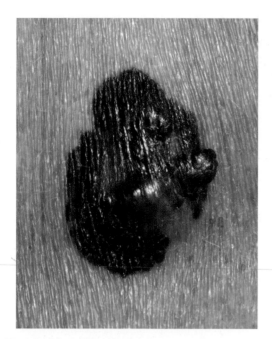

Figure 22.18 Nodular malignant melanoma.

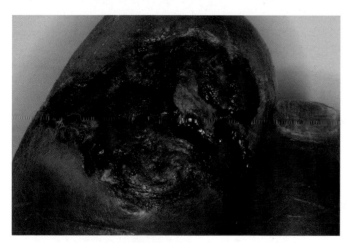

Figure 22.19 Acral malignant melanoma.

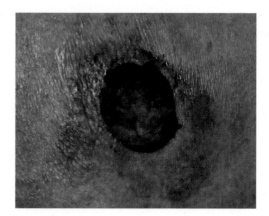

Figure 22.20 Amelanotic malignant melanoma.

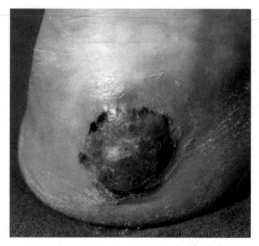

Figure 22.21 Dysplastic malignant melanoma.

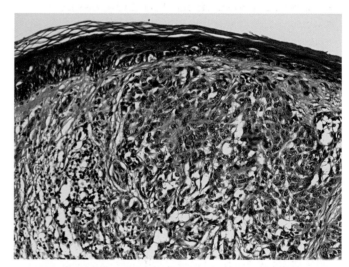

Figure 22.22 Malignant melanoma: histology.

fold adjacent to the nail (Figure 22.19). It is important to distinguish talon noir, in which a black area appears on the sole or heel. It is the result of trauma – for example sustained while playing squash – causing haemorrhage into the dermal papillae. Paring the skin gently with a scalpel will reveal distinct blood-filled papillae, to the relief of doctor and patient alike.

Amelanotic melanoma. As the melanoma cells become more dysplastic and less well differentiated they lose the capacity to produce melanin and form an amelanotic melanoma (Figure 22.20). Such non-pigmented nodules may be regarded as harmless but in fact are highly malignant. A rare form but also highly malignant is the dysplastic form of malignant melanoma (Figure 22.21).

Prognosis

The prognosis depends on the depth to which the melanoma has penetrated below the base of the epidermis seen histologically: the so-called Breslow thickness of the lesion (Figure 22.22). This is measured histologically in millimetres from the granular layer to the deepest level of invasion. A depth of less than 1.5 mm is associated with a 90% 5-year survival, 1.5–3.5 mm with a 75% 5-year survival, and greater than 3.5 mm with only a 50% 5-year survival. These figures are based on patients in whom the original lesion had been completely excised. A recent study in Scotland has shown an overall 5-year survival of 71.6–77.6% for women and 58.7% for men. Ulceration, lymph node involvement and skin metastases are associated with a poorer prognosis.

The greater the Breslow thickness and the greater the Clark's level (see Box 22.2) then the worse the prognosis, lesions confined to the epidermis having better prognosis than those penetrating into the dermis.

Treatment of MM

If an MM is suspected it should ideally be excised in its entirety with just a 2-mm margin for histological analysis. Definitive treatment including wide local excision margins will be guided by the Breslow thickness (determined histologically) as well as any potential risk for lymph node involvement. The higher the Breslow thickness the more likely the draining lymph nodes may contain MM metastases. If a palpable lymph node is found on examination then a fine needle aspiration or lymph node removal for cytology/histology respectively should be undertaken. If no lymph nodes are palpable but the Breslow thickness is ≥1 mm then the patient may be offered sentinel lymph node biopsy (this is the first draining node from the affected MM skin site).

Sentinel lymph node biopsy (SLNB)

The presence or absence of nodal metastases is a significant prognostic indicator. SLNB is therefore currently offered to patients who have a MM of ≥1 mm Breslow thickness. SLNB is usually undertaken simultaneously with the wide local excision. To detect the sentinel nodes lymphoscintigraphy (which maps the lymphatics using technetium-99m) is carried out, plus methylene blue dye is infiltrated around the excision scar and a gamma probe is used to identify positive nodes. All blue nodes and those with more than 10% radioactivity are identified as sentinel nodes. The sentinel lymph node/s are examined histologically for evidence of MM micrometastases. A false negative rate of between 4 and 12% is reported. If the sentinel lymph node is positive for MM then local lymph basin clearance and/or adjuvant therapy in a clinical trial is usually offered to the patient. Unfortunately there is no evidence that undergoing SLNB and lymph basin clearance improves survival but it is the most accurate currently available staging method.

Adjuvant therapies for MM

Patients with evidence of metastases may be offered the opportunity to take part in multicentre studies to receive either trial medicines or placebo. However to date no survival benefit has been demonstrated with any adjuvant treatment for metastatic melanoma, which is disappointing. Treatments using chemotherapy, radiotherapy, immunotherapy, retinoids and biological therapies have all been tried. High-dose interferon alpha 2b (INF-α2b) has, however, been shown to give slightly better disease-free survival but no difference in overall survival rates when compared to observation only. Melanoma vaccines may provide hope for future patients.

Cutaneous lymphoma

Primary invasion of the skin by abnormal T- or B-lymphocytes is relatively rare but is worth mentioning as patients are frequently misdiagnosed for many years.

Cutaneous T-cell lymphomas (CTCLs) are a heterogeneous group of disorders that account for 80% of primary cutaneous lymphomas (B-cell types 20%). The most common form of CTCL is mycosis fungoides (MF), which is more common with increasing age, male sex and black skin. MF has a relatively good overall prognosis but some individuals may have more aggressive disease. Clinically MF may initially resemble eczema, psoriasis or fungal infections. Patients have scaly erythematous patches and plaques on the skin, particularly on the buttock area (Figure 22.23). These may be itchy or asymptomatic. Lesions usually remain fixed and do not respond to mild topical steroids or antifungal creams. These lesions may remain stable for many years but eventually may transform to tumour stage disease when nodules may appear in long-standing plaques or arise *de novo*.

Five per cent of mycosis fungoides patients develop a generalized exfoliative erythroderma with lymphadenopathy and atypical peripheral T-cells (Sézary cells): the so-called Sézary syndrome. This can be considered to be a more aggressive form of MF. A clone of malignant T-cells can be demonstrated in the skin, lymph nodes and blood by T-cell gene rearrangement studies.

Primary cutaneous B-cell lymphomas (CBCLs) arise from a malignant transformation of B-cells at different stages of their development leading to different types including follicular, marginal zone, diffuse large B-cell 'other' and diffuse large B-cell on the leg (the latter has a worse prognosis). Clinically lesions present as firm

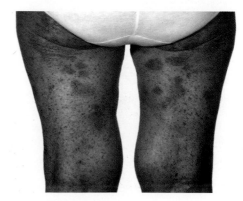

Figure 22.23 Mycosis fungoides.

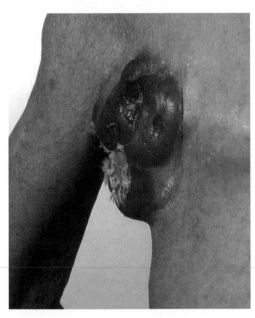

Figure 22.24 Primary cutaneous B-cell lymphoma.

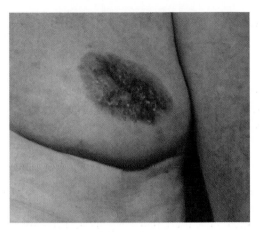

Figure 22.25 Paget's disease of the nipple.

indurated papules, nodules or plaques that may be erythematous, violaceous or brown (Figure 22.24).

If primary cutaneous lymphoma is suspected then the patient should be referred if possible to a local dermatologist or specialist lymphoma unit for assessment and management.

Other cutaneous malignancies

Paget's disease of the nipple presents with unilateral non-specific erythematous changes on the areola/nipple spreading to the surrounding skin. The cause is an underlying adenocarcinoma of the ducts. It should be considered in any patient with eczematous changes in one breast that fail to respond to simple treatment (Figure 22.25). Extramammary Paget's can affect the axillae and groin.

Metastases from internal organs most commonly spread from cancers of the breast, lung, GI tract, renal tract, oral pharynx, larynx and melanoma (originating from the retina, leptomeninges). Early recognition of cutaneous metastases may allow accurate and rapid diagnosis of internal malignancy and expedite possible curative therapies.

Further reading

Agnew KL, Gilchrest BA, Bunker CB. *Skin Cancer (Fast Facts)*. Health Press, Oxford, 2005.

Buchan J, Roberts D. *Pocket Guide to Malignant Melanoma*. Blackwell Science, Oxford, 2000.

Nouri K. *Skin Cancer*. McGraw-Hill Medical, New York, 2007.

CHAPTER 23

Practical Procedures

Raj Mallipeddi

OVERVIEW

- The object of physical treatments is to remove lesions and, if appropriate, to provide material for histological diagnosis.

- Destructive methods of treatment include cryotherapy, electrocautery and laser treatment. Curettage both destroys the lesion and provides fragmented material for histology.

- Cryotherapy involves the use of extreme cold to destroy the affected tissue. Solid carbon dioxide, nitrous oxide and ethyl chloride can all be used but liquid nitrogen is the most effective. It produces inflammation and may cause ulceration.

- Electrosurgery is the use of electric current to destroy tissue by heat in two forms: electrocautery simply using a heated element and electrodessication using a high-frequency alternating current.

- Curettage is suitable for superficial lesions and is usually combined with electrocautery.

- Specimens for histology can be completely excised lesions or samples. Usually only part of the lesion is obtained by incisional, shave and punch biopsies and therefore resulting specimens do not give information on the extent of the lesion.

- Surgical excisions require adequate training and knowledge of the management of skin lesions and correct surgical techniques to completely excise lesions whilst causing the least possible scarring.

This chapter will focus on the more conventional procedures undertaken in general practice.

Cryotherapy

This involves the destruction of tissues by extreme cold (Box 23.1). The tissue is frozen to subzero temperatures, which is then followed by sloughing off dead tissue. Several mechanisms are involved including the osmotic effects of intracellular water leaving the cell and causing dehydration, intracellular ice formation disrupting the cell membrane, and ischaemic damage due to freezing of vessels. Liquid nitrogen is most commonly employed, although various freezing agents are available such as solid carbon dioxide,

Box 23.1 **Cryotherapy – practical points**

- Be confident of the diagnosis before treating and if in doubt perform a biopsy
- Monitor the freeze time, which begins when the target is completely frozen. Spray in short bursts to maintain an iceball and stop when the desired freeze time is over
- Warn patients about potential side-effects including pain, redness, swelling and blistering. An information sheet helps to ensure that the patient is fully aware of these side-effects
- Children do not tolerate cryotherapy well so consider alternative treatments

nitrous oxide and a mixture of dimethyl ether and propane. Unless otherwise stated the rest of this section will relate to liquid nitrogen cryotherapy.

The low temperature of liquid nitrogen (−196°C), ease of storage and relative low cost make it an effective and convenient cryogen. However, its low temperature also results in rapid evaporation and therefore it should be stored carefully in an adequately ventilated area and preferably in a pressurized container.

Application technique

The liquid nitrogen is best applied as a spray using a canister (Figure 23.1).

An alternative method is to use a cotton bud that is immersed in liquid nitrogen and then applied to the lesion being treated, using moderate pressure until frozen. More than one application may be needed. A fresh cotton bud should be used for each patient to diminish the risk of transferring human papillomavirus. However, with this method there in an increase in temperature partly due to poor thermal capacity of the cotton and also warming when the cotton tip is transferred from the liquid nitrogen container to the patient's skin. The freeze time is important, and will vary according to the lesion being treated.

Freeze time is counted from the moment the entire lesion becomes frozen white rather than simply from when spraying begins. Once spraying is complete the rate of thawing of the tissue is an important factor as more tissue destruction occurs with rapid freezing and slow thawing. The 'freeze–thaw' cycle may be repeated to increase the degree of damage and the additional freeze

---

ABC of Dermatology, 5th edition. Edited by P. K. Buxton and R. Morris-Jones.
© 2009 Blackwell Publishing, ISBN: 978-1-4051-7065-9.

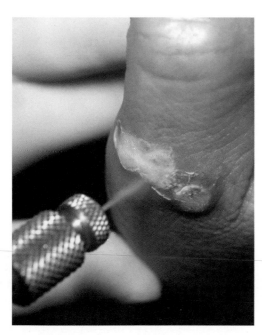

Figure 23.1 Cryotherapy.

has a greater penetration due to improved cold conductivity of the previously frozen tissue. Freeze times and the number of freeze–thaw cycles depend on the type of lesion (i.e. whether benign or malignant) as well as size and thickness.

Risks and precautions

- Patients should be warned about reactions which can occur within the first 48 hours after treatment such as pain, redness, swelling and blistering, so that they are not unduly alarmed. A potent topical steroid cream applied over the affected area for a few days can be used to limit this.
- Ulceration may occur, particularly on the lower limb if there is poor perfusion.
- Although secondary bacterial infection is rare, increased pain, redness or swelling after 2–3 days may be indicative of this.
- Later risks include scarring and, particularly in darker skin types, hypopigmentation or hyperpigmentation. As might be expected these are more of an issue with prolonged treatments.

Skin lesions suitable for freezing

Cryotherapy is usually initiated on the basis of a clinical diagnosis without prior histological confirmation and therefore the clinician must be confident of the diagnosis. If there is any diagnostic doubt, consider a biopsy first or alternative treatment modality where histology can also be obtained. Although there are several other possible treatments, the following lesions are frequently treated with cryotherapy.

Viral warts

A single freeze lasting 10–30 seconds per treatment, which includes a 1–2 mm margin of normal skin, is usually sufficient, although for thick plantar warts in particular, a double freeze–thaw cycle may improve clearance. Often several treatments at 2–3-week intervals

are necessary and cryotherapy may be combined with topical therapies such as salicylic acid preparations for increased efficacy. Paring down the wart with a blade before cryotherapy can also be helpful.

Seborrhoeic keratoses

A single freeze of between 5 and 20 seconds including a 1–2-mm margin of normal skin should be effective for most lesions. A frozen lesion once thawed for a few seconds can also be curetted off. Larger, thicker lesions may require prolonged freezing or repeat freeze–thaw cycles thereby increasing pain and inflammation. In these circumstances it may be better to curette and gently cauterize the area.

Papillomas and skin tags

A single freeze of 5–10 seconds may be sufficient and it is helpful to stabilize the skin tag with metal forceps so that the liquid nitrogen is sprayed obliquely, avoiding non-lesional skin. An alternative method is to treat by compression with artery forceps dipped in liquid nitrogen.

Actinic keratosis

A single freeze of between 5 and 15 seconds including a 1–2-mm margin of normal skin is advised. When necessary, lifting away hard keratin to expose the underlying abnormal epithelium makes the freezing more effective. Rarely a double freeze–thaw cycle may be needed but be aware that a lesion which does not respond to cryotherapy may be a squamous cell carcinoma.

Bowen's disease

This is an intraepidermal (*in situ*) form of squamous cell carcinoma, which can be effectively treated with a single freeze of 30 seconds including a 1–2-mm margin of normal skin. Again, a biopsy is necessary should there be any doubt about the diagnosis and follow-up is essential to make sure the lesion has cleared and is not progressing.

Basal cell carcinoma

If cryotherapy is to be employed, it is best limited to the treatment of the superficial type of BCC, when lesions are primary (i.e. previously untreated), small (<1 cm in diameter) and well defined. The cure rate for other types of BCC is worse with cryotherapy than other forms of treatment such as excision.

Two cycles of freezing lasting between 20 and 30 seconds, including a 3-mm rim of clinically normal skin, with a thaw time of 2 minutes is effective.

Electrosurgery

This term describes the use of electricity to cause thermal tissue destruction. There are two main forms of treatment: electrocautery and electrodessication.

Electrocautery

Heat from an electrically heated element causes thermal damage by direct transfer of heat. Remember in this situation the treating element is hot.

Electrodessication (diathermy or hyfrecation)

High-frequency alternating current energy is converted to heat due to tissue resistance. The treatment electrode is cold as heat generation occurs within the tissue. Electrode contact with skin causes superficial tissue dehydration. A variation of electrodessication is electrofulguration in which the electrode is held 1–2 mm from the skin surface to cause superficial epidermal carbonization. Furthermore, depending on the voltage of current used and electromagnetic waveform, the degree of tissue cutting (electrosection) and coagulation (electrocoagulation) can be modified. If only one treatment electrode is present then alternating current variably enters and exits the tissue, with electrons being randomly dissipated into the environment and this is known as a monopolar procedure. However, if there is also a second indifferent electrode that completes an electrical circuit, the procedure is termed bipolar. With alternating current the treatment electrodes are not truly positive or negative poles, and the terms mono- and biterminal are more accurate.

In routine dermatology electrocautery or electrodessication can be used as the sole treatment for vascular lesions such as spider naevi and telengiectasia, although a vascular laser may produce better results with a lower risk of scarring. However, it is more commonly used for haemostasis during skin surgery (Figure 23.2) or in combination with curettage (see below).

Curettage

This is a simple method of removing superficial lesions, particularly in areas with thick underlying dermis such as the trunk and extremities (Box 23.2). A metal spoon or ring with a sharp edge is used to scrape away the lesion (Figure 23.3). The advantage over cryotherapy is that a sample can be sent for histology although completeness of removal cannot be accurately assessed. Curettage is combined with electrodessication or electrocautery to treat benign lesions such as seborrhoeic keratoses and xanthelasma as well as dysplastic lesions (actinic keratoses and Bowen's disease) and basal

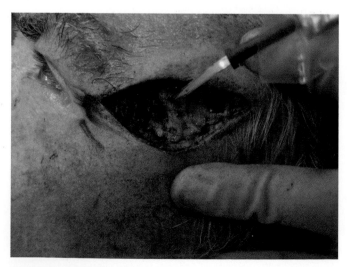

Figure 23.2 Electrodessication during surgery.

> Box 23.2 **Curettage – practical points**
>
> - Use a curette which is of appropriate size for the lesion
> - Stretch the skin with the non-dominant hand and keep firm control of the curette to avoid unintended scraping of normal skin
> - Send the sample for histology but clearly state on the request that it is a curetted specimen
> - Consider shaving off the specimen first to provide a solid sample for diagnosis before commencing curettage and electrocautery. Pathologists prefer this to curetted fragments

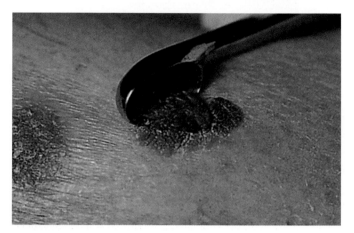

Figure 23.3 Spoon curettage.

cell carcinoma. For curettage to work well the lesion ideally should be softer than surrounding unaffected skin.

Lesions suitable for curetting include:

- seborrhoeic keratoses
- solitary viral warts
- solar keratoses
- cutaneous horns
- small basal cell carcinomas.

Technique

The area under and around the lesion is injected with local anaesthetic. Next using the thumb and index finger of the non-dominant hand ensure that the skin around the lesion is taut, so that there is a firm base on which to curette. Curette off the lesion and then cauterize the base to achieve haemostasis as well as to destroy any remaining tumour. Avoid curetting normal skin. For basal cell carcinomas the process is repeated so that a total of 2 or 3 cycles of curettage and electrocautery/electrodessication is performed.

Risks and precautions

- Patients should be warned that the wound may take to 3–4 weeks to heal and that although the resultant scar will hopefully will be a flat, white patch, it could ultimately become indented (atrophic) in addition to being pink, itchy and raised (hypertrophic) for several months before complete healing.
- Ulceration may occur, particularly on the lower limb if there is poor perfusion.

- The types of basal cell carcinomas best treated with this method are primary, nodular, small (<1 cm diameter), well defined and in non-high risk or cosmetically sensitive sites. Sites generally to be avoided include the area around the eyes, nose, lips, chin, ears and hair-bearing scalp.
- If curettage results in exposure of subcutaneous fat then the procedure should be abandoned and the area excised down to fat and usually sutured. This is because firstly it is not possible to distinguish accurately between soft tumour and fat, and secondly the outcome will be suboptimal in terms of wound healing and scarring, once the fat layer has been breached.

Diagnostic biopsies

Although in many circumstances a diagnosis can be confidently made on clinical examination alone, often it is important to secure a diagnosis with the aid of histopathology. For example, a melanocytic naevus may be proven on histology to be completely benign or by complete contrast a malignant melanoma. There are different methods of performing a diagnostic biopsy, each with its own advantages and disadvantages. The area to be biopsied must be adequately infiltrated with local anaesthesia before commencing the procedure.

Shave biopsy

This is appropriate for sampling or removing lesions which are limited to the epidermis and papillary dermis including seborrhoeic keratoses, nodular basal cell carcinomas and naevi. The skin is held taut and the lesion is gently sliced with either a scalpel blade or double-edged razor blade held horizontal to the skin surface. The angle of the blade controls the depth but the aim should be to reach mid-dermis. Haemostasis can be achieved with electrosurgery or aluminium chloride but firm pressure may suffice. One advantage of this technique is that sutures are unnecessary. However, this technique is not recommended for any suspicious naevus, which should be excised entirely.

Punch biopsy

The biopsy tool comes in sizes varying from 2 to 8 mm (Figure 23.4) and consists of a small cylinder with a cutting rim which is used to penetrate the epidermis by rotation between the operator's finger and thumb. The skin is held taut at 90° to the orientation of the relaxed skin tension lines ('wrinkle lines') so that an oval defect results, which is easier to close (Figures 23.5–23.9). The resulting plug of skin is lifted out with forceps and cut off as deeply as possible. Pressure and/or electrosurgery is required for haemostasis. The advantage over a shave biopsy is that the

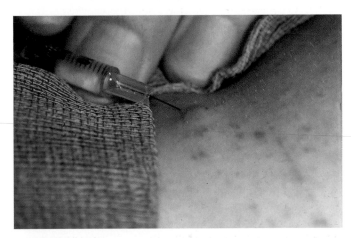

Figure 23.5 Punch biopsy: injecting local anaesthetic.

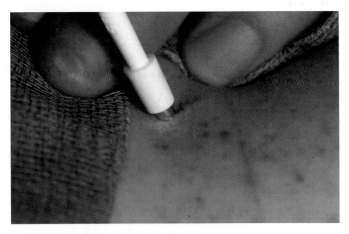

Figure 23.6 Punch biopsy: tool insertion.

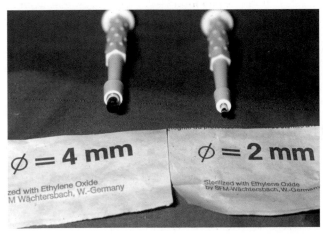

Figure 23.4 Punch biopsy tools.

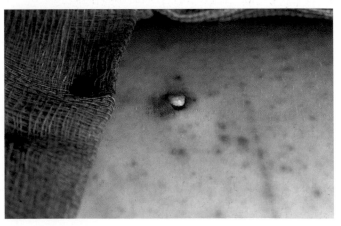

Figure 23.7 Punch biopsy: plug of skin.

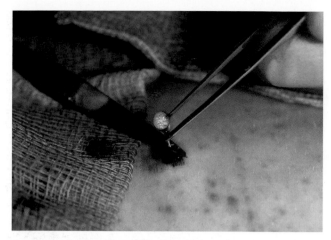

Figure 23.8 Punch biopsy: raising a plug of skin.

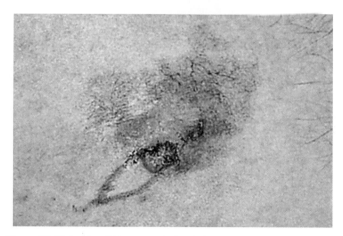

Figure 23.10 Incisional biopsy: marked area for sampling.

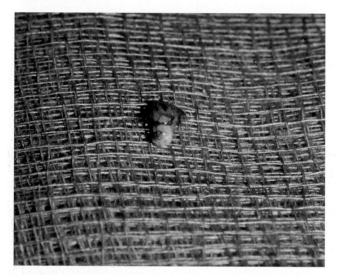

Figure 23.9 Punch biopsy: specimen taken.

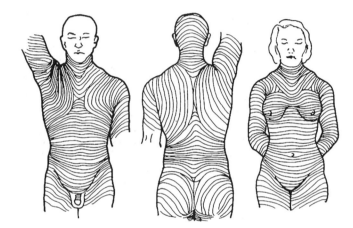

Figure 23.11 Surgical excision: 'skin wrinkle lines' of the trunk.

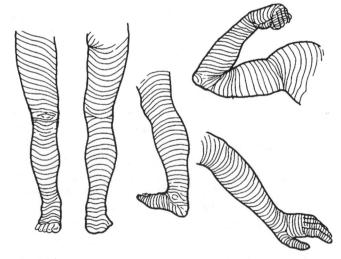

Figure 23.12 Surgical excision: 'skin wrinkle lines' of the limbs.

specimen obtained is full thickness containing epidermis, dermis and fat, but the area sampled is small. Although it depends on the site, punch biopsies 3 mm or less can generally be left to heal by secondary intention whereas those 4 mm or larger are better sutured for cosmesis. The punch biopsy tool can also be used to make holes over cysts and lipomas through which the contents can be extruded.

Incisional biopsy

This is suitable for larger lesions and is taken across the margin of the lesion in the form of an ellipse. It is essential to include deeper dermis, as the significant changes in, for example, granuloma or lymphoid infiltrate may not be near the surface. An adequate amount of normal tissue should be included, so this can be compared with the pathological area and this also means there is enough normal skin to suture the incision together (Figure 23.10).

Surgical excision

Excision of skin lesions is both curative and diagnostic. It may be the best way of making a diagnosis if there are multiple small papules or vesicles, one of which can be excised intact. Incisions should follow tension or wrinkle lines (Figures 23.11–23.13).

In the case of malignant lesions it is particularly important that the whole lesion is adequately excised. The pathologist can report on the adequacy of excision, but this is hard to assess in lesions

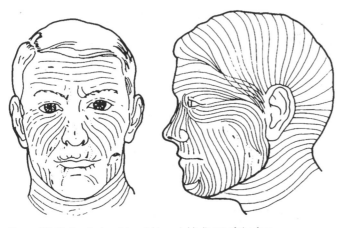

Figure 23.13 Surgical excision: 'skin wrinkle lines' of the face.

Box 23.4 **Suturing**

- Correct suture placement is vital to optimize the cosmetic outcome of a wound (Figures 23.17 & 23.18)
- Following an excision both subcutaneous sutures and epidermal sutures are placed
- Subcutaneous sutures are absorbable such as Vicryl (Polyglactin 910, Ethicon Inc., Somerville, NJ, USA), which take up to 70 days for complete absorption whereas typical epidermal sutures such as nylon and polypropylene are non-absorbable and are removed between 5 days and 2 weeks depending on the site
- Monofilament sutures cause less inflammation and trapping of serum than the braided variety, but are harder to tie securely
- Suture placement should result in wound eversion so that the resultant scar is less noticeable

Box 23.3 **Surgical excision**

- After initially inserting the needle, withdraw the plunger of the syringe to check the needle has not entered the blood vessels. Raising a small 'bleb' of local anaesthetic ahead of the needle point helps to prevent this
- It is important to learn appropriate suturing techniques for different sites of the body and size of lesion
- Warn the patient about the resultant scar and be careful to avoid deformities such as displacement of the eyelid (ectropion)
- Always send an excised lesion for histology as a significant number of lesions considered likely to be benign clinically actually turn out to be malignant on histology

such as multifocal basal cell carcinoma where there are scattered collections of cells. If there is likely to be any doubt about the excision being complete it is helpful to attach a suture to one end of the excised specimen so the pathologist can describe which border, if any, extends over the excision margin.

Technique (Boxes 23.3 & 23.4)

The basic technique consists of making an elliptical incision (Figures 23.14–23.16) with the length three times the width and the angles at the poles about 30° to minimize the formation of standing cones of tissue also known as 'dog ears'. The long axis of the excision should be parallel to the 'wrinkle lines' of the skin or to the Langer lines. Although on most parts of the body these correspond closely, they are not exactly the same, as Langer lines correspond to the alignment of collagen fibres within the dermis. Scars parallel to these tend to heal better and be less obvious. Lesions excised on the sternal area, upper chest and shoulders are more likely to result in keloid scar formation and may be best referred to a dermatological or plastic surgeon.

Local anaesthetic is injected subcutaneously but close to the skin. The incision should be vertical rather than wedge shaped. Before suturing of the wound undermining is often required to reduce wound tension. This involves dissection of the skin subdermally (blunt and/or sharp), although the depth will depend on the body site.

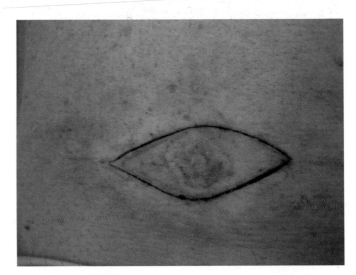

Figure 23.14 Surgical excision of BCC from lower back. Ellipse design including a 4-mm margin.

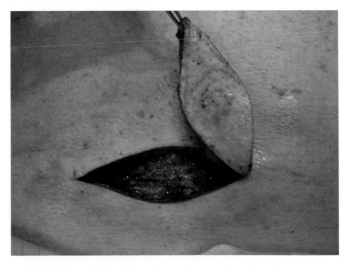

Figure 23.15 Surgical excision of BCC: removal of specimen illustrating the defect.

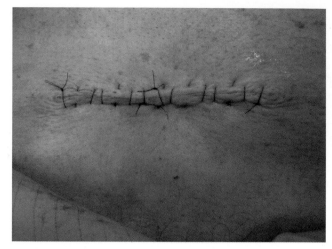

Figure 23.16 Surgical excision of BCC: after suturing showing wound eversion.

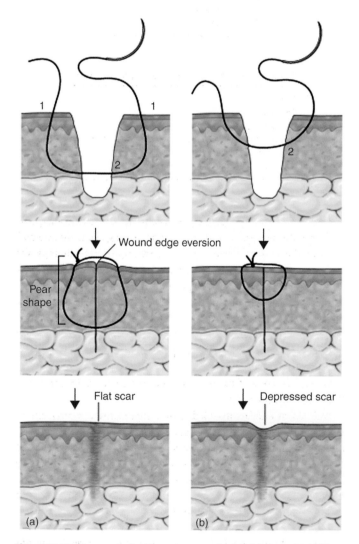

Wound edge eversion

Pear shape

Flat scar

Depressed scar

(a)

(b)

Figure 23.17 Placement of epidermal sutures. From Robinson *et al.* 2005.

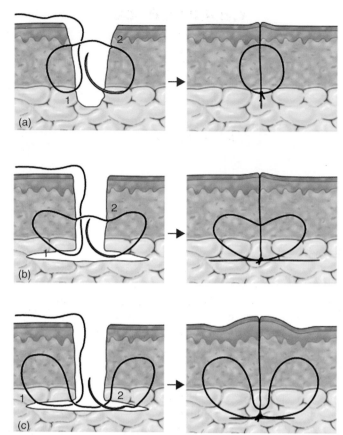

Figure 23.18 Methods of placing buried dermal sutures. From Robinson *et al.* 2005.

Where a wound cannot be closed directly (i.e. from side to side) or if direct closure does not produce the best aesthetic outcome then a cutaneous flap or skin graft may be appropriate. Flaps may be advancement, rotation or transposition. Grafts are defined as full thickness if the entire epidermis and dermis is included, and split thickness if less than the entire dermis is included. These are outside the scope of this book.

Further reading

Lawrence C. *Introduction to Dermatological Surgery*, 2nd edn. Blackwell Science, Oxford, 2002.

Lawrence CM, Walker NPJ, Telfer NR. Dermatological surgery. In: Burns DA, Breathnach SM, Cox NH, Griffiths CEM, eds. *Rook's Textbook of Dermatology*, 7th edn, Vol. 4. Blackwell Publishing, Oxford, 2004: 78.5–78.7.

Robinson J, Hanke CW, Sengelmann RD, Siegel DM. *Surgery of the Skin – Procedural Dermatology*. Elsevier Mosby, Philadelphia, 2005.

Zachary CB. *Basic Cutaneous Surgery: a Primer in Technique*. Churchill Livingstone, New York, 1991.

CHAPTER 24

Lasers, Intense Pulsed Light and Photodynamic Therapy

Alun V Evans

OVERVIEW

- Laser treatment uses high-energy radiation at different wavelengths which can be directed at specific targets.

- Laser treatments should only be undertaken by those with appropriate training.

- It is essential to make sure that patients are carefully selected, are fully informed and have an adequate preoperative assessment.

- A variable level of pain is experienced by patients. Surface, local or general anaesthesia is used as necessary.

- Different types of laser are used to target different tissues in the skin and therefore careful selection of the correct laser is essential. Lasers can target pigment (melanin, tattoo dyes), blood cells, hair follicles, or surface cells (resurfacing).

- Photodynamic therapy (PDT) involves the photoactivation of a topical chemical, usually a derivative of aminolevulinic acid, by light (630-nm range). It is commonly used to treat solar keratoses, Bowen's disease and large superficial basal cell carcinoma.

Table 24.1 The acronym 'LASER'.

L	Light
A	Amplified by
S	Stimulated
E	Emission of
R	Radiation

Table 24.2 Possible complications of laser treatment.

Pain
Erythema
Bruising (vascular lasers)
Pigmentary change (hypo- or hyperpigmentation)
Blistering
Scarring

Laser treatment

Laser science

Lasers emit a beam of light of a single wavelength, which can be selectively absorbed by a target of a certain colour, causing heating and subsequent lysis (Table 24.1). This target is known as a chromophore, from the Greek for 'bearing colour'. The duration of the laser pulse is also set to be selective for the size of the chromophore. Larger targets like hair follicles take longer to heat up and are slower to cool than smaller targets such as melanosomes. Lysis of the chromophore leaves a residue of smaller particles which are subsequently phagocytosed by macrophages. This concept of selective photothermolysis underpins laser science.

Preoperative assessment

Laser treatment should be preceded by a full medical history and dermatological examination.

Laser centres should offer a preoperative consultation by a qualified practitioner who can diagnose and manage skin disease and counsel the patient regarding the most appropriate therapy for their condition. It should always be borne in mind that laser treatment may not represent the optimum management for a patient and that patients are not infrequently referred with the wrong diagnosis. Careful patient selection for laser treatment has been shown to be associated with fewer adverse events, more realistic patient expectations and higher levels of patient satisfaction. The process of patient selection and preparation and an understanding of the cutaneous biology of the lesions to be treated are as important as the laser treatment itself.

Patients should be provided with comprehensive written information relating to laser treatment of their particular condition before obtaining informed consent. The consent form itself should detail possible complications of treatment (Table 24.2). Scarring may be more likely in certain areas such as the chest, shoulders and back. It is sensible to perform a small test patch using the desired settings before starting laser treatment or increasing the energy (fluence).

Patients should avoid direct sunlight and use a high-factor sun block before laser treatment in order to minimize the amount of pigment in the skin and reduce the risk of complications.

Table 24.3 shows which type of cutaneous disorders may be amenable to treatment with which lasers.

ABC of Dermatology, 5th edition. Edited by P. K. Buxton and R. Morris-Jones.
© 2009 Blackwell Publishing, ISBN: 978-1-4051-7065-9.

Table 24.3 Suitable lasers for specific skin disorders.

Cutaneous disorder	Lasers indicated
Vascular lesions	Pulsed dye laser, KTP
Melanocytic lesions	Q-switched Nd-YAG and Ruby
Skin pigmentation	Q-switched Nd-YAG, Ruby and Alexandrite
Ablation and resurfacing	Carbon dioxide
	Erbium-YAG
Hair removal	Q-switched Nd-YAG, Ruby and Alexandrite
Tattoos	Q-switched Nd-YAG, Ruby and Alexandrite

Perioperative anaesthesia

Patients experience varying amounts of pain during laser treatment and anaesthesia must be adjusted to the needs of the individual patient and the procedure being undertaken. Some lasers have cooling devices attached, which provide a degree of anaesthesia, and many patients will undergo treatment without additional pain relief. Topical local anaesthetics (EMLA®, Ametop®) may be applied under occlusion before treatment but for procedures such as resurfacing or extensive port wine stains local or regional anaesthesia will be required. General anaesthesia is reserved for treatment of young children and other special cases.

Postoperative care

All patients should be given a greasy emollient to apply regularly to the treated area for 3 days following treatment. The aim is to maintain the barrier function of the skin where this might have been disrupted by collateral thermal injury of the epidermis. Any blistering implies significant thermal injury to the epidermis and lower fluences should be employed. Patients should also avoid excessive exposure to sunlight for at least 3 months following treatment. Resurfacing procedures require intensive post-operative care by both the laser operator and the patient or carer.

Laser safety

The main dangers posed by lasers arise from the energy contained within the beam which can produce a thermal burn or ignite flammable materials. The eyes of the patient, operator and assistants must be protected using goggles or eye shields specific to the laser being used. Other risks come from the high-voltage electricity and operator-dependent errors in technique. Those intending to operate lasers should have prior appropriate training.

Careful patient selection for laser treatment by highly qualified medical practitioners has been shown to be associated with lower levels and better management of adverse events, more realistic patient expectations and higher levels of patient satisfaction. Preparation and selection of patients and an understanding of skin disease is crucial before selecting a suitable laser, if any. Laser centres should offer a preoperative consultation by a qualified practitioner who can diagnose and manage skin disease and counsel the patient regarding the most appropriate therapy for their condition.

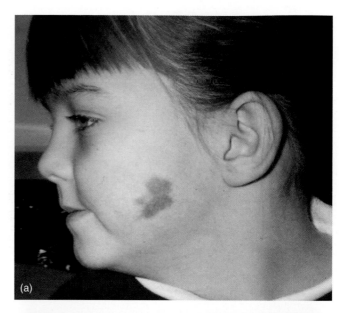

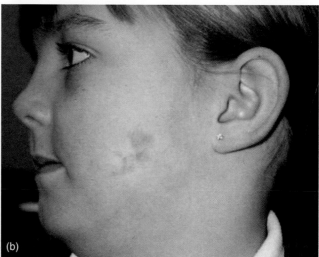

Figure 24.1 Port wine stain (a) before and (b) after treatment with a pulsed dye laser.

Vascular lesions

There are numerous conditions which consist of fixed abnormal blood vessels in the skin including port wine stain (Figure 24.1), spider naevus, telangiectasia and various types of haemangioma. The pulsed dye laser (585–600 nm) or the KTP laser (532 nm) are used to target oxyhaemoglobin within these vessels. The pulse duration is set so that larger vessels are targeted but the smaller normal vasculature of the skin remains intact. Lysis of the abnormal vessels quickly produces a well-demarcated bruise which may be quite prominent and lasts for up to 14 days (Figure 24.2). Repeated treatments, approximately 8 weeks apart, will be necessary for most patients, and lesions such as port wine stains that evolve over time may require ongoing therapy.

Pigmented lesions

A wide variety of pigmented lesions affecting the skin are amenable to laser treatment. The appropriate laser for each lesion can

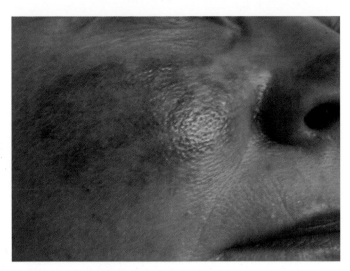

Figure 24.2 Bruising following pulsed dye laser treatment.

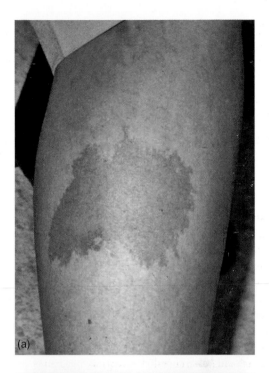

(a)

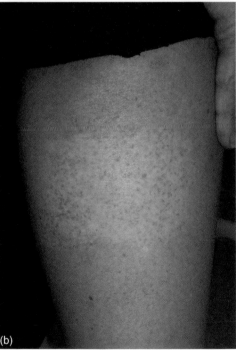

(b)

Figure 24.3 Café au lait macule (a) before and (b) after treatment with a Q-switched Nd-YAG laser.

be selected by considering the cause and location of the abnormal pigmentation.

The commonest pigmented lesions are the result of an abnormal accumulation of melanin within the skin. The melanin is contained within melanosomes which are around 0.4 μm in size. A laser with a very short pulse duration such as the 532-nm Q-switched Nd-YAG or Q-switched ruby lasers will selectively target melanin within the epidermis. Solar lentigos, café au lait macules (Figure 24.3) and ephilides (freckles) can all be treated relatively easily in this fashion. Between one and three treatments are usually required to achieve patient satisfaction. Lesions that repigment over time can be retreated when necessary.

When the melanin is located in the dermis the greater penetration afforded by a longer-wavelength light is required to reach the chromophore. A 1064-nm Q-switched Nd YAG laser is usually employed in the treatment of congenital naevus of Ota, naevus of Ito and Mongolian blue spots.

Naevi (moles) are the result of a proliferation of melanocytes and often cause cosmetic problems. Their pigment may well be amenable to laser treatment but this remains controversial as they have a potential for malignant transformation. This potential can range from being extremely small (e.g. junctional naevi) to an appreciable risk requiring regular dermatological review (e.g. giant congenital melanocytic naevi). The effect of laser treatment on the potential for malignant transformation is unknown. Many would suggest that it is negligible but would still be concerned that litigation might arise from any future malignancies in or around the treated lesion.

A second problem is that these malignancies will usually declare themselves through a local pigmentary change which may be masked by a laser that destroys pigment.

Certain types of melanocytic pigmentation are not amenable to laser treatment. Laser treatment of generalized pigmentary disorders such as that associated with Addison's disease should not be attempted, even in exposed sites, as the lack of uniformity of colour after treatment will lead to dissatisfaction. Melasma (chloasma) is the result of an overproduction of melanin in sun-exposed skin. The response to laser treatment is poor and may worsen the condition.

Post-inflammatory hyperpigmentation is the result of a temporary overproduction of melanin by melanocytes following inflammation. Laser treatment is likely to cause further inflammation and exacerbate the problem.

Various forms of abnormal pigmentation exist in the skin which are due to substances other than melanin. Certain drugs cause localized pigmentation of the skin which may be amenable to laser treatment. Amiodarone and minocycline produce pigmentation

Table 24.4 Laser selection by colour for tattoo removal.

Blue/black	Q-switched Nd-YAG 1064 nm
	Q-switched Ruby 694 nm
	Q-switched Alexandrite 755 nm
Red	Q-switched Nd-YAG 532 nm
Green	Q-switched Ruby 694 nm
	Q-switched Alexandrite 755 nm

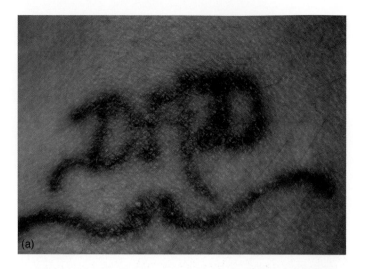

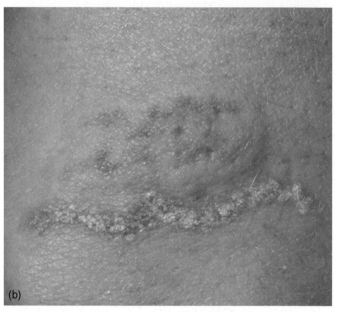

Figure 24.4 Tattoo undergoing laser removal. (a) Before treatment. (b) Fading of tattoo and 'laser snow' following Q-switched Nd-YAG laser treatment.

which may be selectively targeted by the Q-switched Nd-YAG, Ruby and Alexandrite lasers.

Haemosiderin is an iron-containing pigment that is deposited in the skin following extravasation of red blood cells. This is very common on the lower legs but treatment with laser is not indicated.

Tattoos

The art of inserting exogenous pigments into the dermis of the skin for decorative effect has been practised for thousands of years. The subsequent granulomatous reaction permanently fixes the pigment in the skin, although this fixation often outlasts the desire to retain the tattoo.

If the colour and consequently the absorption spectrum of the tattoo pigment differs sufficiently from the surrounding skin then it may be amenable to laser treatment. The appropriate wavelength is selected based on the colour of the tattoo (Table 24.4).

There is no uniformity in the constituents or the application of tattoo pigment and thus no uniformity in response to treatment. Some tattoos show significant fading after only one treatment whereas others can prove far more resistant. In general, amateur tattoos will fade faster than professional ones which may require 10 or more treatments. Care should be taken in the selection of treatable tattoos and the patient must be given a realistic assessment of what is achievable for their tattoo. Responsible laser operators may deem some large multicoloured tattoos untreatable from the outset.

Laser treatment of tattoos creates microscopic steam bubbles in the skin, sometimes referred to as 'laser snow' (Figure 24.4) which disappears in a matter of minutes. Initially there will be no apparent difference in colour but over the next few months macrophages will phagocytose the newly exposed pigment particles and the tattoo will gradually fade. Treatment is therefore carried out on a 2–3-monthly basis.

Hair removal

Laser hair removal is carried out using the Alexandrite, Ruby or Nd-YAG laser, the latter being more suitable for darker skin types. The chromophore is melanin in the hair and thermal energy dissipates to and damages the surrounding follicular cells effecting longer-term hair removal. Thus white, grey, blonde or red hair is unresponsive to treatment, and equally care must be taken where the skin is pigmented. Erythema in the treated area can be expected for up to 48 hours. Around six treatments will be required for a satisfactory response.

Laser resurfacing

The carbon dioxide laser (10600 nm) and the Erbium-YAG laser (2940 nm) have water as their chromophore. All components of the human body contain water and the action of these lasers on the skin cannot truly be described as selective. Rather they are a destructive entity used to vaporize tissue. They may be applied as a narrow continuous beam to cut tissue which has the advantage of achieving reasonable haemostasis as one proceeds, enabling convenient excision of unwanted tissue, e.g. keloids.

Alternatively 'resurfacing' of the skin is achieved by photothermolysing the epithelial surface of the skin to a reasonably predictable depth in one or more passes with subsequent healing. This method can improve the appearance of superficial lesions, for example, acne scarring, wrinkles or epidermal naevi.

A satisfactory result will only be achieved by careful patient selection and scrupulous attention to pre- and postoperative wound

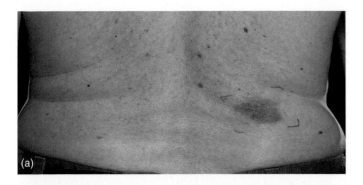

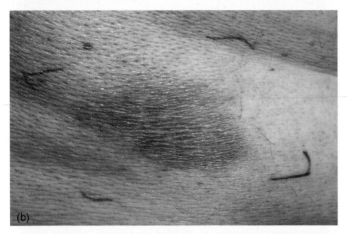

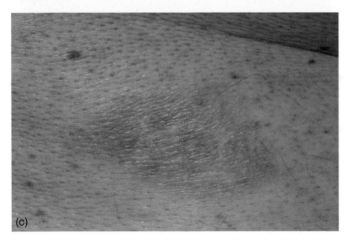

Figure 24.5 Superficial basal cell carcinoma on the lower back. (a,b) Before treatment with Hetvix photodynamic therapy (PDT). (c) Six months after PDT. Figures courtesy of Dr Andrew Morris, University Hospital of Wales, Cardiff.

care. Considerable training is required to operate these lasers successfully and they should only be operated by those with appropriate expertise.

Intense pulsed light

Non-laser light sources such as intense pulsed light (IPL) have been advocated as cheaper alternatives for the treatment of various skin abnormalities including vascular and pigmentary disorders. They emit light over a range of wavelengths and employ filters to achieve some selectivity. Technology is improving but so far they lack the efficacy of monochromatic lasers.

Photodynamic therapy

Photodynamic therapy (PDT) in dermatology involves the topical application of a photoactivated toxin such as aminolevulinic acid or methyl aminolevulinate to a lesion followed after 4 hours by exposure to light, usually in the 630-nm range. The effective penetration at this wavelength is 1–3 mm and PDT is used to treat solar keratoses, Bowen's disease and superficial basal cell carcinoma (Figure 24.5). However, the treatment is painful for the patient and expensive in terms of staff time and consumables. Equivalent results can be usually be achieved with cryotherapy, topical 5-fluorouracil or curettage and cautery. Therefore the use of PDT is generally limited to larger lesions in poorly healing sites.

PDT has also been advocated for use in acne, but antibiotics and isotretinoin provide cheaper and more effective alternatives. It may have a role where patients are unable or unwilling to pursue more conventional treatments.

Further reading

Lanigan S. *Lasers in Dermatology*. Springer-Verlag, London, 2000.

Tanzi EL, Lupton JR, Alster TS. Lasers in dermatology: four decades of progress. *J Am Acad Dermatol* 2003; **49**: 1–31.

Website of the New Zealand Dermatological Society: dermnetnz.org/procedures/lasers.html

CHAPTER 25

Dressings and Bandages

Judy Davids

OVERVIEW

- Natural wound healing may be enhanced by the correct selection and application of dressings and/or bandages.
- Detailed assessment of skin wounds is important to guide the type of dressings required.
- Understanding the properties and functions of different dressings enables the practitioner to make the most appropriate choice for each wound.
- Correct application of bandages is essential to ensure they are neither too tight nor too loose.
- Patient preferences, comfort and compliance are critical to successful wound healing.
- Excellent channels of communication are needed between all the different practitioners caring for the patient's skin.
- The patient's quality of life can be markedly enhanced by optimal wound care.

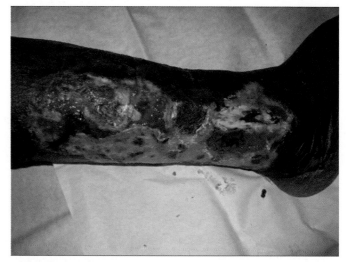

Figure 25.1 Wound with loss of the epidermis and dermis.

Introduction

Effective wound management requires an understanding of the process of wound healing and the knowledge of the properties of the dressings and bandages available. The wound care practitioner is confronted with a diverse range of products from the simple to the sophisticated, each made from a variety of materials including foams, films, hydrogels and hydrocolloid whereas bandage fabrics include cotton, linen, viscose, elastic, neoprene and even rubber. Many dressings are non-adhesive and consequently require a bandage to hold them in place. Hence the skin care practitioner needs a good understanding of the principles and properties of both dressings/bandages and wounds for optimum management. This chapter provides a practical approach to wound management rather than a detailed look at the physiology of the wound healing process.

Wounds

A wound is a physical break in the skin that may consist of a tear, cut, erosion, puncture or ulcer where the top layer of the skin is lacking (Figure 25.1). When the skin's barrier function is breached tissues are vulnerable to fluid, blood and heat loss, and may allow invasion of micro-organisms and foreign materials into the skin.

The science of wound healing is progressing rapidly and considerable advances have been made in the development of new products in wound healing. These include growth factors, skin substitutes, and gene and stem cell therapy. There are ongoing clinical trials on the effectiveness and ultimate use of these novel products in wider clinical practice, but this chapter will focus on products currently available to most practitioners.

When assessing any wound there are multiple factors that need to be taken into consideration in addition to the possible underlying aetiology (Box 25.1).

Wound types

In order to manage wounds optimally they are classified into four different types according to the appearance of the wound bed.

1 *Necrotic wounds.* Dead (ischaemic) tissue is usually black and covered with devitalized epidermis.
2 *Sloughy wounds.* These are often yellow due to the accumulation of cellular debris, fibrin, serous exudate, leucocytes and bacteria on the wound surface.

ABC of Dermatology, 5th edition. Edited by P. K. Buxton and R. Morris-Jones.
© 2009 Blackwell Publishing, ISBN: 978-1-4051-7065-9.

Box 25.1 **Wound-related factors to be considered in selecting an ideal dressing**

- The type of wound
- The size of the wound
- The location of the wound
- The stage of healing
- The tissue involved
- The amount of exudate
- The condition of the surrounding skin
- The patient's general health and environment

Box 25.2 **Key factors adversely affecting wound healing**

- Disease processes e.g. diabetes and cancer
- Advancing age
- Psychological factors e.g. stress and anxiety, sleep disturbances
- Malnutrition
- Dehydration
- Smoking
- Drug therapy
- Poor wound management
- Poor surgical technique

Box 25.3 **Principles for selecting an ideal dressing**

- To provide a moist environment to promote healing
- To manage excess wound exudate
- To allow gaseous exchange
- To protect the wound from pathogenic organisms
- To protect the wound from trauma and contamination
- To minimize and contain odour
- To provide a constant wound interface temperature
- To be non adherent and easily removed
- To be non-toxic, non-allergenic and non-sensitizing
- To reduce pain
- To promote debridement
- To protect the surrounding skin
- To cause minimum distress and discomfort during dressing change
- To improve the quality of life
- To be cosmetically acceptable to the patient
- To be cost-effective and available in hospitals and the community

3 *Granulating wounds* are characteristically deep pink or red with a highly vascular irregular granular appearance.

4 *Epithelializing wounds.* Cells migrate from the wound edges to start the process of re-epithelialization which is seen as pink tissue in the wound bed.

Regardless of wound type any wound may be additionally infected due to colonization by micro-organisms. If organisms proliferate above a certain threshold then the wound may develop a clinical infection characterized by pain, oedema, erythema, odour, purulent exudates, abscess formation and local heat. See Box 25.2 for factors that affect wound healing.

Dressings

Modern dressings are described as interactive. In other words, depending on their composition and structure dressings can interact with the wound to enhance healing. Dressings may be used to absorb exudates, combat odour and infection, relieve pain, encourage debridement and overall promote healing. When selecting a dressing the practitioner must undertake a holistic assessment of the patient including their nutritional status and the nature of the wound itself, and decide on what properties are required of the dressing to assist rapid healing. It is important to appreciate that the nature of the wound will change during the healing process and therefore the most suitable dressing required will also change with time (Box 25.3).

Types of wound dressings

The process of dressing selection is determined and influenced by a variety of factors. These include patient-focused issues and the types of dressings available (Table 25.1).

Non- or low adherent (NA or LA) dressings (Figure 25.2)

These are used for superficial, lightly exuding wounds. Their major function is to maintain a moist wound bed and allow exudate to pass through to a secondary dressing. Examples include the following.

- Knitted viscose dressings with an open structure to facilitate the free passage of exudates (e.g. Tricotex®).
- Perforated film absorbent dressings. The film is perforated to allow the exudate into the absorbent layer (e.g. Melolin®, Release®).
- Silicone dressings. These are a conformable silicone-covered mesh (e.g. Mepitel®).
- Paraffin tulle dressings consisting of an open-weave cotton or viscose and cotton-mix dressing impregnated in yellow or white soft paraffin (e.g. Jelonet® and Paratulle®).

Semipermeable adhesive film dressings

These consist of a thin layer of transparent polyurethane coated with an acrylic adhesive (allowing gaseous exchange), but are impermeable to micro-organisms. Films are flexible and therefore suitable for difficult anatomical sites such as across joints. They can be used for primary prevention of skin breakdown at sites of friction or exposure to moisture. In addition, they can be used on superficial pressure sores, donor sites and post-operative wounds and as a secondary dressing for other products. These dressings are not recommended for deep, infected or exuding wounds. Removal of these dressings can be traumatic to the surrounding skin and it is therefore recommended to follow the manufacturers' instructions. Examples include Opsite®, Tegaderm®, Bioclusive® and C-View®.

Hydrogel dressings (Figure 25.3)

These consist of insoluble polymers which are hydrophilic and can absorb excess fluid or produce a moist environment at the wound surface. They can be used on dry, sloughy and necrotic wounds which allow rehydration of dead tissue and autolytic debridement. Hydrogel dressings may also be suitable for pressure sores,

Table 25.1 Wound types and suitable dressings.

Wound type		Characteristics	Examples of suitable dressings
Epithelializing		Clean, superficial, low to medium exudate, pink in colour	Low and non-adherent dressings, knitted viscose, paraffin gauze, film dressings
Granulating		Clean, low to medium exudate, red in colour with granular appearance	Alginates, hydrocolloids, foams
Sloughy		Medium to high exudate, yellowish-grey in colour, partially or completely covered in slough	Hydrogels, alginates, spun hydrocolloids
Necrotic wounds		Black, dry, eschar devitalized tissue	Hydrogels, hydrocolloids
Infected wounds		Painful, moderate to high exudate, malodorous, crusting	Silver-impregnated dressings, hydrogels, spun hydrocolloids
Blistering		Clean, superficial, low to medium exudate	Non-adherent dressings

leg ulcers and surgical wounds; however they should not be used for wounds producing high levels of exudates or where gangrene is present. Hydrogel dressings usually require a secondary dressing to keep them in place. These dressings need to be changed every 1–3 days. Examples include Intrasite gel®, Granugel®, Sterigel® and Nugel®.

Hydrocolloid dressings (Figure 25.4)
These contain gel-forming agents such as carboxymethylcellulose and gelatin applied to a flexible film. They are waterproof, self-adhesive and reported to reduce pain, and can absorb wound exudate to form a gel in the wound bed which promotes moist wound healing. The waterproof nature of the dressings allows patients to bathe or shower and dressings can be left in place for up to 7 days.

Hydrocolloid dressings rehydrate and promote debridement of sloughy, necrotic wounds such as leg ulcers, pressure sores, donor sites and moderately exudative wounds. They should not be used to manage heavily exuding wounds, diabetic foot ulcers and any wound infected with anaerobic organisms. Examples include Comfeel®, Granuflex®, Tegasorb® and Hydrocoll®.

Hydrofibre dressings (Figure 25.5)
These are composed of sodium carboxymethylcellulose spun into fibres which can absorb and retain significant amounts of exudate

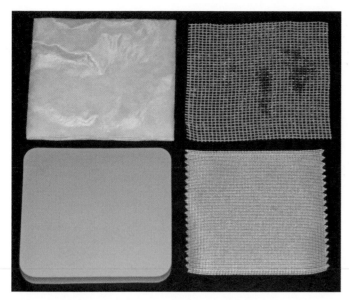

Figure 25.2 Non-adherent dressings (from top left clockwise: Melolin, Jelonet, Lyofoam, knitted viscose).

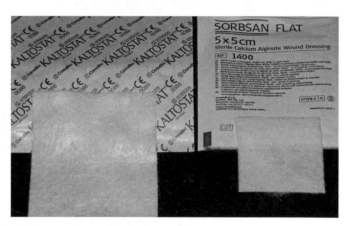

Figure 25.5 Hydrofibre dressing absorbs exudate.

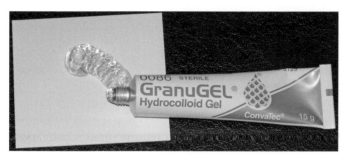

Figure 25.3 Hydrogel dressing.

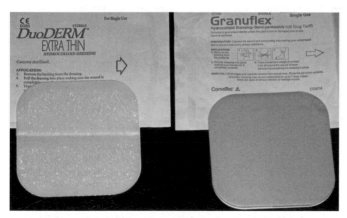

Figure 25.4 Hydrocolloid dressings.

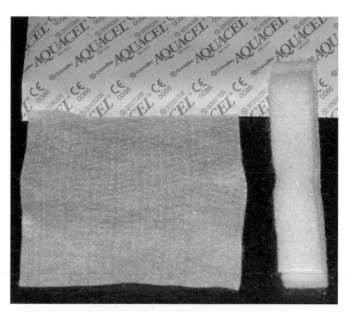

Figure 25.6 Alginate dressings.

Alginate dressings (Figure 25.6)

These consist of sodium and calcium salts of alginic acid in a sterile fibrous dressing. They are derived from brown seaweeds (Phaeophycecae family) and absorb exudates to form a moist hydrogel. Sorbsan® and Tegagel® are available in sheet and rope forms and are useful in the management of highly exudating wounds and filling cavities. Kaltostat® has haemostatic properties and is therefore useful for bleeding wounds. Alginates are easily removed by irrigating the wound with saline. Sinuses and diabetic foot ulcers must be lightly packed to allow for drainage.

Polyurethane foam dressings (Figure 25.7)

These contain hydrophilic, absorbent polyurethane foam and may have an outer waterproof, bacteria-proof backing. They transmit moisture and oxygen to provide thermal insulation at the wound bed. These dressings are useful in the management of low/moderate exudative wounds and may require a secondary dressing. Foam dressings are available for cavity wounds. Polyurethane dressings can protect the skin around the wound from subsequent

by vertical wicking. The exudate is then converted into a gel sheet on the wound. Hydrofibre dressings are therefore suitable for any wound with heavy exudates, slough and wet necrosis. A secondary dressing is required to keep hydrofibre dressings in place. Dressing change should be undertaken every 1–7 days depending on any underlying wound infection. Aquacel® is currently the only hydrofibre dressing available.

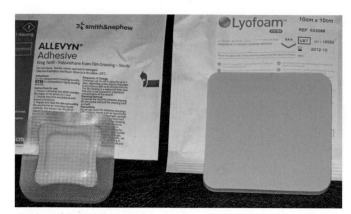

Figure 25.7 Polyurethane foam dressings.

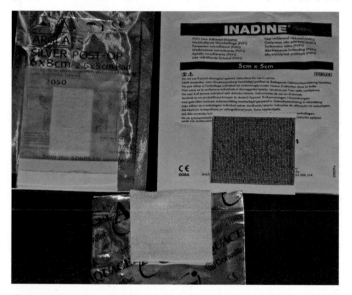

Figure 25.8 Antimicrobial dressings impregnated with iodine and silver.

damage and can be left in place for 5 days. Examples include Lyofoam® (shiny side applied to skin), Allevyn® and Tielle®.

Antimicrobial dressings (Figure 25.8)

Secondary bacterial infection of wounds is always of concern to wound practitioners, but with hospital-acquired infections and antibiotic resistance on the increase the demand for antimicrobial dressings has increased. Silver has been used for many years as an antimicrobial agent for the treatment of burns in the form of sulphadiazine cream. New dressings impregnated with silver are available for a variety of wounds that are either colonized or infected. Examples include Actisorb Silver®, Aquacel Ag®, SilvaSorb® Silverlon® and Urgotul SSD®.

Iodine has the ability to lower bacterial growth in chronic wounds and is active against Gram-positive and -negative organisms. Caution is required for patients with thyroid disease due to possible systemic uptake of iodine. Examples include Inadine® and betadine®.

Metronidazole gel can be applied to infected wounds, particularly those colonized with anaerobic organisms. The gel helps with

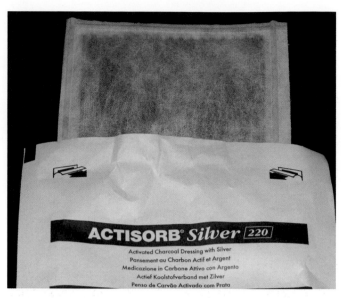

Figure 25.9 Odour-absorbing dressing containing activated charcoal.

odour control and is especially useful in managing fungating malignant wounds.

Odour-absorbing dressings (Figure 25.9)

Charcoal dressings filter and absorb malodorous chemicals from wounds, they can be used as a primary or secondary dressing and they are indicated in all malodorous wounds.

The activated charcoal loses its function to absorb odours when it is saturated with exudate and requires regular changing. Examples include Actisorb®, Clinisorb® and Kaltocarb®.

Cavity dressings (Figure 25.10)

Traditionally, cavity wounds were packed with ribbon gauze but are now commonly dressed with alginate fibre in the form of rope or ribbon. These dressings are used to lightly pack wound cavities to encourage healing from the wound bed in an upwards direction. In addition foam chips in pouches of varying sizes are also available that can be placed inside cavities to absorb exudate and stimulate granulation. Examples include Aquacel ribbon®, Allevyn Cavity®, Kaltostat rope® and Sorbsan Ribbon®.

Larvae therapy (Figure 25.11)

Therapeutic maggots are the larvae of the green bottle fly (*Lucillia seriata*) which are used to debride sloughy and necrotic wounds without attacking healthy granulation tissue. In the UK larvae are supplied by the Biosurgical Research Unit at the Bridgend Hospital in South Wales where they are bred under sterile conditions and dispatched by a courier. Larvae are applied twice weekly until the wound is debrided and granulation tissue exposed, after which a conventional dressing should be used until the wound has healed.

Honey dressings (Figure 25.12)

Honey is an ancient treatment for infected wounds which has recently been reintroduced for wound management particularly where conventional agents have failed. The antimicrobial properties

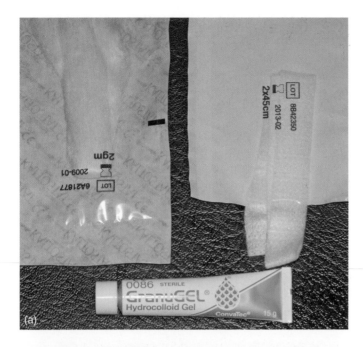

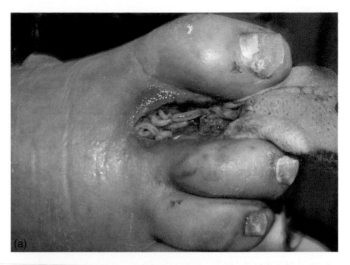

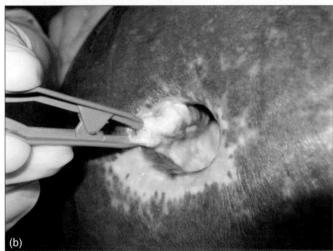

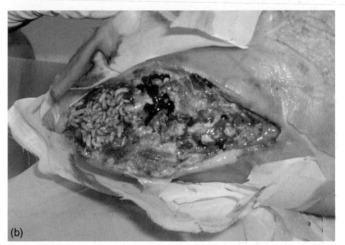

Figure 25.11 Larvae therapy on (a) toes and (b) amputation stump.

Figure 25.10 (a) Cavity dressings (ropes, ribbons and gel). (b) Rope *in situ* in a deep pressure sore.

of honey include the release of low levels of hydrogen peroxide. Examples of honey dressings include Activon Honey Tulle® and Advancis®.

Negative pressure dressings (Figure 25.13)
The application of controlled levels of negative pressure (with a vacuum pump) to wounds has been shown to accelerate debridement and promote healing. Negative pressure assists with the removal of interstitial fluid, reduces localized oedema and increases blood flow. These dressings must be applied by an experienced practitioner.

Adverse effects of dressings
- Maceration of the surrounding skin.
- Irritant contact dermatitis.
- Allergic contact dermatitis.

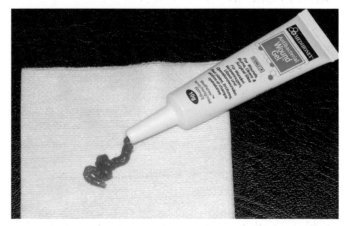

Figure 25.12 Honey dressing.

Bandages

Bandages have been used for thousands of years, going back to the time of the ancient Egyptians who applied woven fabric with considerable skill to mummify their dead. With the discovery of natural rubber in the mid-19th century, the first elasticated bandages were

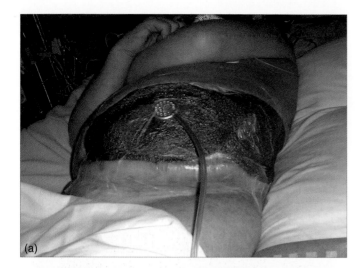

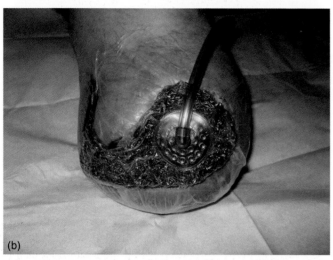

Figure 25.13 Vacuum pump dressing on (a) the abdomen and (b) an amputation stump.

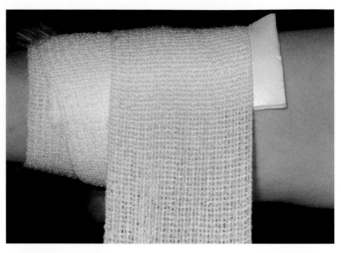

Figure 25.14 Type I retention bandages holding a non-adherent dressing in place.

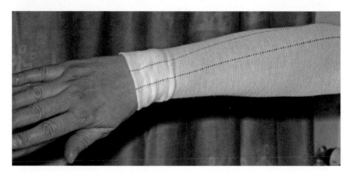

Figure 25.15 Type II light support bandage made from elasticated viscose.

produced for the management of varicose veins. These bandages were made of natural fibres through a weaving process as a simple retention bandage to provide support and protection.

Bandage application is a necessary skill required by most nursing and some medical practitioners during their working life. Therefore it is essential that training in bandage application is adequate in order that bandages may be applied correctly and safely to patients.

Definitions relating to bandaging

- *Extensibility*: determines the length produced when an extending force is applied.
- *Elasticity*: the ability to return to its original length once the extending force is removed.
- *Compression*: the force applied to produce a desired clinical effect.
- *Support*: the retention and control of tissue without the application of compression.
- *Conformability*: the ability to follow the contours of a limb and is largely due to the extensibility and density of the fabric. Knitted bandages are more conformable than woven bandages.

Classification of bandages

Type I (Figure 25.14)

Lightweight conforming bandages used for the retention of light dressings. These bandages should conform to limbs and joints without causing restriction. Examples are Slinky®, J-fast® and Stayform®.

Type II (Figure 25.15)

Light support bandages are manufactured from cotton, polymide, viscose and elastane. They are used for the retention of dressings, mild support in the treatment of strains and sprains, and to prevent oedema. They are not suitable for compression but can be used in the treatment of venous ulceration with arterial disease. Type II include crepe-type bandages such as Soffcrepe®, Elastocrepe®, Leukocrepe and Comprilan®.

Type III

Compression bandages are used to apply compression to control oedema and reduce swelling in the treatment of venous or lymphovenous disease of the lower limbs. They are subdivided into four categories according to their ability to provide set levels of compression.

Type IIIa

Light compression bandages providing low levels of pressure up to 20 mmHg at the ankle. They are indicated in the management of early, superficial varices but are not suitable for controlling or reducing oedema. Examples include K-Plus®, Tensolastic® and Elset®.

Type IIIb

Moderate compression bandages may be used to manage varicosities during pregnancy, for the prevention/treatment of ulcers and for control of mild oedema. These exert levels of compression of 30 mmHg at the ankle.

Type IIIc

High compression bandages may be used for applying 40 mmHg pressure at the ankle. These bandages can be used to manage large varices, leg ulcers and limb oedema. Examples include Tensopress®, Setopress® and Surepress®.

Type IIId

These extra-high performance compression bandages apply 50 mmHg pressure at the ankle and therefore can sustain high pressure for extended periods to grossly oedematous limbs. Examples include Varico® and Elastic Web® bandage.

Tubular bandages

These are cotton bandages used extensively in dermatology in the treatment of atopic eczema and patients with erythroderma. They can be applied to limbs, cut and fashioned into a body suit and used as dry or wet wraps.

Wet wraps are moist bandages applied to the body over emollients and/or topical steroids to acute active or chronic lichenified eczema. Wet wraps are cooling, reduce itching, prolong emollient effects, enhance topical steroid potency and protect the skin from trauma though scratching. Wet wraps are not indicated for long-term use with a topical steroid and should be avoided if the skin is infected.

Dry wraps are applied in a similar fashion to cover the skin. They enhance the effect of topical agents and protect the skin and the patient's clothing.

Manufacturers are now producing cotton garments (Figure 25.16) for the same purpose, making it easier for parents and patients to apply the materials and therefore manage skin disease.

Medicated paste bandages (Figure 25.17)

These bandages are made from flat open-weave cotton bandages impregnated with appropriate medicaments. They are widely used in a variety of dermatological conditions such as venous ulceration, nodular prurigo, psoriasis, lichen simplex and chronic lichenified eczema. They should be avoided if the skin is macerated or exudative.

Paste bandages are used to soothe, occlude, protect the skin from scratching and enhance the effect of topical applications. Examples include Calaband® (zinc paste with calamine), Tarband® (zinc paste with coal tar), Ichthaband® (zinc and icthamol) and Steriband® (zinc paste bandage).

Medicated bandages need to be applied skilfully to prevent constriction and to allow for shrinkage, and need to be changed when they are drying out. They require a secondary bandage to keep it in

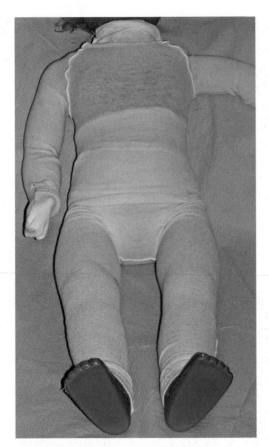

Figure 25.16 Cotton garments for wet/dry wrapping.

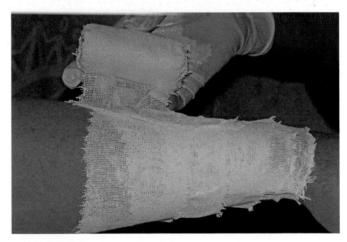

Figure 25.17 Medicated bandage with zinc paste and calamine.

place and protect the patient's clothing. Hypersensitivity reactions can develop to the medicaments.

Application of bandages

The correct application of bandages is of paramount importance. Applied too loosely, the bandage will be ineffective and applied too tightly the bandage may cause constriction resulting in tissue damage and necrosis. In extreme cases this can lead to amputation.

Research has shown that there is a great variation in the consistency of the tension in the application of bandages between

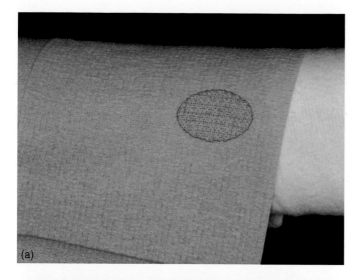

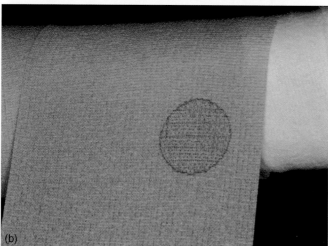

Figure 25.18 Markings on bandages to ensure consistent tension. (a) Incorrect tension (oval). (b) Correct tension (circle).

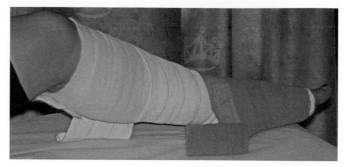

Figure 25.19 Type III compression bandaging. Four layers applied to the leg can be seen as follows from the knee downwards: 1st layer orthopaedic wool; 2nd layer cotton crepe; 3rd layer elastic extensible bandage; 4th layer cohesive bandage.

6 High compression requires an ankle/brachial pressure index (ABPI) of more than 0.8.

The four-layer compression system for ankle circumference 18–25 cm

Orthopaedic wool (Figure 25.19). The purpose is to absorb exudate, protect bony prominences and redistribute the pressure around the limb. Apply from the base of the toes to the knee overlapping 50%. Pad the tender areas on the dorsum of the foot, the Achilles tendon and the shin.

Cotton crepe. This layer adds absorbency and smoothes the wool layer. Apply from the base of the toes, in even tension with 50% overlap to ensure a smooth surface for the application of the elastic layers.

Elastic, extensible bandage. The first compression layer with sub-bandage pressure of 17 mmHg at the ankle. Anchor the bandage at the base of the toes with two turns and 50% extension, continue with a 'figure of 8' around the ankle and extend up the limb with 50% overlap and 50% extension of the bandage.

Cohesive bandage. This is the second compression bandage of the system and adds the remaining 23 mmHg at the ankle to give 40 mmHg. The cohesiveness assists in the retention of the bandages. The bandage is applied in a spiral technique with 50% stretch and 50% overlap.

In patients with 'champagne'-shaped legs, apply with a 'figure of 8' method to prevent slippage of the bandage.

Modifications

In patients with ankle circumference less than 18 cm and greater than 25 cm, the four-layer system can be modified to produce the correct pressure at the ankle as follows:

- where less than 18 cm, apply two or more layers of orthopaedic wool
- where 25–30 cm, use wool, a high compression bandage and cohesive bandage
- where more than 30 cm, wool, elastic-conformable, high-compression and cohesive bandages can be used.

practitioners. To overcome this problem, some bandages have a design printed on the bandage at regular intervals which changes shape when the correct extension is applied (Figure 25.18).

Preparation for compression bandaging

1 A limb assessment to identify any deformities, oedema and alteration of the limb contour which may need consideration when applying the bandage. Measure the ankle circumference to ensure the correct compression bandages are used.
2 Wound assessment at baseline by measurements or photography to monitor progress.
3 Dressings. Appropriate, non-adherent, absorbent dressings to overcome exudate, odour and pain.
4 Pain assessment. Eighty per cent of patients with venous ulcers complain of pain which requires appropriate management to enable them to tolerate the compression.
5 Patient preparation. Patient understanding and commitment to compression therapy is vital to the success of the treatment and patient concordance.

Two-layer compression

This system consists of a layer of orthopaedic wool and a high-compression bandage applied from the base of the toes in a spiral with 50% overlap and 50% extension. Short-stretch compression bandages are applied at full stretch over an orthopaedic wool bandage.

Rubber sensitivity

There is a continuing high incidence of contact sensitivity in patients with venous leg ulcers which has implications for their management. Contact dermatitis to rubber limits the type of compression bandages that can be used. Cotton short-stretch bandages are recommended for these patients. Apply a tubular cotton gauze bandage directly to the skin. Next apply the wool layer as before and then the short stretch at full extension with a figure of 8 around the ankle and continue with a spiral overlapping 50% at full extension up the leg.

Patient information

Patient compliance is as vital to wound healing as the dressings and bandages themselves. To ensure that the patient complies adequately with their wound management the following should be considered.

- Ensure the patient understands their treatment regime.
- Devise a treatment plan to suit the patient's lifestyle.
- Provide an information leaflet explaining aftercare.
- Peripheral circulation to the toes should be checked after application of bandages.
- In the event of excessive pain or discomfort caused by the bandages patients should be advised to contact the treatment unit.

- Patients should be advised not to be alarmed by breakthrough exudates.
- Bandages should be kept dry by providing aids to use in the bath/shower.
- Encourage a good balance between rest and exercise.
- Advise patients not to remove bandages themselves.
- Provide the patient with a contact telephone number to ring for advice.

The efficacy of dressings and bandages to heal wounds and treat skin complaints depends on selection of the correct products for the particular situation. Ideally there should be good channels of communication and clinical consistency between primary/secondary care and wound management specialists. Team work should ensure the optimum management of the patient's skin, promote rapid healing, provide an excellent local service, reduce the cost of wound care and enhance the patient's quality of life.

Further reading

Charles H. Does leg ulcer treatment improve patients' quality of life? *J Woundcare* 2004; **13**(6): 209–13.

Jones V, Grey JE, Harding K. ABC of wound healing: wound dressings. *BMJ* 2006; **332**: 777–80.

Moffat C. Know how. Four-layer bandaging. *Nurs Times* 1997; April 16–22; 93(16):82–3.

Myers BA. *Wound Management: Principles and Practice*, 2nd edn. Pearson/Prentice Hall, New Jersey, 2004.

www.worldwidewounds.com

CHAPTER 26

Formulary

Karen Watson

Introduction

The treatment of skin disease has evolved dramatically over recent years. Historically, patients were admitted for intensive nursing with extemporaneously prepared combinations of topical steroids, tars, pastes and bandaging. Today however, there is a much greater emphasis on outpatient treatment. Quality control and cost issues have seen a reduction in the number of extemporaneous products available, and there have been exciting new developments in both topical and systemic treatment.

Topical therapy

The skin has the advantage of being readily amenable to treatment with topical therapy. Relatively high concentrations of medication can be applied to the skin safely, with good efficacy and comparatively few side-effects. Several factors govern the choice of topical treatment, such as formulation, frequency of application, site and severity of skin disease and patient ability to apply local therapy. Complications tend to be local irritant or allergic reactions.

The choice of topical treatment depends on the disease process, pharmaceutical properties of the drug, site of application and cosmesis.

Emollients

Emollients are important in the treatment of dry, scaly and inflammatory skin conditions as they help to reduce transepidermal water loss from a damaged epidermal barrier. They soften dry skin by filling in the spaces left by desquamating keratinocytes.

The constituents of an emollient or topical base have significant properties. Lipids for example, cover the stratum corneum to prevent evaporation of water. White and yellow soft paraffin and liquid paraffin are extracted from crude oil. They are stable, inert hydrocarbons, which form the basis of most commercially available ointments and emollients. Emulsifying agents are used to stabilize emulsions, which are immiscible mixtures of aqueous and oily constituents, and penetration enhancers, such as urea and propylene glycol may be used to increase penetration of an active component

through the skin. Humectants are compounds with a high affinity for water, which are able to draw water into the stratum corneum and have useful emollient properties.

The properties of various formulations of topical therapy are outlined in Table 26.1.

Bath emollients and soap substitutes are as important as regular emollients in the treatment of dry skin conditions. Soaps are detergents, which irritate the skin, remove intercellular lipids and break down the stratum corneum barrier. They should therefore be avoided whenever possible.

Topical immunomodulatory treatments

Topical corticosteroids

The development of topical corticosteroids revolutionized the treatment of skin disease in the 1950s and 60s, and they have been used to treat a wide range of inflammatory dermatoses since. The mechanism of action is complex. The steroid diffuses through the stratum corneum, through the cell membranes and to the cytoplasm of the keratinocytes. Here, it binds to the glucocorticoid receptor, activating the receptor. The ligand-bound receptor enters the nuclear compartment and interacts with glucocorticoid response elements (GREs). This results in the modulation of gene transcription. Furthermore, the ligand-bound receptor may also inhibit other transcription factors. The overall effect is to suppress inflammatory cytokines, inhibit T-cell activation and reduce cell proliferation.

Topical corticosteroids are classified according to their potency, which seems to be related to their affinity for the glucocorticoid receptor. This classification allows determination of the relative strength and potential side-effects of therapy, so that the most appropriate treatment is chosen for a given skin disorder and site.

Table 26.2 outlines a number of topical steroids and their relative potency.

Topical corticosteroids have a number of side-effects and should therefore be applied sparingly. However, fear of potential complications can often result in under-treatment. Side-effects include:
- skin atrophy
- telangiectasia
- striae (Figure 26.1)
- ecchymoses
- hirsutism

ABC of Dermatology, 5th edition. Edited by P. K. Buxton and R. Morris-Jones.
© 2009 Blackwell Publishing, ISBN: 978-1-4051-7065-9.

Table 26.1 Comparison of formulations for topical therapy.

Formulation	Characteristics	Advantages	Disadvantages
Ointments	Oil-based. Provide occlusive film over skin and help to retain water. Aid skin hydration and penetration of topical treatment	Tend not to require preservatives as lack of water in preparation prevents microbial growth	Greasy and cosmetically less appealing to use
Creams	Emulsions containing water and oil. May be composed of oil in water or water in oil (oily creams). Aid skin hydration, but generally less effectively than ointments	Cosmetically acceptable	Contain preservatives, which may cause sensitization
Lotions	Watery suspensions, often containing alcohol	Easily spread over a large area. Evaporation of water or alcohol has a drying, cooling effect. Cosmetically acceptable. Useful for hair-bearing areas, such as the scalp	Contain preservatives and therefore have sensitizing potential. Alcohol may cause stinging
Gels	Semisolid emulsion in alcohol base. Useful for suspending insoluble drugs. Good absorbent properties	Tend to dry on skin. Useful for hair-bearing areas. Cosmetically acceptable, especially for use on the face	Relatively high irritant and sensitizing potential

Table 26.2 Relative potency of topical corticosteroids.

Generic name	Proprietary name	Potency
Hydrocortisone 1%	Efcortelan®	Mild
Hydrocortisone acetate 1% and fusidic acid 1%	Fucidin H®	Mild
Hydrocortisone 1%, nystatin 100 000 units/g and oxytetracycline 3%	Timodine®	Mild
Clobetasone butyrate 0.05%	Eumovate®	Moderate
Alclometasone diproprionate 0.05%	Modrasone®	Moderate
Betamethasone valerate 0.1%	Betnovate®	Potent
Mometasone furoate 0.1%	Elocon®	Potent
Diflucortolone valerate 0.1%	Nerisone®	Potent
Betamethasone diproprionate 0.05% and salicylic acid 3%	Diprosalic®	Potent
Betamethasone valerate 0.1% and fusidic acid 3%	Fucibet®	Potent
Clobetasol proprionate 0.05%	Dermovate®	Superpotent
Clobetasol proprionate 0.05%, neomycin sulphate 0.5% and nystatin 100 000 units/g	Dermovate NN®	Superpotent

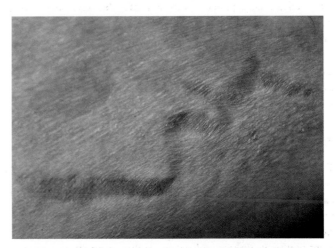

Figure 26.1 Liberal application of a potent topical steroid resulting in striae formation.

- folliculitis
- steroid-induced rosacea
- perioral and periorbital dermatitis (Figures 26.2 & 26.3)
- absorption, and suppression of the hypothalamic–pituitary axis.

Calcineurin inhibitors

Topical tacrolimus and pimecrolimus were originally developed for the treatment of eczema. They inhibit calcineurin, a calcium- and calmodulin-dependent serine/threonine phosphatase, and suppress T-cell activation. Topical tacrolimus has also been used in the treatment of actinic dermatitis, alopecia areata, oral and genital lichen planus, pyoderma gangrenosum, cutaneous graft versus host disease and vitiligo, with varying degrees of success. Pimecrolimus is less potent than topical tacrolimus and is used predominantly in the treatment of eczema in children. It helps reduce flares and the requirement for a topical corticosteroid.

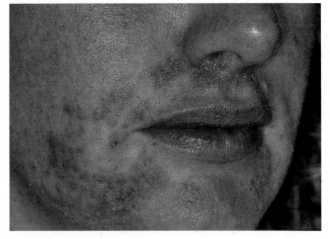

Figure 26.2 Perioral dermatitis caused by local application of topical steroids.

Topical antimicrobials

A number of topical antimicrobial preparations are available, some of which are summarized in Table 26.3.

Miscellaneous topical therapy used in the treatment of psoriasis

These are outlined in Table 26.4.

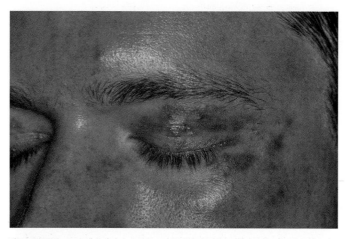

Figure 26.3 Periorbital dermatitis caused by local application of topical steroids.

Topical antiproliferative agents

Topical 5-fluorouracil

5-Fluorouracil is an antimetabolite which blocks DNA synthesis by inhibiting thymidylate synthetase. It is used topically to treat actinic keratoses, Bowen's disease and superficial actinic keratoses. Its main adverse effects include local erythema and irritation. Continued application may result in considerable inflammation and erosions.

Topical diclofenac

Diclofenac is a non-steroidal anti-inflammatory drug available in a 3% gel formulation for the treatment of actinic keratoses. The mechanism of action is unclear. It is generally well tolerated, although there may be some localized inflammation.

Topical imiquimod

Topical imiquimod is a recently developed preparation, used to treat conditions such as genital warts, vulval intraepithelial neoplasia (VIN), extramammary Paget's disease, actinic keratoses, superficial BCCs and lentigo maligna. It stimulates the

Table 26.3 Topical antimicrobials used in the treatment of superficial infections.

	Preparation	Indications	Complications
Topical antibiotics	Fusidic acid (Fucidin ointment®)	Staphylococcal infections	Resistance
	Mupirocin (Bactroban ointment®)	Gram-positive and some Gram-negative organisms Treatment of nasal staphylococcal carriage	Resistance
	Silver sulphadiazine (Flamazine®)	Pseudomonal infection and some prophylaxis against staphylococcal infection	Minimal absorption and renal impairment when applied to extensive burns
	Retapamulin (Altargo®)	Staphylococcal and streptococcal infections	Application site irritation
Topical antibiotics used in the treatment of acne	Tetracyclines Erythromycin Clindamycin	Acne May be used in combination with keratolytics such as benzoyl peroxide	Resistance May stain clothing yellow
Topical antifungals	Allylamines Terbinafine cream (Lamisil cream®)	Fungicidal against dermatophyte infections	Ineffective against dermatophyte infections of the nails and scalp
	Imidazoles Clotrimazole (Canesten®) Econazole Ketoconazole Miconazole	Fungistatic Active against *Candida* and *Pityrosporum* May be used in combination with topical steroids Used in the treatment of intertrigo, pityriasis versicolor and some dermatophyte infections	Concurrent use of topical steroid may mask infection
	Amorolfine (Loceryl lacquer®)	Fungistatic Used in the treatment of onychomycosis Some activity against *Scytalidium* Synergistic activity with systemic antifungals	Poor cure rates in dermatophyte infections affecting the nail matrix when used as sole therapy
Topical antivirals	Aciclovir cream (Zovirax®)	Used to treat labial and genital herpes simplex	Needs to be applied as early as possible in the episode for maximum benefit
Antiparasitic agents	Permethrin	5% cream used in the treatment of scabies and pubic lice. 1% rinse used to treat head lice	Require two treatments 1 week apart
	Malathion	Used in the treatment of scabies, head lice and pubic lice	Alcoholic lotions can irritate skin and can exacerbate eczema Resistance

Table 26.4 Miscellaneous preparations used in the treatment of psoriasis.

Preparation	Mode of action	Indications	Complications
Crude coal tar and coal tar solution Derived from the distillation of organic matter	Unclear Tar has antiproliferative effects on the epidermis	Psoriasis Used in combination with ultraviolet radiation with additive effects	Messy to use Potent odour Scrotal squamous cell carcinoma
Dithranol Available in cream formulation or in Lassars paste in concentrations from 0.1% to 3%	Unclear Dithranol has potent antiproliferative effects	Psoriasis Short contact regimens used in outpatient settings	Local reactions and irritation of normal surrounding skin Skin staining
Vitamin D3 analogues: Calcipotriol (Dovonex®), and tacalcitol (Silkis®) Combination of calcipotriol and betamethasone (Dovobet®)	Regulate cell growth, differentiation and immune function	Psoriasis	Hypercalcaemia Irritation Prolonged use of betamethasone and calcipotriol may precipitate the formation of pustules on withdrawal

innate immune system and also promotes the development of antigen-specific cell-mediated responses via Toll-like receptor 7. It causes considerable inflammation with oedema, erosions and occasional ulceration.

Miscellaneous agents

Keratolytics

Keratolytic agents are topical preparations used in the treatment of hyperkeratosis and acne. They help soften the skin and aid the removal of scale. They may also have anticomedogenic activity, although they can cause local irritation with erythema and dryness. Examples include salicylic acid and vitamin A derivatives such as tretinoin and adapalene.

Sunscreens

The aim of sunscreens is to block both UVA and UVB penetration of the skin and thereby inhibit the ageing and carcinogenic effects of UV radiation. Compounds used to achieve sun protection may either reflect and scatter UV light or absorb it. Examples of physical agents blocking UV include zinc oxide, titanium dioxide and ferrous oxide. They tend to be used in combination with light absorbers such as para-aminobenzoic acid (PABA) and benzophenones. The sun protection factor (SPF) of a sunscreen is an indication of the level of protection from UVB. An SPF over 15 is considered to confer good UVB protection when the sunscreen is applied adequately. UVA protection is measured on a 1–5 star basis, although there is little standardization.

Cosmetic camouflage

Cosmetic camouflage plays an important role in the treatment of patients with disfiguring conditions such as scarring, dyspigmentation and port wine stains. Proprietary preparations are readily available, and the Red Cross provides a volunteer-led service for patients.

Phototherapy

Phototherapy involves the treatment of skin disease with ultraviolet (UV) radiation alone and photochemotherapy UV irradiation in combination with a psoralen (PUVA). Both are used extensively in dermatological practice to treat a wide range of skin disorders. Phototherapy involves the use of artificial UVB irradiation delivered by fluorescent lamps. UVB consists of electromagnetic energy of wavelength 290–320 nm and represents that part of the spectrum that is largely responsible for sunburn. UVA consists of energy of wavelength 315–400 nm. Both PUVA and narrow-band UVB phototherapy are now widely used for the treatment of psoriasis, atopic eczema, polymorphic light eruption, mycosis fungoides and vitiligo, amongst others.

Systemic therapy

Drugs used for infectious disorders

Antibacterial drugs

Antibiotics are used widely in dermatology for conditions ranging from acne to impetigo to cellulitis, and may be required for prolonged courses over a period of weeks to months. There are a number of considerations to be taken into account when choosing an antibiotic, such as host and drug factors, and causative pathogen. Host factors include underlying disease, age, previous adverse reactions and pregnancy. Swabs should always be performed for microbiology, culture and sensitivity to confirm the causative pathogen and to identify resistance. Drug parameters include interaction with concomitant therapy, side-effect profile, dosage, route of administration and cost. Table 26.5 illustrates some of the antibiotics used in dermatology, their mode of action, indications and complications.

Antifungal drugs

Most cutaneous fungal infections can be effectively treated with topical therapy. However, systemic treatment is required for fungal infection of the nails and hair. Terbinafine and griseofulvin are used to treat tinea capitis and onychomycosis caused by dermatophytes, and itraconazole is also effective in the treatment of pityriasis versicolor. Terbinafine is an allylamine that binds to plasma proteins and is found in high concentrations in the hair, nails and stratum corneum. It is fungicidal. In tinea capitis it appears to be more effective

Table 26.5 Antibiotics used in dermatology, their method of action, indications and complications.

Antibiotic group	Method of action	Antibiotic	Indications	Complications
Penicillins	Inhibition of bacterial cell wall synthesis Activation of autolytic bacterial enzymes Bactericidal	Penicillin	Gram-positive infections (e.g. *Streptococcus*) Cellulitis Erysipelas	Hypersensitivity reactions which may be severe Dose reduction in renal impairment
	B lactamase-resistant penicillin	Flucloxacillin	B lactamase-producing organisms (e.g. *Staphylococcus aureus*) Cellulitis Impetigo	Hypersensitivity reactions
Macrolides	Penetration of bacterial cell wall and inhibition of RNA-dependent protein synthesis by reversible binding to ribosomes	Erythromycin	Gram-positive infections Penicillin allergy Cellulitis Erysipelas Impetigo Acne Erythrasma	Nausea, diarrhoea
		Clarithromycin	Gram-positive and Gram negative cover Erysipelas	Fewer gastrointestinal side-effects
Tetracyclines	Inhibition of protein synthesis by ribosomal binding	Oxytetracycline Minocycline Doxycycline Lymecycline	Gram-positive and Gram-negative organisms Mycobacteria Acne Rosacea Perioral dermatitis Bullous pemphigoid Lyme disease Fish tank granuloma	Nausea, vomiting Brown discolouration of teeth and delayed bone growth in children. Therefore contraindicated in children under 12 years Hypersensitivity reactions Blue-black pigmentation of nails and skin

against endothrix organisms such as *Trichophyton tonsurans* than ectothrix infections such as *Microsporum canis*. Although it is not licensed for use in children, several studies have shown it to be safe and effective. It is used daily for 4 weeks in the treatment of tinea capitis and the dose is calculated according to the weight of the patient. Prolonged courses of 3 or more months are required in the treatment of onychomycosis involving the nail matrix.

Griseofulvin has fungistatic activity and is widely used for the treatment of tinea capitis in children, in which it requires a 6-week course. However, its use is rapidly being overtaken by terbinafine and itraconazole, which tend to be better tolerated and have a broader spectrum of activity. Griseofulvin is ineffective against pityriasis versicolor or yeast infections such as *Candida albicans*.

Itraconazole is a triazole used in pulsed therapy or continuously for the treatment of onychomycosis, tinea capitis particularly in young infants, and pityriasis versicolor resistant to topical therapy.

Antiviral drugs

Systemic antivirals are available for the treatment of human herpesvirus (HHV) infections such as herpes simplex virus type 1 and type 2 (resulting in herpes labialis and genital lesions respectively) and varicella zoster virus (VZV), causing chicken pox and herpes zoster (shingles).

Aciclovir is a well-established antiviral drug used in the treatment of HHV. It inhibits viral DNA polymerase and irreversibly inhibits viral DNA synthesis. The dose and duration of treatment depends on the diagnosis; primary genital herpes simplex infection generally requires a prolonged course whilst herpes zoster and chicken pox in adults require a high dose. It tends to be most effective if therapy is started early in the disease, during the prodrome. For frequently recurrent HSV infection, low-dose prophylactic treatment may be useful. Intravenous administration is usually necessary in severely ill patients, particularly those who are immunocompromised or those with eczema herpeticum, who are at risk of disseminated HSV infection.

Alternative antivirals include valaciclovir and famciclovir, which are licensed for the treatment of herpes zoster and primary and recurrent genital herpes. Their advantage is that they are administered three times daily whereas aciclovir is taken five times daily. They are, however, more expensive.

Antiparasite drugs

Scabies and pediculosis are usually adequately treated with topical therapy. However, Norwegian (crusted) scabies or scabetic infection and pediculosis that has failed to settle with multiple courses of conventional topical preparations may be amenable to treatment with ivermectin. Ivermectin causes paralysis and death of parasites and a single dose is usually all that is required. It is available on a named-patient basis only.

Larva migrans and larva currens tend to respond well to topical therapy, but may also be treated with short courses of systemic albendazole or ivermectin.

Systemic immunomodulatory drugs

Corticosteroids

Systemic corticosteroids are used in the treatment of a wide range of inflammatory dermatoses. They are effective immunosuppressant and anti-inflammatory agents, but have a number of side-effects. These include hyperglycaemia, hyperlipidaemia, hypertension, sodium and fluid retention, atherosclerosis, suppression of the hypothalamic–pituitary axis (HPA), growth retardation, osteoporosis, avascular necrosis of bone, alteration of fat distribution, myopathy, increased incidence of infection, re-activation of tuberculosis, peptic ulceration, glaucoma, cataracts, striae and psychiatric disorders. The indications, risks, benefits, potential adjuvant steroid-sparing therapy and gastrointestinal and bone protection should therefore be carefully considered. However, systemic corticosteroids are particularly useful in controlling immunobullous disorders, eczema, vasculitis, drug eruptions, connective tissue disorders, sarcoidosis, erythroderma, lichen planus and neutrophilic dermatoses amongst others. They are relatively contraindicated in psoriasis as withdrawal of the steroid may precipitate an exacerbation or generalized pustular psoriasis.

Patients treated with corticosteroids should be monitored closely for side-effects, and they should be weaned off therapy slowly over a period of time, depending on the dose and duration of treatment. Patient education is important for those on long-term treatment. They should be provided with a steroid treatment card, which outlines important information for patients and carers.

Methotrexate

Methotrexate is an antimetabolite and is a potent inhibitor of the enzyme dihydrofolate reductase. It competitively and irreversibly binds to dihydrofolate reductase with a much greater affinity than its natural substrate folic acid, thereby preventing the conversion of dihydrofolate to tetrahydrofolate. This is an important step in the synthesis of thymidylate and purine nucleotides needed for DNA and RNA synthesis, and results in inhibition of cell division.

Methotrexate is very useful in the treatment of psoriasis and psoriatic arthropathy. It is thought to act as an immunomodulator by inhibiting DNA synthesis in lymphocytes rather than having an antiproliferative effect. It is primarily used to treat psoriasis, but is also used in sarcoidosis, bullous pemphigoid, vasculitis and morphoea.

Methotrexate is taken as a once a week dose, the dose being carefully titrated by 2.5-mg increments. It has a number of side-effects including bone marrow suppression, hepatotoxicity, nausea and vomiting, pulmonary fibrosis and teratogenicity, and patients must therefore be monitored closely. Procollagen III may be measured as a marker of liver fibrosis. Folic acid 5 mg once daily is taken simultaneously, but not on the day of methotrexate administration. This reduces nausea and hepatotoxicity. Acute methotrexate overdose or toxicity may be treated with folinic acid, which bypasses the metabolic effects of methotrexate.

Methotrexate also has a number of potentially serious drug interactions.

Azathioprine

Azathioprine is an antimetabolite that inhibits DNA and RNA synthesis, and also the differentiation and proliferation of lymphocytes. It is an immunosuppressant and is often used in conjunction with corticosteroids as it has steroid-sparing effects. Azathioprine is an effective treatment in a wide range of dermatological conditions, such as severe atopic eczema, chronic actinic dermatitis, immunobullous disorders, systemic lupus erythematosus and dermatomyositis. Although it is usually well tolerated, it has a number of side-effects including bone marrow suppression, nausea and vomiting, hypersensitivity reactions, hepatotoxicity, macrocytosis, pancreatitis and diffuse hair loss. Bone marrow suppression may be predicted in susceptible patients who have low levels of the enzyme thiopurine methyl transferase (TPMT), and who are therefore unable to metabolize the drug efficiently. Unfortunately the other side-effects of azathioprine do not seem to correlate with TPMT activity.

Ciclosporin

Ciclosporin is an immunosuppressant drug derived from the fungus *Tolypocladium inflatum*. It suppresses the induction and proliferation of T-lymphocytes and inhibits the production of inflammatory cytokines. It is effective in the treatment of severe psoriasis (including erythrodermic psoriasis and palmoplantar pustulosis), atopic eczema and severe drug eruptions such as toxic epidermolytic necrolysis (TEN). Its advantages include rapid onset of action (1–2 weeks) and lack of bone marrow suppression. However, it has a number of side-effects such as renal toxicity, hypertension, hypertrichosis, tremor and gingival hyperplasia. There is also an increased risk of malignancy. Ciclosporin therefore tends to be used for short periods to treat severe flares of disease, or as part of a rotational regimen. It is metabolized by cytochrome P450 and interacts with a number of other drugs.

Mycophenolate mofetil

Mycophenolate mofetil (MMF) is an immunosuppressant agent, which acts by selectively and irreversibly inhibiting inosine monophosphate dehydrogenase, resulting in the depletion of intracellular guanine nucleotides. It seems to have a selective effect on activated T-lymphocytes. In dermatology it is mainly used for the treatment of immunobullous disorders and pyoderma gangrenosum. Side-effects are predominantly gastrointestinal with nausea, vomiting and diarrhoea. The elderly tend to be more susceptible to the adverse effects of MMF, which also include bone marrow suppression, infection, fatigue, headaches and weakness.

Systemic retinoids

Retinoids are derived from vitamin A and include acitretin, isotretinoin and bexarotene. They activate nuclear receptors and regulate gene transcription. They have anti-inflammatory, antikeratinizing, antisebum, anti-tumour and antiproliferative effects. Acitretin is used in the treatment of psoriasis, Darier's disease, pityriasis rubra pilaris, ichthyosis and keratodermas, and in transplant recipients who are at high risk of developing cutaneous malignancies. Isotretinoin is the drug of choice for treating severe nodulocystic acne and timely initiation of treatment is aimed at preventing significant scarring. It may also be used in hidradenitis suppurativa, dissecting cellulitis of the scalp and severe recalcitrant papulopostular rosacea. Bexarotene is reserved for the treatment of cutaneous T-cell lymphoma.

Systemic retinoids have a number of side-effects, the most important of which is teratogenicity. Women of child-bearing age must use a robust form of contraception for at least a month before and during treatment. Isotretinoin and bexarotene have a relatively short elimination half-life and contraception needs to be continued for at least a month after discontinuation of therapy. Acitretin has a very much longer half-life and pregnancy needs to be avoided for at least 2 years after treatment has stopped.

The side-effect profile of systemic retinoids is summarized in Table 26.6.

Antihistamines

Histamine has numerous effects on the skin, causing itching, vasodilatation and increased vascular permeability predominantly through its action on H1 receptors. Antihistamines reversibly block H1 receptors. First-generation antihistamines tend to be sedating and include chlorpheniramine, hydroxyzine and promethazine amongst others. Second-generation antihistamines tend to be non-sedating, have a slower onset and longer duration of action. They include cetirizine, loratidine, fexofenadine, levocetirizine and desloratidine. They play a central role in the treatment of urticaria and angio-oedema, type 1 hypersensitivity reactions and anaphylaxis, pruritus, cutaneous mastcytosis and acute insect bite reactions. They tend to be well tolerated, although side-effects include drowsiness, anticholinergic activity and arrhythmias. Topical

Table 26.6 Side-effects of systemic retinoids.

Teratogenicity
Depression
Cheilitis
Hypercholesterolaemia
Hypertriglyceridaemia
Elevation of transaminases
Hepatitis
Pancreatitis
Myopathy
Reduced night vision
Dry eyes
Epistaxis
Facial erythema
Photosensitivity
Hair loss
Diffuse interstitial skeletal hyperostosis (DISH)
Premature epiphyseal closure
Leucopenia*
Agranulocytosis*
Hypothyroidism*

*Predominantly a risk with bexarotene.

antihistamines should be avoided because of the risk of developing allergic contact dermatitis.

Miscellaneous drugs

Dapsone

Dapsone is a sulphonamide, traditionally used in the treatment of leprosy. Its mode of action is unclear, but it is particularly useful in the treatment of disorders where neutrophils or IgA immune complexes play a role, for example dermatitis herpetiformis, bullous pemphigoid, mucous membrane pemphigoid, linear IgA disease and pyoderma gangrenosum. Side-effects include dose-related haemolysis and haemolytic anaemia, which are more common in those individuals with glucose-6-phosphate dehydrogenase (G6PD) deficiency. G6PD should therefore be measured before starting treatment. Other adverse effects include agranulocytosis, methaemoglobinaemia, hypersensitivity syndrome and peripheral neuropathy.

Antimalarials

Hydroxychloroquine, mepacrine and chloroquine are used to treat systemic lupus erythematosus, discoid lupus erythematosus, subacute cutaneous lupus erythematosus, sarcoidosis, polymorphic light eruption and porphyria cutanea tarda. Their mode of action is thought to involve interruption of antigen processing and inhibition of inflammatory cytokines. Chloroquine can cause irreversible retinopathy, and mepacrine is unlicensed in the UK. Hydroxychloroquine therefore tends to be the antimalarial of choice in the treatment of dermatological disorders. It is well tolerated although retinal toxicity is a rare complication. Visual acuity should be monitored for those patients on long-term therapy.

Biological therapies

Biological therapies or 'biologicals' are a novel treatment modality used in dermatology predominantly in the treatment of psoriasis. There are two main groups:
- anti-tumour necrosis factor (TNF-α) agents such as infliximab, etanercept and adalimumab
- agents directed at targeting T-cells or antigen presenting cells, such as efalizumab.

These agents are used in the treatment of moderate to severe psoriasis, and the body of evidence of biologics used in psoriasis lies with infliximab, etanercept and efalizumab. The advantage of biological therapies is that they are well-tolerated, effective treatments. Infliximab for example, is associated with 90% clearance in 10 weeks. However, biologicals are expensive and their long-term side-effects are unknown.

Further reading

Smith C, Ormerod A, Chalmers R, Reynolds N, Anstey A, Griffiths C *et al*. British Association of Dermatologists. Guidelines for use of biological interventions in psoriasis. *Br J Dermatol* 2005; **153**: 486–97.

Wakelin SH. *Handbook of Systemic Drug Treatment in Dermatology*. Manson, London, 2002.

Wolverton SE. *Comprehensive Dermatologic Drug Therapy*. WB Saunders, Philadelphia, 2001.

Index

Note: Page numbers in *italics* refer to figures, those in **bold** refer to tables and boxes

acanthosis nigricans 70, **71**
aciclovir 101, 102, 198
  allergy *29*
  topical **196**
acitretin 199–200
  psoriasis **18**, 23
acne 84–90
  antibiotic therapy **196**
  causes 84–6
  cleansers 88
  corticosteroid-induced 86
  diet 85–6
  dissecting folliculitis 140
  fluid retention 85
  hormones 84–5
  ice pick scars 87
  infantile 87
  inheritance 76
  oestrogens 85, 86
  oil folliculitis 86
  oral contraceptives 84–5, 86
  photodynamic therapy 183
  rosacea differential diagnosis 90
  seasonal effects 86
  treatment 88–90, 200
    photodynamic therapy 183
    systemic 89–90
    topical 88–9, **196**
  types 86–8
acne conglobata 87–8
acne excoriée 87
acne fulminans 87–8
acne keloidalis 86
acne keloidalis nuchae 94–5
acne vulgaris 86–7
acrodermatitis of Hallopeau 146
acrodermatitis pustulosa 15
acromegaly 69
  hyperpigmentation 70
actinic keratoses 163–4
  cryotherapy 173
  curettage 174
  photodynamic therapy 183
  squamous cell carcinoma 166
actinic lentigines 167
acute generalized exanthematous pustulosis
  (AGEP) 45–6, 50

adalimumab 23, 200
adapalene 197
Addison's disease 69, 148
  pigmentation 181
adrenaline, urticaria management 39
agyria 69
AIDS 108
  see also HIV infection
albendazole 199
albinism
  genetic abnormality **76**
  oculocutaneous 41
alefacept 17
alginate dressings 187
allergic reactions, insect bites 122–3
allergies
  contact dermatitis 28, 29, 30
  drug reactions 67
  metal 7
  occupational conditions 9, 32
  photosensitive 7
alopecia
  diffuse 139
  lymphocytic disorders 140, *141*
  neutrophilic disorders 140–41
  non-scarring 138–9
  postfebrile 139
  scarring 140–41
    secondary causes **141**
  tinea capitis 139–40
  traction 138
alopecia areata 138–9
  nails 149
amiodarone, skin pigmentation 48, 181–2
amphotericin B 131
amyloid deposits 74
anagen 137
anaphylaxis 200
Ancylostoma caninum (dog hookworm) 127
androgen suppression 142
androgenetic alopecia 139
  alopecia areata differential
    diagnosis 138
androgenic hormones, acne 84–5
angiolipoma 160
angiomas 68
angio-oedema 36–7, 38–9
  clinical history 36–7
  hereditary 38–9
  investigations 39

  management 39, 200
  with respiratory distress 39
ankle, compression bandaging 191–3
ankle–brachial pressure index (ABPI) 28
annular lesions 6
antiandrogens, acne treatment 89
antibiotics 197, **198**
  acne treatment 89
  bacterial infections 94
  eczema management 34
  folliculitis decalvans 140–41
  leprosy 130
  mycetoma 133
  nail infections 149
  rosacea treatment 91
  topical **196**
anticoagulation, vasculitis 62
antifungals 116, 117, 118, 120, 197–8
  histoplasmosis 133
  mycetoma 133
  nail infections 119
  seborrhoeic dermatitis 143
  tinea capitis 140
  topical **196**
antihistamines 200
  drug rash 47
  pruritus 35
  urticaria management 39
antimalarials 200
antimicrobial dressings 188
antimicrobials
  topical 195, **196**
  see also antibiotics
antimonials, pentavalent 131
antinuclear antibodies 62, 63
antiparasitic agents **196**, 198–9
antiproliferative agents, topical 196–7
anti-tumour necrosis factor α (TNF-α) 200
antiviral agents 198
  topical **196**
  see also aciclovir
apocrine hidrocystomas 159
aqueous cream 33
arterial ulcers 82
athlete's foot 117–18
atopic eczema 1, 6, 7, 25
  ciclosporin therapy 199
  distribution *26*
  genetics 77
  inheritance 76, 77

atopic eczema (*Contd.*)
  pathophysiology 24–5
  risk factors 26
  scalp 143
atrophie blanche 80
atrophy 4, 5
Auspitz sign 11
autoimmune disorders
  blistering 53–9
  nails 149
azathioprine 34, 199
azelaic acid
  acne treatment 88
  rosacea treatment 91

bacillary angiomatosis 97–8, 126
bacterial infections 8, 92–9
  antibiotics 94
  clinical presentation 92, **93**
  deep 95–7
  folliculitis 94, 95
  HIV infection 111–12
  investigations 92, 94
  management 94
  mycetoma 132–3
  periungual skin pustules 146
  superficial 94–5
  tropical 128–31
baldness, male-pattern 139
bandages 189–93
  application 191–3
  classification 190–91
  compression 190–91
  definitions 190
  medicated paste 191
  patient compliance 193
  support 190
  tubular 191
bandaging, compression 191–3
Bartonella 97–8
  HIV infection 111
  transmission 126
basal cell carcinoma 164–6
  cryotherapy 173
  curettage 174, 175
  management 165–6
  morphoeic 165
  nodular 164, *165*
  photodynamic therapy 183
  pigmented 165
  risk factors 164
  superficial 165
  surgical excision 177, *177–8*
  trichoblastoma differential diagnosis 161
  types 164–5
Bazin's disease 97, *98*
Beau's lines 11, 145–6, 151
Becker's naevus 142, 156, *157*
bee stings 124
benzoyl peroxide, acne treatment 88
betamethasone, calcipotriol combination **197**
bexarotene 199, 200
biliary cirrhosis, xanthomas 72–3
biological therapy 200
  psoriasis 23
biopsy
  diagnostic 175–6

incisional 176
sentinel lymph node for malignant
    melanoma 170
Blashko's lines, mosaic defects 76–7
blastomycosis 133
blistering/blistering disorders 53–9
  management 58–9
  Stevens–Johnson syndrome 54, 68
  wounds **186**
blisters 8, *8–9*, 53
  development 54
  distribution 54–5
  durability 54
  duration 54
  insect bites **54**, 121, *122*
  management 58–9
  see also bullae
body lice 126
Borrelia burgdorferi 123
  erythema chronicum migrans 68
Bowen's disease 164
  cryotherapy 173
  curettage 174
  photodynamic therapy 183
  squamous cell carcinoma 166
Breslow thickness for malignant
    melanoma 169–70
bullae 3, *4*, 8, *9*
  insect bites 121, *122*
bullous disorders, autoimmune 53–9
bullous pemphigoid 5
  Beau's lines 146
  clinical features 55, *56*
  dapsone treatment 200
  histopathology *58*
  immunofluorescence *59*
  management 58
  pathophysiology 53
  skin biopsy **58**
  urticated plaques 55

C1 inhibitor deficiency 39
cachexia, skin conditions 71
café au lait patches 70
  laser treatment 181
calcineurin inhibitors 194
calcipotriol, psoriasis treatment 19, **197**
calcium, skin deposits 63
Campbell de Morgan spots 158, *159*
canaliform nail dystrophy of
    Heller *146*
Candida albicans 110–11
  chronic paronychia 119
  nail infections 150
  periungual skin pustules 146
Candida infections 119–20
carbon dioxide cryotherapy 172
catagen 138
cat-scratch disease 98
cavernous haemangiomas 158
cavity dressings 188, *189*
CD4 cell count 108
cellulitis 9, 96
  dissecting of scalp 200
  tropical infection 128
cetirizine 200
cherry haemangioma 158, *159*

chicken pox 101–2
  blistering **54**
  see also varicella zoster virus
children
  atopic eczema 25
  fungal infections 116
  nail transverse splits 146
  napkin psoriasis 15, *16*
  scabies 124, *125*
chloasma 69
  laser treatment contraindication 181
chloroquine 200
chlorpromazine
  hyperpigmentation 70
  skin pigmentation *48*
chromoblastomycosis 133
chronic actinic dermatitis (CAD) 43
ciclosporin A
  eczema 34
  psoriasis 18, 23, 199
Cladosporium werneckii 132
Clark classification for malignant melanoma **170**
cleansers 88
coal tar
  acne 86
  psoriasis 18, 19, 20, **197**
  UV treatment combination 21
coeliac disease 2
  dermatitis herpetiformis 57, 72
cold sore *see* herpes labialis
compression bandages 190–91
compression bandaging 191–3
congenital angiomas 68
congenital hyperpigmentation 70
congenital melanocytic naevi 155
  giant 167
connective tissue disease 60
  investigations **61**
  mixed 66
contact dermatitis 6–7, 8, 28–30
  allergic 28, 29, 30
    occupational 32
  blistering **54**
  clinical features 28–9
  drug rash 47
  immunological response 30, *31*
  investigations 32
  irritant 30, *31*
    occupational 31
  paraphenylenediamine 143
  rubber 193
contagious conditions 6–7
corticosteroids *see* steroids
Corynebacterium 111
Corynebacterium minutissimum 95
  tinea corporis differential diagnosis 118
cosmetic camouflage 197
cotton garments 191
cowpox 103
Coxsackievirus A 106–7
CREST syndrome 62, 63
Crodylobia anthropophaga (tumbu fly) 134
Crohn's disease 72
cryotherapy 172–3
  actinic keratoses 163
Cryptococcus neoformans 110
curettage 174–5

cutaneous B-cell lymphoma, primary 170–71
cutaneous larva migrans 127
    treatment 199
cutaneous mastocytosis 200
cutaneous T-cell lymphoma (CTCL) 170, 200
cutting oils 86
cytokines, proinflammatory 17

danazol 39
dapsone 200
Darier's disease 149
    genetic abnormality **76**
    nails 146
deep vein thrombosis 80
deep venous obstruction 80
delayed hypersensitivity reaction *see*
        hypersensitivity reactions, type IV (delayed)
delusions of parasitosis 121–2
Demodex mite 110
Dercum's disease 160
dermatitis 24–35
    actinic 30, *31*
        chronic 43
    hand 29
    irritant 145
    management 33–5
    occupational 31–2
    perioral *195*
        rosacea differential diagnosis 90–91
    periorbital 29, *196*
    photodermatitis 30–31
    phytophotodermatitis 30, 42
        blistering **54**
    seborrhoeic 117
        HIV infection 109
        pityriasis versicolor differential
            diagnosis 119
        scalp 142–3
    see also contact dermatitis
dermatitis artefacta 83
dermatitis herpetiformis 2, 8
    clinical features **55**, 57
    dapsone treatment 200
    skin biopsy **58**
    systemic disease associations 72
dermatofibroma 156–7
dermatographism 39
dermatology day treatment units
        (DDTUs) 18–19, 20
Dermatology Life Quality Index (DLQI) 2, 18
    acne 88
dermatomyositis 65–6
    hyperpigmentation 70, **71**
dermatosis papulosa nigra 154, 159
desloratidine 200
desquamation 6
diabetes mellitus
    neuropathic ulcers 82
    skin manifestations 73–4
    trophic ulcers 83
diabetic dermopathy 73
diathermy loop cautery, wart treatment 104
diclofenac 164
    topical 196
dicophane 86
diet, acne 85–6
diltiazem, skin pigmentation *49*

dimethyl ether and propane cryotherapy 172
discoid lupus erythematosus 65
    alopecia 140
    antimalarials in treatment 200
    characteristics *64*
dithranol
    alopecia areata 139
    psoriasis 19, **197**
    UV treatment combination 21
DNA viruses 100
Dracunculus medinensis (dracunculiasis) 136
dressings 185–9
    adverse effects 189
    alginate 187
    antimicrobial 188
    cavity 188, *189*
    honey 188–9
    hydrocolloid 186, *187*
    hydrofibre 186–7
    hydrogel 185–6, *187*
    low-adherent 185
    negative pressure 189, *190*
    non-adherent 185, *187*
    odour-absorbing 188
    patient compliance 193
    semipermeable adhesive film 185
drug rash with eosinophilia and systemic
        symptoms (DRESS) 46, 50, *51*
drug rashes 8, *9*, 45–52
    clinical features 46–7
    fixed drug eruptions 47–8
        blistering **54**
    generalized 45–6, 49–52
    HIV infection 113–14
    immune-mediated 45
    investigations 47
    localized 45, 46–7
        types 47–8, *49*
    management 47
    mucous membrane involvement **46**
    non-immune-mediated 45
    onset 47
    pathophysiology 45–6
    photosensitive drug eruptions 48
    skin biopsy 47
drug reactions
    allergic 67
    hyperpigmentation 69, 70, 181–2
    immunobullous disorders 55, 57, 58
    photodermatitis 30
    psoriasis 9, 18
dry wraps 191
dye allergy *29*
dysplastic naevus syndrome 167

ecthyma 97
eczema 8, 24–35
    asteatotic 26, *27*
    Beau's lines 146
    classification **24**
    clinical features 24
    discoid 26, *27*
    endogenous 25–8
        investigation 27–8
    exogenous 28–32
    hyperpigmentation 70
    infected 34

inflammatory linear verrucous epidermal
        naevus differential diagnosis 162
    management 33–5
    nail bed 149
    nails 148–9
        changes 145
    nummular lesions 4
    pathology/pathophysiology 24–5
    pompholyx 26, *27*
    seborrhoeic 90
    varicose 28
    venous 26–7
    see also atopic eczema
eczema herpeticum 25–6, *101*
efalizumab 17, 23, 200
Ehlers–Danlos syndrome 72
    genetic abnormality **76**
electrocautery 173, 174
electrodessication 174
electrosurgery 173–4
emollients 194
    eczema 33
    pruritus 35
    psoriasis 19, 20
emulsifying ointments 33
endocarditis 126
endothelial growth factor receptor (EGFR)
        inhibitors 47
endothrix 116
eosinophilia, eczema 28
eosinophilic folliculitis 110
ephilides 181
epidermal naevus 162
epidermis
    atrophy 4, *5*
    changes 8
    eczema 25
    erosion 5
    excoriation 6
epidermoid cysts 160–61
epidermolysis bullosa 8
    dystrophic **76**
    gene therapy 76
    genetic abnormality **76**
    junctional **76**
    simple **76**
epidermolytic hyperkeratosis, genetic
        abnormality **76**
Epidermophyton 116
epithelializing wounds 185, **186**
epithelium, photothermolysis 182
Epstein–Barr virus (EBV) 106
    HIV infection 112
erosion 5
erysipelas 95–6
    tropical infection 128
erythema
    hyperpigmentation 71
    inflammation 9
    of nailbed 68
    palmar 72
    psoriasis 12
    systemic disease associations 67–8
    toxic 49
erythema annulare 68
erythema chronicum migrans 123
    systemic disease associations 68

erythema gyratum repens 68
erythema induratum 97, 98
erythema infectiosum 106
erythema marginatum 68
erythema multiforme 1, 46, 50–51, 67–8
   blistering **54**
erythema nodosum 1, 9
   drug-induced 48
erythrasma 95
   HIV infection 111
   tinea corporis differential diagnosis 118
erythroderma, drug-induced 49
erythroplasia of Queyrat 164
etanercept 17, 23, 200
ethinyloestradiol, acne treatment 89
excoriation 6

face, fungal infections 116–17
famciclovir 198
familial venous valve incompetence 80
favus 132
fexofenadine 200
fibroblasts, gene therapy 76
fibroepithelial polyps 155, 159
fibrokeratoma, periungual 152
fifth disease 106
filaggrin gene mutations 76
filariasis 134–6
finasteride, androgenetic alopecia 139
fish tank granuloma 97
fissures 6
fixed drug eruptions 47–8
   blistering **54**
   hyperpigmentation 70
flaps, surgical excision 178
fluid retention, acne 85
5-fluorouracil cream 163, 196
folliculitis
   bacterial 94, 95
   dissecting 140
   Gram negative 88
   hot-tub 94
folliculitis decalvans 140–41
food proteins, contact urticaria 32
foot
   fungal infections 117–18
   palmoplantar keratoderma **76**
   palmoplantar pustulosis 146
   poroma 153
   tinea pedis 117–18
   toe nail trauma 150–51
formulary 194–200
   systemic therapy 197–200
   topical therapy 194–7
freckles 155
   laser treatment 181
fungal infections 115–20
   deep 120, 132–3
   diagnosis **115**
   face 116–17
   feet 117–18
   general features 116
   hands 117–18
   HIV infection 110–11
      deep 120
   investigations 115–20
   mycetoma 132–3

nails 119, 145, 147, 150
   periungual skin pustules 146
   scalp 116–17
   superficial 131–2
   tropical 131–3

gene therapy 76
genetic disorders 75–7
   complex 77
   photosensitivity 41
   single gene 76–7
Gianotti–Crosti syndrome 106
glomus tumours, nail 151
gluten-free diet, dermatitis herpetiformis 57, 59
Goeckerman regimen 21
grafts, surgical excision 178
granulating wounds 185, **186**
granuloma annulare 73, *74*
griseofulvin 197, 198
Guinea worm 136

H1-receptor blockers 39
H2-receptor blockers 39
habit-tic picking of nails 151
haemangioma
   cherry 158, *159*
   laser treatment 180
haemochromatosis 69
haemosiderin deposition 69, 182
hair 137–42
   excessive 141–2
   fungal infection 132
   growth cycle 137–8
   laser removal 182
   loss 138–9
   types 137
halo naevi 156, *157*
halogenated hydrocarbons, acne 86
hand, foot and mouth disease 106–7
hands
   fungal infections 117–18
   palmoplantar keratoderma **76**
   palmoplantar pustulosis 146
head lice 125–6
henna tattoo *29*
Henoch–Schönlein purpura 61, 62
hepatitis, erythema multiforme 51
herpes labialis, eczema herpeticum association 25
herpes simplex virus (HSV) 8, 100–101
   blistering **54**
   erythema multiforme 51
   HIV infection 112
   periungual skin pustules 146
   treatment 198
herpes zoster (shingles) 101–102
   HIV infection 112
herpesviruses 100–2
   HIV infection 112
   treatment 198
hidradenitis suppurativa
   dissecting folliculitis 140
   isotretinoin treatment 200
highly active antiretroviral therapy
   (HAART) 108
hirsutism 141–2
Histoplasma capsulatum (histoplasmosis) 110,
   133

history-taking 1
HIV infection 100, 108–14
   bacterial infections 111–12
   drug rashes 113–14
   early stages 109
   fungal infections 110–11
      deep 120
   histoplasmosis 133
   infections 110–13
   infestations 113
   Kaposi's sarcoma 112–13
   late-stage 109
   mycobacterial disease 112
   primary 108–9
   scabies 113
   seroconversion illness 109
   skin disorders 109–14
   stages 108–9
   syphilis coinfection 99, 111
   viral infections 112–13
HLA-B27 17
honey dressings 188–9
human leukocyte antigens (HLA), psoriasis 16,
   17, 77
human papilloma virus (HPV) 100, 104
   HIV infection 113
   squamous cell carcinoma 166
Hutchinson's sign 148, 168–9
hydrocolloid dressings 186, *187*
hydrofibre dressings 186–7
hydrogel dressings 185–6, *187*
hydroxychloroquine 200
hyperpigmentation 68–70
   congenital conditions 70
   HIV infection 113–14
   hormonal 69, *70*
   laser treatment 181
   malignancy 70–71
   neoplastic 70
   post-inflammation 181
hypersensitivity reactions
   type I 45, 200
   type II 45
   type III 45
   type IV (delayed) 30, 45
      polymorphic light eruption 42–3
hyperthyroidism 69
hypertrichosis 142
hypopigmentation, genetic/hormonal 68
hypoproteinaemia, alopecia 139

ichthammol
   psoriasis 19
   venous ulcers 82
ichthyosis, acquired **71**
ichthyosis, X-linked recessive **76**
ichthyosis vulgaris 76
IgA deposition, Henoch–Schönlein purpura
   61, 62
Imiquimod®
   actinic keratoses treatment 164
   topical 196–7
   wart treatment 104
immune complexes, circulating in
   dermatomyositis 66
immune reconstitution inflammatory syndrome
   (IRIS) 112

immunobullous disorders 53–9
  clinical features 55–8
  differential diagnosis 53–4
  drug reactions 55, 57, 58
  immunofluorescence studies 58, 59
  investigations 58, *59*
  management 58–9
  pathophysiology 53–5
  skin biopsy 58
immunofluorescence
  immunobullous disorders 58, *59*
  vasculitis 61
immunoglobulin E (IgE) 28
immunological disorders 8
immunomodulators
  eczema management 33
  systemic 199
immunosuppressants
  alopecia areata 139
  eczema management 34
  systemic lupus erythematosus 65
  vasculitis 62
immunotherapy, wart treatment 104
impetigo 8, 94
  ecthyma 97
  HIV infection 111
  Staphylococcus **54**
  tropical 128
induration 8
infants
  acne 87
  atopic eczema 25
  scabies 124, *125*
infections
  diabetes mellitus 73
  drug formulary 197–9
  leg ulcers 81–2, 83
  nails 150, 152
  onycholysis 150
  venous ulcers 81–2
  wounds **186**
  see also bacterial infections; fungal infections;
    viral infections
infestations 124–7
  HIV infection 113
  tropical 134–6
inflammation 9
  hyperpigmentation 181
  nails 152
    loss 146
inflammatory disorders 8, 60–66
inflammatory linear verrucous epidermal naevus
    (ILVEN) 162
infliximab 17, 23, 200
Ingram regimen 21
injection abscess 97
insect bites 121–4
  allergic reactions 122–3
  blistering **54**, 121, *122*
  bullae *4*, 121, *122*
  clinical features **121**
  management of reactions 200
  parasite transmission 123
  persistent reaction 121, *122*
  prevention 123
  risk factors **121**
insect stings 124

intense pulsed light 183
interferon α (IFN-α), psoriasis 17, 23
interferon α2b (IFN-α2b) 170
intertrigo, *Candida* 119
iodine 188
iron deficiency
  alopecia 139
  koilonychia 146
irritant reactions, contact dermatitis 28, 29
isotretinoin 199–200
itraconazole 197, 198
ivermectin 199

jaundice, obstructive 72
jewel sign 58
joint disease, psoriasis 16, *17*

Kaposi's sarcoma 112–13
Keloid scars 86, 87
keratin, nails 144
keratinocytes
  eczema 25
  gene therapy 76
  lichen planus 64
  psoriasis 11, *12*, 17
  squamous cell carcinoma 166
keratoacanthoma 166
keratoderma, palmoplantar **76**
keratolytic agents 197
keratoses
  actinic 163–4, 166
    cryotherapy 173
    curettage 174
    photodynamic therapy 183
  seborrhoeic *2*, 153
    cryotherapy 173
    curettage 174
kerion 116, *117*, 139, *140*
Klippel–Trenaunay syndrome 158
Koebner's phenomenon 9, 13, *14*, 18, 64
koilonychia 146–7

labial lentigines 155
LAMB syndrome 155
lanugo hair 137
larva currens 199
larva migrans *see* cutaneous larva migrans
larval therapy 188, *189*
laser resurfacing 182–3
laser snow 182
laser treatment 179–83
  perioperative anaesthesia 180
  pigmented lesions 180–82
  port wine stains 158
  postoperative care 180
  preoperative assessment 179
  principles 179
  rosacea 91
  safety 180
  vascular lesions 180
latex glove allergy 29, 32
Laugier–Hunziker syndrome 155
leg ulcers 78–83
  arterial 82
  assessment 78
  hydrogel dressings 186
  infection 81–2, 83
  inflammatory conditions 82, *83*

malignancy 81, 83
  neuropathic 82
  polyarteritis nodosa 82
  prevalence 78
  vasculitic 82
  venous 78–82
leishmaniasis, cutaneous 130–31
lentigines 155
  actinic 167
  laser treatment 181
lentigo maligna melanoma 168
LEOPARD syndrome 155
leprosy 128–30
  borderline 130
  diagnosis 129–30
  lepromatous 129
  spectrum of clinical disease 129
  treatment 130, 200
  tuberculoid 129
leukonychia 147, 149
leukotriene receptor antagonists 39
levocetirizine 200
lice 125–7
lichen planopilaris 140, *141*
lichen planus 1, 64
  hyperpigmentation 70
  koilonychia 147
  nails 149
lichen sclerosus 63
lichen simplex *4*, 26
lichenification 4
  hyperpigmentation 70
lichenoid drug eruption 49, *50*, 64
light eruption, polymorphic 7
light spectrum *40*
linear IgA disease
  clinical features **55**, 57–8
  dapsone treatment 200
  skin biopsy **58**
lipodermatosclerosis 80
lipomas 160
liquid nitrogen 172–3
  actinic keratoses treatment 163
  wart treatment 104
liver disease 72
  porphyria cutanea tarda 72–3, 74
Loa loa (loiasis) 134, 135–6
loratidine 200
lupus
  drug-induced 48
  pterygium formation *150*
lupus erythematosus 64–5
  nails 149
  rosacea differential diagnosis 90
  see also discoid lupus erythematosus; systemic
    lupus erythematosus (SLE)
lupus vulgaris 97
Lyme disease 123
  erythema chronicum migrans 68
lymphoedema 80
  filariasis 134, 135
lymphoma
  cutaneous 170–71
  hyperpigmentation 70, **71**

macular purpura 50
macule 2–3

madura foot 132–3
malabsorption
    hyperpigmentation 70
    skin conditions 71
Malassezia furfur 117, 118
malignancy
    hyperpigmentation 70–71
    leg ulcers 81, 83
    paraneoplastic pemphigus 57
    venous ulcers 81
    see also skin tumours, malignant
malignant change 2
malignant melanoma 2, 148, 167–70
    acral 168–9
    adjuvant therapies 170
    amelanotic 169
    Breslow thickness 169–70
    Clark classification **170**
    dysplastic 169
    metastases 170
    nodular 168, *169*
    prognosis 169–70
    risk factors 167
    sentinel lymph node biopsy 170
    superficial spreading 168
    treatment 170
    types 168–9
mandibular nerve zoster *102*
Marjolin's ulcer 81, 83, 166
measles 100, 105
medicated paste bandages 191
melanin *3*
    inflammation 181
    laser treatment 181
    lentigines 155
    loss 68
    nail plate deposition 148
melanocytes 68
    lentigines 155
    melanocytic naevi 155
    naevi 167
melanocytic naevi 155–6
    acquired 155–6
    congenital 155
        giant 167
melanonychia 148
melanosomes, laser treatment 181
melasma 69, *70*
    laser treatment contraindication 181
mepacrine 200
metabolic disorders 8
    photosensitivity 41–2
metal allergy 7
metastases
    from internal organ malignancy 171
    malignant melanoma 170
methicillin-resistant *Staphylococcus aureus*
    (MRSA) 97
methotrexate 199
    eczema 34
    psoriasis **18**, 22–3
metronidazole
    rosacea treatment 91
    wound healing 188
microangiopathy, diabetic dermopathy 73
Microsporum 116

Microsporum canis 139–40, 198
milia 159, *160*
milker's nodules 103
minimal erythema dose (MED), UV treatment 21
minocycline
    hyperpigmentation 70
    skin pigmentation 48, 181–2
minoxidil, alopecia treatment 139
mixed connective tissue disease 66
Moh's micrographic surgery, basal cell
    carcinoma 165
moles 155–6, 167
    atypical 167
    malignant melanoma progression 168
    multiple 167
    protruberant benign 153
molluscum contagiosum 100, 103
    HIV infection 113
Mongolian blue spot 70, 155, *156*
morphoea 62–3
mosaicism 76–7
mucous membrane pemphigoid
    clinical features **55**, 56
    dapsone treatment 200
    management 58
    skin biopsy **58**
mycetoma 132–3
mycobacteria, atypical 97
mycobacterial disease 97
    HIV infection 112
Mycobacterium leprae (leprosy) 128
Mycobacterium marinum 97
Mycobacterium tuberculosis (tuberculosis) 97
mycophenolate mofetil 34, 199
Mycoplasma infection, erythema multiforme 51
mycosis fungoides 170
    hyperpigmentation 70–71
myiasis, subcutaneous 134
myxoedema, pretibial 75
myxoid pseudocysts 151, *152*

naevi 167
    ABCDE for malignant potential **167**
    adjacent to nail 151
    Becker's 156, *157*
    blue 156
    compound 155–6
    dysplastic 167
        multiple 168
    epidermal 162
    halo 156, *157*
    intradermal 156
    junctional 155, *156*
    melanocytic 155–6
        giant 167
    spider 68, 72, 158, *159*
        electrosurgery 174
        laser treatment 180
    Spitz 156, *157*
    strawberry 158
naevus flammeus neonatorum 157
naevus sebaceus 161
nail(s) 144–52
    alopecia areata 149
    attachment changes 144–7
    autoimmune disorders 149

    Beau's lines 11, 145–6, 151
    clubbing 147, 151
    colour changes 147–8
        acral melanoma 168–9
    dermatomyositis 66
    dystrophy 11, *13*, 139
        alopecia areata 149
        canaliform of Heller *146*
    eczema 148–9
    friable 149
    fungal infections 119, 145, 147, 150
        treatment 197, 198
    glomus tumours 151
    growth 144
    habit-tic picking 151
    infection 149–50, 152
    inflammation 152
    lesions adjacent 151–2
    lichen planus 149
    longitudinal splits 146
    longitudinal streaks 148
    loss 146
    lupus erythematosus 149
    myxoid pseudocysts 151, *152*
    oily spot 145, 148
    pemphigoid 149
    pemphigus 149
    pitting 11, *13*, 144, *145*, 148, 149
    psoriasis 11, *13*, 13–14, 147, 148
    shape changes 144–7
    shedding 146, 151
    splinter haemorrhages 11, 151
    spoon-shaped deformity 146–7
    structure 144
    systemic diseases 151, 152
    transverse ridges 145, 148
    transverse splits 146
    treatment of conditions 152
    whitening 147
    see also onycholysis; paronychia
nail bed
    colour changes 147
    cyanosis 151
    eczema 149
    erythema 68
    warts 151
20-nail dystrophy 149
nail plate
    atrophy 149
    colour changes 147
    melanin deposition 148
    thickening 145
necrobiosis lipoidica 73
necrotic wounds 184, **186**
necrotizing fasciitis 74
negative pressure dressings 189, *190*
nematodes, cutaneous larva migrans 127
neonatal lupus erythematosus 65
neoplasia, hyperpigmentation 70
neurofibromatosis 72
    hyperpigmentation 70
neuropathic ulcers 82
nickel allergy
    periorbital dermatitis 29
    pompholyx eczema 26
Nikolsky's sign 46, 51, 96

nitrous oxide cryotherapy 172
nodules 3
    benign skin tumours **154**, 160–61
nummular lesions 4, *5*

obesity, hyperpigmentation 70
occlusive therapy, eczema 33–4
occupational conditions 7, 9
    dermatitis 31–2
oculocutaneous albinism 41
odour-absorbing dressings 188
oestrogens, acne 85, 86
oil folliculitis 86
Onchocerca volvulus (onchocerciasis) 134, 135
onycholysis 145
    chronic 145
    infections 150
    psoriasis 11, *13*, 13–14, 148
onychomadesis 146, 151
onychomycosis 119, 145, 147
    dermatophyte 150
    treatment 197, 198
ophthalmic zoster *102*
oral contraceptives, acne 84–5, 86
    treatment 89
oral hairy leukoplakia 112
orf 103–4

Paget's disease of the nipple 28, 171
palmoplantar keratoderma **76**
palmoplantar pustulosis 146
papillomas
    cryotherapy 173
    skin tags 166
papules 3
    benign skin tumours **154**, 159–60
Paracoccidioides brasiliensis 133
paraphenylenediamine, contact dermatitis 143
parapsoriasis, hyperpigmentation 71
parasite transmission by insect bites 123
parasitosis, delusions 121–2
Parkes–Weber syndrome 158
paronychia, chronic 119, 145
parvovirus B19 106
patch testing 32
patient assessment 9
patient compliance, wound healing 193
pediculosis 198–9
pellagra, hyperpigmentation 70
pemphigoid 8
    cicatricial 56
    see also bullous pemphigoid; mucous
        membrane pemphigoid
pemphigoid gestationis 74
    clinical features 55–6
    management 58
    skin biopsy **58**
pemphigus 8
    nails 149
    paraneoplastic 57
pemphigus vulgaris
    clinical features **55**, 56–7
    histopathology *59*
    immunofluorescence *59*
    management 59
    pathophysiology 53

scalp 143
    skin biopsy **58**
periungual fibrokeratoma 152
periungual skin, pustules 146
Peutz–Jeghers syndrome
    hyperpigmentation 70
    labial lentigines 155
    systemic disease association 72
phenytoin, hyperpigmentation 70
photodermatitis 30–31
photodynamic therapy 164, 183
photoporphyria 74
photoprotective behaviour 41, 42, 43–4
photosensitivity 40–44
    drug eruptions 48
    drug reactions 42
    exogenous substances 42
    genetic disorders 41
    idiopathic disorders 42–3
    metabolic disorders 41–2
    reactions 7
phototherapy *see* ultraviolet (UV) treatment
photothermolysis of epithelium 182
phytophotodermatitis 30, 42
    blistering **54**
piebaldism 68, *69*
Piedraia hortae (piedra) 132
pigmentation
    changes in systemic disease 68–70
    drug-induced 48, *49*
    HIV infection 113–14
    laser treatment 181
    see also hyperpigmentation
pilar cysts 161
pilomatrixoma 161
pimecrolimus 33, 195
pituitary tumour, hyperpigmentation 70
pityriasis alba 25, *26*
pityriasis amiantacea 142
pityriasis rosea 119
pityriasis versicolor 118–19
plant exposure
    chronic actinic dermatitis 43
    phytophotodermatitis 30, 42, **54**
plaque 3, *4*
    benign skin tumours **154**, 161–2
    see also psoriasis, plaque
podophyllin, wart treatment 104
poikiloderma, hyperpigmentation 71
polyarteritis nodosa 61
    leg ulcers 82
polycystic ovarian syndrome 142
polymorphic light eruption 42–3
    antimalarials in treatment 200
polyurethane foam dressings 187–8
pompholyx eczema 26, *27*
poroma 161
    foot 153
porphyria 8, 41–2, 74
    blistering **54**
    hepatic 41–2
porphyria cutanea tarda 41
    antimalarials in treatment 200
    liver disease 72–3, 74
port wine stain 68, 158
    laser treatment 180

poxviruses 102–4
practical procedures 172–8
prednisolone
    dermatomyositis 66
    eczema management 34
    systemic lupus erythematosus 65
pregnancy 74
    see also pemphigoid gestationis
Propionibacterium acnes 84, 88
prurigo, nodular 110
pruritic urticarial papules and plaques of
        pregnancy (PUPPP) 74
pruritus 34–5
    ani 35
    dermatitis herpetiformis 57
    HIV infection 110
    hyperpigmentation **71**
    management 34–5, 200
    with skin changes 34
    vulvae 35
pseudoacanthosis nigricans,
        hyperpigmentation 70
pseudofolliculitis 94–5
pseudofolliculitis barbae 94
Pseudomonas, nail infections 150
Pseudomonas aeruginosa, hot-tub
        folliculitis 94
pseudopelade of Brocq 140
pseudoxanthoma elasticum 72
    genetic abnormality **76**
psoralens 21–2
    photodermatitis 30
psoriasis 11–17
    arthropathy 16, 17, *17*
    HIV infection 109
    Beau's lines 146
    biological therapy 23, 200
    causes 17
    clinical appearance 11–12
    coal tar **197**
    drug-induced 9, 18
    erythema 12
    erythrodermic 15–16
        management **18**
    family history 12
    flexural 15, *16*
        management **18**
    genetics 77
    guttate 9, 14, *15*, 18
        management **18**
    HIV infection 109
    inheritance 76
    management 18–23
    nails 11, *13*, 13–14, 147, 148
        oily spot 145, 148
    napkin 15, *16*
    oily spot of nails 145, 148
    onycholysis 11, *13*, 13–14, 148
    palmar/plantar 22
        management *15*, **18**
    patient assessment 9
    plaque 1, *4*, 11, *13*
        management **18**
        pattern 13–16
    precipitating factors 9
    proinflammatory cytokines 17

psoriasis (*Contd.*)
 pustular 4, 12, 15
  management **18**
  periungual skin 146
 scaling 11, 13
 scalp 20, 142, 143
  scaling 13
 systemic treatment **18**, 22–3
 T cells 17, 18
 topical treatment 19–20, 143, **197**
 trigger factors 12–13, 18
 UV treatment **18**, 20–22
Psoriasis Disability Index (PDI) 18
psoriasis susceptibility locus
  (PSORS1) 17, 77
pterygium formation 149, *150*
pubic lice 126
punch biopsy 175–6
pustules 4, *5*
 periungual skin 146
 psoriasis 12, 15
  management **18**
pustulosis, palmoplantar 146
pyoderma faciale 88
pyoderma gangrenosum
 dapsone treatment 200
 leg ulcers 82, *83*
 systemic disease associations 71–2
pyogenic granuloma 153, 158–9

radioallergosorbent testing (RAST) 28
 urticaria 39
radiotherapy
 basal cell carcinoma 166
 squamous cell carcinoma 167
rashes 1, 6–9
 diagnosis 6–7
 distribution 7
 endogenous/exogenous 7
 morphology 8–9
 recurrence 7
 symmetry 7
 viral diseases 105–7
Raynaud's phenomenon 62, 63
red man syndrome 49
Reiter's syndrome 17
reticulate change 6
retinoids
 alopecia areata 139
 oral
  acne treatment 89–90
  rosacea treatment 91
 side-effects 200
 squamous cell carcinoma prophylaxis 167
 systemic 199–200
 topical in acne treatment 89
retroviruses 108
Rickettsia prowazekii transmission 126
rickettsial infections 98–9
ringworm, scalp 116
RNA viruses 100, 108
Rocky Mountain spotted fever 98–9
rosacea 90–91
roseola infantum 106
rubber
 allergy 29

contact dermatitis 193
 sensitivity with venous ulcers 193
rubella 105–6

salicylic acid 197
 acne treatment 88
 psoriasis **18**, 20, 143
salmon patches 157
sand fleas 134
saphenous vein insufficiency 80
sarcoidosis 75
 antimalarials in treatment 200
Sarcoptes scabiei 124–5
scabies 6–7, 124–5, **126**
 crusted 124–5
 HIV infection 113
 management 125, **126**, 198–9
scalp
 atopic eczema 143
 diseases 142–3
 dissecting cellulitis 200
 fungal infections 116–17
 pemphigus vulgaris 143
 pityriasis amiantacea 142
 psoriasis 20, 142, 143
 ringworm 116
 scaling in psoriasis 13
 seborrhoeic dermatitis 142–3
Schamberg's disease 69
sclerodactyly 63
scurvy, hyperpigmentation 70
sebaceous gland hyperplasia 159–60
seborrhoeic dermatitis 117
 HIV infection 109
 pityriasis versicolor differential
   diagnosis 119
 scalp 142–3
seborrhoeic keratoses *2*, 153
 cryotherapy 173
 curettage 174
sentinel lymph node biopsy, malignant
   melanoma 170
shave biopsy 175
shingles 101–2
 HIV infection 112
silver dressings 188
sixth disease 106
SKALP/elafin gene 17
skin *2, 3*
 barrier function 92
 examination 2
 Fitzpatrick classification of types 40–41
 flora 92
 systemic diseases 67–77
 wrinkle lines *176–7*
skin grafting, venous ulcers 82
skin prick testing, urticaria 39
skin tags 154–5, 159
 cryotherapy 173
skin tumours, benign 153–62
 bleeding 153
 diagnosis 153
 differential diagnosis **154**
 nodules **154**, 160–61
 painful 160
 papules **154**, 159–60

pigmented 153–**7**
 laser treatment 180–82
 plaques **154**, 161–2
 vascular **154**, 157–9
  laser treatment 180
skin tumours, malignant 164–71
 surgical excision 176–7
skin tumours, premalignant 163–4
sloughy wounds 184, **186**
smallpox 102–3
spider bites 123–4
spider naevi 68, 72, 158, *159*
 electrosurgery 174
 laser treatment 180
Spitz naevi 156, *157*
squamous cell carcinoma 2, 166–7
 Bowen's disease 164
 management 166–7
 ulcer presentation 83
staphylococcal scalded skin syndrome 96–7
Staphylococcus aureus
 discoid eczema 26
 impetigo 94, 111, 128
 nail infections 149
 periungual skin pustules 146
Staphylococcus impetigo **54**
steroids, oral
 eczema management 34
 urticaria 39
steroids, systemic 199
 acne induction 86
 dermatomyositis 66
 drug-induced vasculitis 50
 immunobullous disorders 58, 59
 vasculitis 62
steroids, topical 194–5
 acne induction 86
 alopecia areata 138–9
 discoid lupus erythematosus 65
 drug rash 47
 eczema 33
 fingertip units 20
 immunobullous disorders 58
 mechanism of action 194
 potency 20, 33, 194, **195**
 pruritus ani/vulvae 35
 psoriasis **18**, 19–20
 scalp diseases 143
 side effects 194–5, *196*
 vasculitis 62
Stevens–Johnson syndrome 46, 51
 blistering **54**, 68
 erythema multiforme 51
 HIV infection 114
stibogluconate 131
stork marks 157
strawberry naevi 158
Streptococcus
 erysipelas 95–6, 128
 nail infections 149
 tropical infections 128
streptococcus, group β haemolytic 14
Streptococcus pyogenes
 cellulitis 96
 impetigo 94
striae formation *195*

string of beads sign 58
Strongyloides 127
Sturge–Weber syndrome, port wine
    stain 158
subacute lupus erythematosus 65
  antimalarials in treatment 200
subungual exostosis 151, *152*
subungual hyperkeratosis 11, 144, 148
sulphur products, scalp psoriasis 20
sunlight
  acne effects 86
  actinic keratoses 163
  avoidance 41, 42, 43–4
  malignant melanoma risk 167–8
  photodermatitis 30, *31*
  polymorphic light eruption 42–3
  urticaria 38
    solar 38, 43
sunscreen use 41, 42, 43–4, 197
  discoid lupus erythematosus 65
  melasma 69
  protection level 44
  rosacea treatment 91
support bandages 190
surgical excision 176–8
  flaps/grafts 178
suturing **177**, *178*
swimming pool granuloma 97, *98*
syphilis 99
  HIV infection 111
syringomas 159
systemic diseases 67–77
  angiomas 68
  erythemas 67–8
  gut 71–3
  nail changes 151, 152
  pigmentation changes 68–70
  sarcoidosis 75
  thyroid disease 75
  see also diabetes; malignancy
systemic lupus erythematosus (SLE) 2, 64–5
  antimalarials in treatment 200
systemic sclerosis 62–3

T cells
  contact dermatitis 30, *31*
  psoriasis 17, 18
tacalcitol 19
tacrolimus 33, 195
talon noir 169
tattoos 182
telangiectasias
  electrosurgery 174
  laser treatment 180
  liver failure 72
  systemic sclerosis 62, 63
telogen 138
telogen effluvium 139
  alopecia areata differential diagnosis 138
terbinafine 197, 198
terminal hair 137
terminology 2–6
testosterone, serum levels 142
tetracyclines, acne treatment 89
T-helper (T$_H$) lymphocytes, eczema 24–5
thiopurine methyl transferase 199

thyroid disease 75
tick bites 123
tinea capitis 116, *117*
  alopecia 139–40
  alopecia areata differential diagnosis 138
  treatment 197–8
tinea corporis 118
tinea imbricata 131, *132*
tinea incognito 117
tinea nigra 132
tinea pedis 117–18
toe nail trauma 150–51
topical therapy formulations 194–7
toxic epidermal necrolysis 46, 51–2
  blistering **54**
  ciclosporin therapy 199
  HIV infection 113, *114*
toxic erythema 49
trachyonychia 149
trauma
  nails 150–51
    loss 146
  onycholysis 145
trench fever 126
Treponema pallidum (syphilis) 99, 111
tretinoin 197
trichoblastoma 161
trichoepitheliomas 159, *160*
Trichophyton 116
Trichophyton concentricum 131
Trichophyton rubrum nail infection 150
Trichophyton schoenleinii 132
Trichophyton tonsurans 116, *117*, 139–40
  antifungals 198
Trichosporum beigelli 132
trichotillomania 140
  alopecia areata differential diagnosis 138
trophic ulcers 73, 83
tropical dermatology 128–36
  bacterial infections 128–31
  fungal infections 131–3
  infestations 134–6
trunk, fungal infections 118–19
tuberculids 97, *98*
tuberculosis
  cutaneous 97
  erythema multiforme 51
tubular bandages 191
tumbu fly 134
tumour necrosis factor α (TNF-α), psoriasis
  17, 23
tumours *see* skin tumours
Tunga penetrans (tungiasis) 134
typhus transmission 126

ulceration 5
  venous eczema 27
  see also leg ulcers; venous ulcers
ultraviolet A (UVA) radiation 40
  sunscreens 197
ultraviolet A with psoralen (PUVA) treatment 197
  alopecia areata 139
  eczema management 34
  psoriasis **18**, 21–2
ultraviolet B (UVB) radiation 40
  sunscreens 197

ultraviolet B (UVB) treatment **18**, 21, 197
  eczema 34
  polymorphic light eruption 43
ultraviolet (UV) light
  avoidance 43
  exposure 40
  malignant melanoma risk 167–8
  skin tolerance 40
ultraviolet (UV) treatment 197
  acne 89
  dosage 21
  minimal erythema dose 21
  psoriasis **18**, 20–22
  risks 20
urticaria 1, 36–8, 39
  cholinergic 37–8
  classification 37–8
  clinical history 36–7
  contact 32
  drug-induced
    localized contact 47
    widespread 49
  investigations 39
  management 39, 200
  non-physical **36**, 37
  ordinary 37, *38*
  pathophysiology 36
  physical **36**, 37
  pressure 38
  with respiratory distress 39
  solar 38, 43

valaciclovir 101, 198
varicella zoster virus 100, 101–2
  blistering **54**
  treatment 198
varicose eczema 28, 80
varicose veins 79
variola 102–3
vasculitis 60–62
  causes **61**
  diagnosis 61
  drug-induced 50
  leg ulcers 82
  management 62
  pathophysiology 61
  purpuric 72
  urticarial 37, 39
vellus hair 137
venous eczema 26–7
venous stasis 79
venous ulcers 78–82
  bandages 81
  blood vessels 79
  clinical features 80–81
  dressings 81
  eczema treatment 82
  incompetent valves *79*, 80
  infection 81–2
  malignant change 81
  pathology 78–80
  risk factors 80
  rubber sensitivity 193
  skin grafting 82
  treatment 81–2
vesicles 3, *4*, 8, *8–9*

viral infections 8, 100–107
   periungual skin pustules 146
   poxviruses 102–4
   rashes 105–7
   transmission 100
   warts 104
   see also named viruses; wart viruses; warts
vitamin A derivatives 197, 199–200
   see also retinoids
vitamin D analogues, psoriasis **18**, 19, **197**
vitiligo 68, *69*
   autoimmune thyroid disease 75
   pityriasis versicolor differential diagnosis 119

wart viruses 104
   HIV infection 113
warts
   cryotherapy 173
   nail fold/bed 151
   seborrhoeic 153
      pedunculated 154–5
   treatment 104
wasp stings 124
wet wraps 191
Wickham's striae 64
wounds 184–5
   blistering **186**

   healing 193
   infection **186**
   larval therapy 188, *189*
   types 184–5, **186**
Wuchereria bancrofti 134

xanthelasma 174
xanthomas
   biliary cirrhosis 72–3
   diabetes mellitus 74
xeroderma pigmentosum 41
   genetic abnormality **76**

yellow nail syndrome 147, *148*